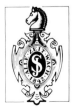

Peter A. Revell

Pathology of Bone

With 171 Figures

Springer-Verlag
Berlin Heidelberg New York Tokyo

Peter A. Revell, BSc, MB, BS, PhD, MRCPath
Senior Lecturer in Morbid Anatomy
Institute of Pathology
The London Hospital
Bone and Joint Research Unit
The London Hospital Medical College
Whitechapel, London, UK

ISBN 3-540-15418-3 Springer-Verlag Berlin Heidelberg New York Tokyo
ISBN 0-387-15418-3 Springer-Verlag New York Heidelberg Berlin Tokyo

Library of Congress Cataloging-in-Publication Data
Revell, P. A. (Peter Allen), 1943–
Pathology of Bone
Includes bibliographies and index. 1. Bones—Diseases. I. Title. [DNLM: 1. Bone and Bones—pathology.
WE 200 R451p] RC930.4.R48 1985 616.7′1 85–17167
ISBN 0–387–15418–3 (U.S.)

© Springer-Verlag Berlin Heidelberg 1986
Printed in Great Britain

Filmset and printed by BAS Printers Limited, Over Wallop, Hampshire.

2128/3916/543210

I dedicate this book to my wife,
children and parents.

Preface

When I first developed an interest in the pathology of bone I found that there were relatively few books on the subject available. Much of my information had either to be obtained from searching the journals or from senior colleagues in the field, who, I should add, were always more than willing to teach me. With this memory in mind, I have endeavoured to produce a book which I hope is of a convenient size and yet will hold sufficient information to be of use mainly to the pathologist faced with a bone problem. This is not intended to be an all-embracing source of knowledge on the subject; indeed, such a task could not be undertaken by a single author in these days of the rapid increase in information even in small subspecialist areas within bone pathology. Although this book is written mainly for the pathologist, it is hoped that it may also be of interest and value to orthopaedic surgeons, rheumatologists and radiologists.

Most of the illustrations are original and many of the drawings are my own. There has been a long tradition of interest in bone pathology at The London Hospital, which has resulted in a wealth of material being available to me from the archives of the Department of Morbid Anatomy. A few of the photographs are those of Prof. H. Turnbull; the observant reader will detect these, since the scales used are not metric.

I have varied the approach, using more tables in some chapters to distil large amounts of information into a small space, but still (I hope) providing a sufficient number of references for the reader to pursue topics further. I offer my apologies to any colleague or author who has not been quoted or feels his views have not been represented, and hope that he will understand the nature of my task.

The opening chapter describes normal bone, its structure and function and is followed by chapters dealing with abnormal skeletal development and inborn biochemical and metabolic disorders. These topics are all treated quite briefly but perhaps in a way which will enable the reader to identify the nature of a diagnostic problem and move into the relevant literature. Before a series of chapters on metabolic bone disease, Paget's disease, hyperostosis and osteopenia, I have given an account of quantitative methods as applied to bone histology. Various aspects of a rather more orthopaedic nature have been drawn together in a chapter on necrosis and healing in bone, which is followed by one on osteomyelitis. There are several extremely good books dealing with bone tumours, so that the final chapter is not written as a comprehensive account of this subject but merely to illustrate points about the general approach to bone tumours and describe common tumours or those which may be confusing to the non-specialist. Radiology is an essential part of bone pathology, and I have tried to include this as much as possible either in text descriptions or in photographs.

Acknowledgements

A number of figures have been published previously, and permission to reproduce them is gratefully acknowledged. Source details are as follows:

Fig. 1.13a: Ali SY, Wisby A, Gray JC (1978) Metab Bone Dis Relat Res 1: 97–103

Fig. 1.13b: Cecil RNA, Anderson HC (1978) Metab Bone Dis Relat Res 1: 89–95

Fig. 2.1: Revell PA (1981) In: Berry CL Paediatric pathology. Springer-Verlag, Berlin Heidelberg New York, pp 451–485

Figs. 4.5 and 4.6: Revell PA (1983) J Clin Pathol 36: 1323–1331

Fig. 4.11: Olah AJ (1976) In: Bone histomorphometry. Armour Montagu, Paris, pp 55–61

Fig. 4.12: Delling G, Luehmann H, Baron R, Mathews CHE, Olah AJ (1980) Metab Bone Dis Relat Res 2 (Suppl): 419–427

Fig. 5.11: Cunningham J, Fraher LJ, Clemens TL, Revell PA, Papapoulos SE (1982) Am J Med 73: 199–204

Fig. 6.15: Rebel A, Basle M, Pouplard A, Malkani K, Filmon R, Lepatezour A (1980) Arthritis Rheum 23: 1104–1114

Fig. 7.6: Revell PA, Pirie CJ (1981) Rhumatologie 33: 99–104

Fig. 9.14: Blaha JD, Inseler HP, Freeman MAR, Revell PA, Todd RC (1982) J Bone Joint Surg [Br] 64: 326–335

Thanks are due to Dr. M. Turner and Dr. O. Khan of the Department of Radiology, The London Hospital, for providing some of the radiographs (Figs. 8.3, 11.1, 11.2 and 11.11).

It is a pleasure to acknowledge the encouragement given by my colleagues Prof. Colin Berry and Dr. David Pollock, particularly in the early stages of the project. I owe a deep debt of gratitude to Mrs. Elizabeth Hart and Mrs. Sandra Beattie for their hard work and long suffering in providing the necessary secretarial help to complete this book. I thank Mr. Michael Jackson, Medical Editor of Springer-Verlag for his patience and understanding throughout.

London, June 1985   P. A. Revell

Contents

Chapter 1

Normal Bone

Structure of bones

The components of the skeleton may be divided into broad categories for general descriptive purposes. The long or tubular bones have a shaft of compact bone surrounding a central cavity which contains cancellous bone together with bone marrow and fat. The cortical bone is thickest in the mid-portion of the shaft, while the cancellous bone is relatively diminished in amount in this region, being more pronounced in density towards the bone ends. The tubular bones comprise the long tubular bones of the limbs (humerus, radius, ulna, femur, tibia and fibula) and the short tubular bones in the hands and feet (metacarpals, metatarsals and phalanges). Tubular bones are divisible into three main regions, namely the epiphyseal and metaphyseal parts and the diaphysis (see Fig. 1.1). It is important to recognise the site at which particular pathological processes occur with respect to these three

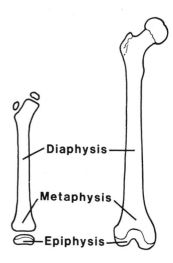

Fig. 1.1. Diagram of femur of a child and an adult to show the positions of the epiphysis, metaphysis and diaphysis

regions, as this may provide important clues as to the type of lesion with which the pathologist is dealing. This is particularly the case with bone tumours and tumour-like conditions.

The flat bones comprise the ribs, sternum, much of the cranium and the scapula (Fig. 1.2). The cranial vault, for example, consists of inner and outer tables of dense cortical bone between which is spongy cancellous bone containing bone marrow (the diploë).

The small bones of the wrist and ankle are sometimes known as 'short bones' or epiphysoid bones, the latter because they form from cartilaginous precursors by ossification from the centre outwards, like epiphyses. They are composed predominantly of spongy cancellous bone with a thin rim of cortical bone.

Certain other bones (the innominate bones, the vertebral column and parts of the skull) do not fit into the above categories when they are each considered as a single bone. A vertebra, for example, comprises the vertebral body and the arches. The vertebral body resembles a tubular bone with a central cancellous portion surrounded by a thin cortical shell and with cartilaginous plates superiorly and inferiorly in continuity with the intervertebral discs. The vertebral arch is formed, however, of more flattened bone with dense cortices and relatively little intervening spongy bone.

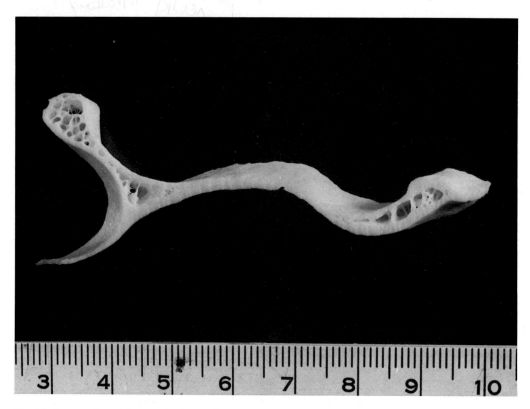

Fig. 1.2. Cross-section of the scapula of an adult, an example of a flat bone

Histological types of bone

Bone as a tissue is divisible into two main types, namely lamellar and non-lamellar bone, the latter being sometimes also known as 'coarse fibred' or 'woven' bone. In lamellar bone, the collagen fibres are arranged in parallel layers or sheets (lamellae; Fig. 1.3) which are readily apparent when viewed by polarisation microscopy (Fig. 1.4). Lamellar bone is present in both structural types of adult bone, namely cortical (or compact) bone and cancellous

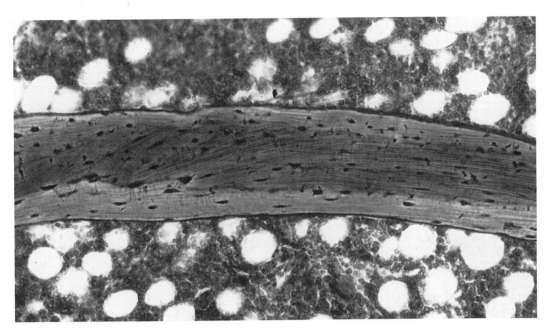

Fig. 1.3. Trabecular bone showing the lamellar structure with parallel layers of collagen fibres. (H&E × 400)

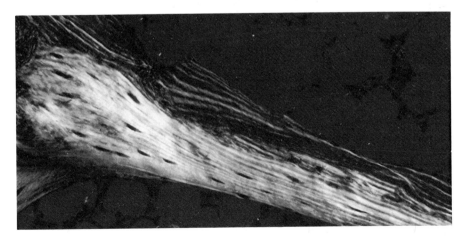

Fig. 1.4. Trabecular bone viewed by polarisation microscopy to show parallel arrangement of birefringent lamellae. (× 400)

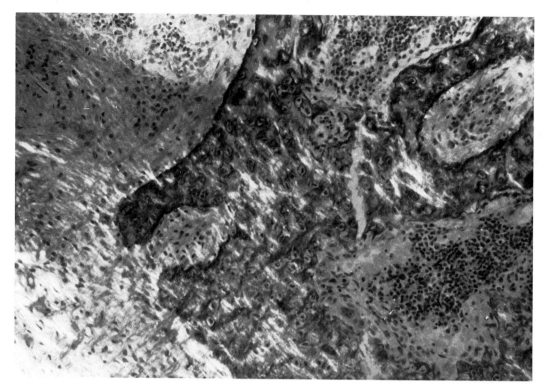

Fig. 1.5. Randomly orientated coarse fibres in woven bone viewed under partially crossed fibres. (H&E × 150)

(spongy or trabecular bone). Non-lamellar (woven) bone is seen in the bones of fetuses and young children, for example in the developing cortex of long bones and the osseous tissue first deposited on the calcified cartilage matrix in endochondral ossification. It is characterised by the presence of randomly orientated coarse fibres which are clearly visible by polarisation microscopy (Fig. 1.5).

Cortical bone

Cortical bone is often taken as the typical histological appearance of bone, but it is important to remember that cancellous bone, with its large surface area, the populations of cells on this surface, and its close relationship to the bone marrow, is the site where pathological changes frequently occur and are most readily recognised. Cortical bone has the familiar structure of Haversian systems or osteons (Fig. 1.6). Haversian canals are round or oval in cross-section and contain blood vessels. They are surrounded by concentrically arranged lamellae and generally run in a longitudinal direction, though they give off branches which join with adjacent Haversian canals. The osteocytes are arranged circumferentially around the central canal in parallel with the lamellae and are interconnected by fine canaliculi containing processes of the osteocyte cytoplasm. Irregular areas of lamellar bone are present between the

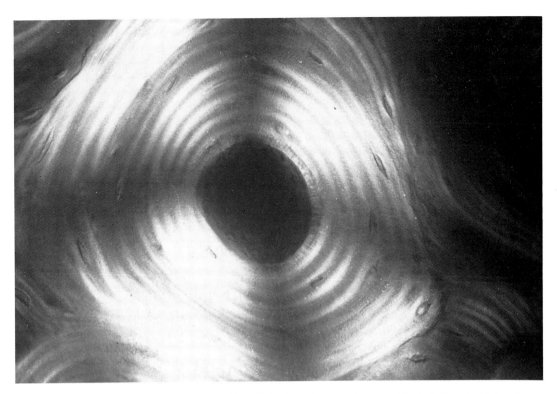

Fig. 1.6. Haversian system in cortical bone viewed by polarisation microscopy in an unstained plastic embedded section. (×600)

Haversian systems and are known as the interstitial lamellae. They represent the remnants of previously formed Haversian systems which have been disrupted in the course of the remodelling which occurs continually in cortical bone. Each osteon is separated from its neighbour and from interstitial lamellae by a cement line which stains darkly with haematoxylin. Straight and smoothly curved cement lines mark resting stages in osteon formation. Irregularly shaped indented lines indicate sites of new bone formation where there has been previous resorption and are sometimes referred to as 'reversal' lines. The outermost and innermost layers of cortical bone contain no Haversian canals, and the lamellae are arranged parallel with the periosteal and endosteal surfaces to form the so-called circumferential lamellae. They are not prominently developed in human bone, but nevertheless are easily recognised when the observer is aware of their existence. The outer surface of the cortical bone is covered by the periosteum, a thin vascular membrane-like layer with collagen fibres which tend to lie parallel with the bone surface. The periosteal membrane blends with the fibres of ligaments and muscle insertions. In fetal life there is a distinctive inner osteoblastogenic layer to the periosteum, but in adult life this is no longer a distinctive separate component, though flattened spindle-shaped cells regarded as resting osteoblasts are still present close to the bone. The periosteum is absent at the sites of attachment of ligaments directly into bone, for example at tuberosities, the linea aspera of the femur and other similar sites.

Cancellous bone

Cancellous or spongy bone is made up of a series of interconnecting plates of bone, each perforated by holes, rather than bars. This is best appreciated in macerated thin slices of bone (Fig. 1.7). This structure, as well as providing a large surface area for the metabolic activities of bone, also gives mechanical strength without the disadvantage of undue weight. The thickest and strongest trabeculae are arranged in that direction which is subjected to the greatest mechanical forces. The cancellous bone of the vertebral body, for example, shows preferential orientation of the bone plates in the vertical and horizontal planes, and the amount of bone is greatest towards the upper and lower surfaces of the vertebral body (Amstutz and Sissons 1969). Each bone trabecula, as visualised by light microscopy, is composed of lamellar bone. The surface of the spongy bone is covered by an attenuated layer of flattened cells, the resting osteoblasts.

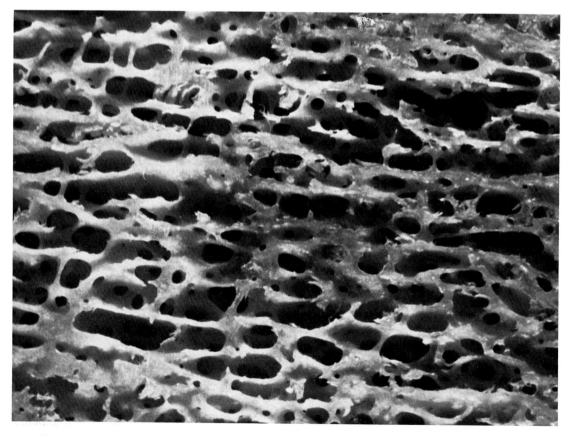

Fig. 1.7. High-power dissection microscope appearance of cancellous bone, showing connecting plates perforated by holes. (Macerated specimen × 13)

Normal development of the skeleton

The skeleton is mesenchymal in origin and formed by either intramembranous or endochondral ossification, depending on the particular bone. The processes of ossification are well described at the basic level in standard textbooks of histology. The structure of the growth plate is described elsewhere in this chapter (see p. 9), since a knowledge of the different zones in this region is important in the study of the developmental abnormalities, which are discussed in Chapter 2.

Similarly, detailed descriptions of the embryology of different parts of the skeleton are available elsewhere, and only the briefest outline is given here. Segmentation of the paraxial mesoderm into somites occurs towards the beginning of the fourth week in the developing embryo, and the ventromedial parts of the somites make up 'sclerotomes', from which the axial skeleton is derived. The mesenchymal vertebral column forms around the framework of the notochord, and rudimentary vertebral bodies are formed as separate cell masses from the sclerotomes. Concentrations of mesenchyme extend dorsally to surround the nerve tube and form a rudimentary neural arch. The mesenchymal tissue is converted firstly into cartilage (Fig. 1.8) and then bone, with the appearance of ossification centres in the vertebral bodies and neural arches. Notochord which is encased in the ossified vertebral bodies disappears, while that between the bones persists in the nucleus pulposus of the intervertebral discs. All the vertebrae consist of osseous tissue at birth, but cartilage persists at the junction of the neural arch with the vertebral body, in the transverse

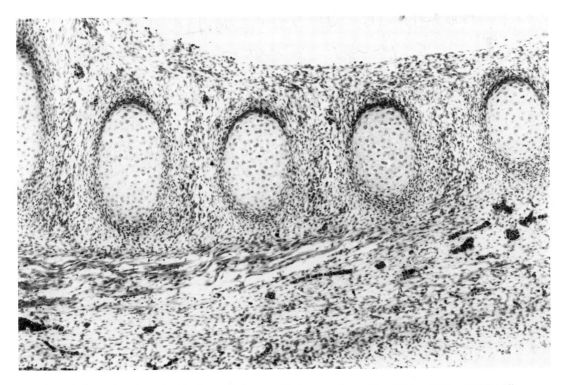

Fig. 1.8. Early formation of vertebral bodies as cartilage models in mesenchyme; 2 cm CR length fetus. (H&E × 80)

and spinous processes and at the epiphyseal plates. Union of the osseous parts of each vertebra commences in early childhood and is completed by 14 or 15 years of age.

The skull is formed in two distinct parts—a basal chondrocranium and the calvaria. The chondrocranium develops as a parachordal part, containing embedded notochordal remnants, and a prechordal part, which lies anterior to the notochord. The calvaria is formed by intramembranous ossification (Fig. 1.9). Bone trabeculae are formed when osteogenesis has become established in the ossification centres and the intertrabecular spaces become filled with bone marrow. The anterior and posterior fontanelles, present at birth, are covered by fibrous tissue and close by a process of ossification. This occurs 2 months after birth in the case of the posterior fontanelle and during the second postnatal year in the case of the anterior fontanelle. The surface area of the vault is increased by the addition of bone along the lines of the sutures during the first 7 years of life.

The limbs arise as outgrowths from the side of the embryo and comprise a mesenchymal core covered by ectoderm. Proliferation of the mesenchymal cells brings about lengthening of the limb in a proximodistal direction, and the mesenchyme is transformed into precartilage, then cartilage, models of the future bones of the pentadactyl limb structure (Fig. 1.10). Each cartilage model is surrounded by perichondrium, which becomes vascularised, leading to the development of a ring of osseous tissue around the middle of the cartilage model by the process of endochondral ossification. The cuff of bone

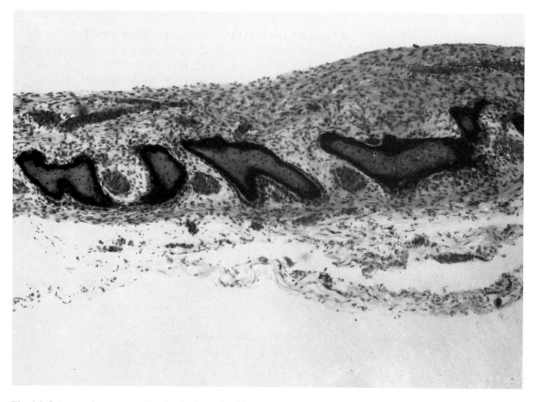

Fig. 1.9. Intramembranous ossification in the parietal bone of a fetus. (H&E × 250)

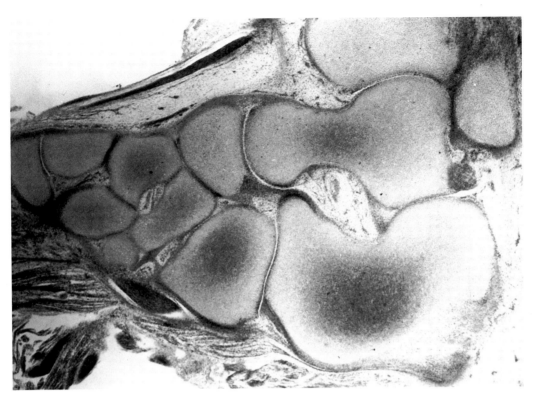

Fig. 1.10. Foot of a 10-week-old fetus showing the presence of cartilage models of the future bones of the ankle. (H&E × 75)

forming the cortex advances towards the ends of the bone in advance of the medullary bone, which becomes partly resorbed to form the marrow cavity. A transverse band of cartilage becomes delineated towards the edge of the bone to form the epiphyseal plate, which is the principal site of longitudinal growth in developing long bones. Epiphyses develop from the ends of the cartilage model beyond the epiphyseal plate, and this epiphyseal cartilage is penetrated by canals carrying small blood vessels derived from the perichondrium. After a variable period of time, depending on the particular bone, an ossification centre appears in the vascularised epiphysis. The ossification centre grows centrifugally, and at the same time the epiphysis is increased in size by further cartilage formation. Fusion of the ossified epiphyses with the shaft is associated with the disappearance of the intervening cartilage plate, which becomes replaced by bone.

Growth plate

The growth plate has been divided into various zones according to their morphology and function (Fig. 1.11). Just beneath the secondary epiphysis is the reserve zone, and adjacent to this are the proliferation and the hypertrophic zones. The latter is itself sometimes subdivided into zones of maturation, degeneration and provisional calcification.

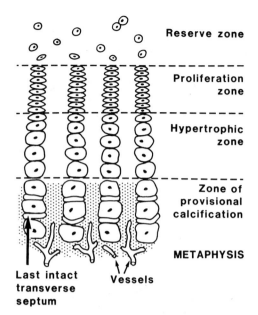

Fig. 1.11. Diagram to show the different zones of the growth plate. (see also Fig. 1.12)

Reserve zone

An alternative name given to the reserve zone is the 'resting zone', even though the cells at this level are not resting. They are spherical in shape and are present singly or in pairs. They are separated by more extracellular matrix than in other zones, and contain glycogen, more lipid and less alkaline and acid phosphatase, glucose-6-phosphate dehydrogenase, lactic dehydrogenase and other enzymes than in other zones (Kuhlman 1960, 1965; Brighton et al. 1973). The chondrocytes show little or no proliferative activity, and the function of the reserve zone has not been clearly defined. There is no evidence to support the idea that it provides the source of chondrocytes.

Proliferation zone

The flattened cells in the proliferation zone are arranged in longitudinal columns (see Fig. 1.12). They contain glycogen and have been shown by electron microscopy to have large amounts of endoplasmic reticulum which increases in amount by nearly three times from the top to the bottom of this zone (Brighton et al. 1973). Autoradiographic studies of tritiated thymidine incorporation have shown that the cartilage cells in the proliferation zone are the only ones that divide (Kember 1960). It is the topmost cell of each column which acts as the source of those lower down. Production of cartilage cells is responsible for the increase in length of a tubular bone, but the cartilage columns themselves, of course, do not increase in length, being converted at their metaphyseal ends into bone.

Hypertrophic zone

The flattened chondrocytes on the metaphyseal side of the cartilage columns are changed into large spherical cells in the hypertrophic zone (Figs. 1.11, 1.12). The cells increase in size by about five times within this zone (Brighton et al. 1973), and lower down the cells lose the intracytoplasmic glycogen which is present in the upper half of the hypertrophic zone (Pritchard 1952; Brighton et al. 1969). There is progressively increasing vacuolation of the cells, which is extensive at the bottom of the zone, where there is fragmentation of the cell membranes and of the nuclear envelope (Brighton 1978). Electron microscopy has demonstrated the presence of electron-dense granules in the mitochondria of growth plate chondrocytes, and these granules have been shown to contain calcium and phosphorus by X-ray spectroscopy (Martin and Matthews 1969, 1970; Sutfin et al. 1971). The mitochondria and cell membranes of the chondrocytes in the upper part of the hypertrophic zone are

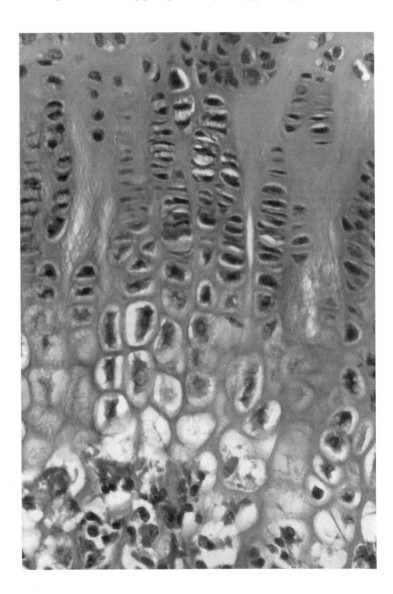

Fig. 1.12. Light microscope appearance of growth plate showing part of reserve zone (*top*), proliferation, hypertrophic and provisional calcification zones, together with part of the metaphysis (*bottom*) (cf. Fig. 1.11). (H&E × 800)

loaded with calcium, and this is progressively lost from these sites through this zone until there is no calcium present at the bottom of the zone (Brighton and Hunt 1974, 1976). Biochemical estimations show the upper part of the hypertrophic zone to have the highest content of alkaline and acid phosphatases, glucose-6-phosphate and lactic dehydrogenases and phosphoglycoisomerase, phosphate, calcium, magnesium and lipid (see Brighton 1978). Degradation of proteoglycan is probably brought about by lysosomal enzymes, the chondrocytes at this level containing higher concentrations than at any other in the growth plate. The initial calcification which occurs in the growth plate occurs within the longitudinal septa of the matrix. The septum becomes calcified by the growth and confluence of crystals in the bottom of the hypertrophic zone, which is also frequently called 'the zone of provisional calcification'. Matrix vesicles (see p. 13) are small extracellular structures distinguishable at the ultrastructural level and thought to be produced by the chondrocytes. They occur in greatest concentration in the hypertrophic zone (Anderson 1969) and are considered to play a central role in the process of mineralisation. The functions of the hypertrophic zone may be defined as the preparation of matrix for calcification and its subsequent calcification.

Metaphysis

The metaphysis begins immediately distal to the last intact transverse septa at the bottom of the cartilage cell columns. The upper part of the metaphysis immediately adjacent to the growth plate shows the presence of small vessels invading the calcified cartilage. Plump oval active osteoblasts are present in the upper part of this region and within a few cells show evidence of forming bone within and upon the calcified cartilage. The area of vascularised calcified cartilage is sometimes termed the primary spongiosum while the zone in which there is bone formed on the cartilage bars is the secondary spongiosum. The initially formed woven bone of this region is replaced by lamellar bone in the process of internal remodelling. Osteoclasts (and chondroclasts) are present within the metaphysis, resorbing both calcified cartilage and the fibre bone in the remodelling process. They are also present at the periosteal surface of the metaphysis, where they are responsible for the external remodelling which results in the narrowing of the bone to the diaphyseal region.

Ossification groove and perichondrial ring

The details of the structure of the growth plate given above are reasonably well known. The peripheral structures in this region are less well so. The periphery of the growth plate is encircled by a wedge-shaped groove of cells termed the ossification groove and a band of fibrous tissue and bone known as the perichondrial ring.

The ossification groove contains oval cells, which are considered to pass from the groove into the cartilage at the level of the beginning of the reserve zone. The function of the groove is thought to be to contribute chondrocytes to the growth plate for its increase in diameter (Tonna 1961). The perichondrial ring is a dense fibrous band encircling the growth plate at the level of the bone–cartilage junction. It is continuous at one end with the group of fibroblasts and collagen fibres of the ossification groove and at the other end with the periosteum and metaphyseal subperiosteal bone. The perichondrial ring provides a mechanical support for the otherwise weak bone–cartilage junction of the growth plate (Chung et al. 1976; Shapiro et al. 1977).

Mineralisation of bone

Elevated serum levels of alkaline phosphatase are regarded as indicating active tissue mineralisation in the absence of liver disease or other similar reasons for raised levels. Many years ago, it was proposed that alkaline phosphatase hydrolysed phosphate esters and produced excess free inorganic phosphate, raising the calcium and phosphate ion product at centres undergoing calcification to a level sufficient to bring about apatite deposition.

It has become clear that the process of mineralisation involves a much larger number of interrelated factors and mechanisms, and these may be divided into three general areas for consideration, namely:

1. The local elevation of calcium and phosphate ion levels to those at which there would be spontaneous precipitation of mineral
2. The presence of substances which would provide sites for the nucleation of mineral
3. The presence of substances preventing mineral formation and their removal or inactivation to allow subsequent calcification

The properties of nucleating systems have been reviewed by Posner et al. (1978), and the reader is referred to this article. Studies of calcium-binding proteins in the mineralisation process have shown that complexes of phospholipid with calcium and phosphate, certain phosphoproteins and bone collagen all may have important roles. Lipids are demonstrated in association with the calcification process by Irving (1963) and Enlow and Conklin (1964). Acid phospholipids have been extracted from calcified cartilage, bone and dentine (Wuthier 1968; Irving and Wuthier 1968; Shapiro 1970; Katchburian 1973; Odutugo and Prout 1974). Calcium-phospholipid-phosphate complexes associated with mineralisation are probably derived from membrane components of the tissue (Boskey 1978) and may play an important role in calcification (Vogel and Boyan-Salyers 1976; Wuthier 1976; Boskey and Posner 1977; Vogel et al. 1978).

Matrix vesicles

The concept of calcification in membrane-bound vesicles was introduced in the early 1970s, and these entities have subsequently become known as 'matrix vesicles' (Fig. 1.13). They are minute (less than 100 nm in diameter) extracellular particles first identified as 'cytoplasmic fragments' (Anderson 1967) and 'osmiophilic bodies' (Bonucci 1967). The early electron microscopic and biochemical work on these structures is reviewed by Anderson (1976). Ultrastructural studies showed that matrix vesicle formation was confined to areas of

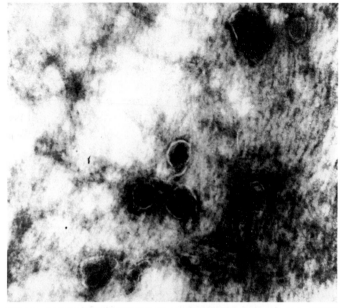

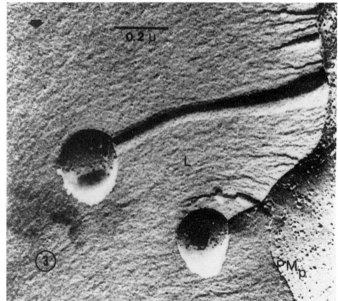

Fig. 1.13a,b. Matrix vesicles. **a** High-power view of electron-dense matrix vesicles with negatively stained double membrane in epiphyseal cartilage. (Sodium silicotungstate, × 10 000.) **b** Matrix vesicles formed as buds at the tip of fine processes from a chondrocyte plasma membrane (*PM*). (Freeze fracture × 75 000; bar = 0.2 μm)

matrix which eventually calcified. The first identifiable needles of apatite mineral were deposited within or close to the membranes of these vesicles (Anderson 1969).

Most investigators believe that matrix vesicles form as buds from the plasma membrane of proliferating or hypertrophic chondrocytes (Anderson 1969; Glauert and Mayo 1973; Rabinowitch and Anderson 1976; Cecil and Anderson 1978). Matrix vesicles are rich in 5-AMP-ase (Ali et al. 1970) and sphingomyelin (Peress et al. 1974), both of which are concentrated in plasma membrane. Dissenters from these views have suggested that matrix vesicles are extruded lysosomal dense bodies (Thyberg and Friberg 1972) or that they are derived from cell organelles rather than the cell membrane (Spycher et al. 1969; Bachra 1970; Kashiwa and Homorous 1971; Sayegh et al. 1974; Silberman and Frommer 1974).

The membranes of matrix vesicles provide an enclosed environment for the accumulation of calcium and phosphate ions, which are precipitated initially as amorphous calcium phosphate and later as apatite. The membranes are enriched with phospholipid, which serves as a trap for calcium ions (Peress et al. 1974) and are also a source of alkaline phosphatase, pyrophosphatase and ATPase (Ali et al. 1970; Matsuzawa and Anderson 1971). These enzymes may play a dual role in calcification, firstly by hydrolysing ester phosphate to provide phosphate ions and secondly by hydrolysing inhibitors of mineral crystal formation such as pyrophosphate and ATP (Fleisch and Bisaz 1962; Betts et al. 1975; Termine and Conn 1976).

The process of nucleation of crystals from ions in solution occurs by two different methods. In homogeneous nucleation, randomly aggregated ions form nuclei large enough to grow into crystals, while in heterogeneous nucleation, the ions aggregate on a substrate to form nuclei and subsequently grow into crystals. It is likely that heterogeneous nucleation is the chief mechanism in biological systems, and the possible nucleating agents have already been mentioned above (viz. phospholipids, phosphoproteins and collagen). The first mineral phase in the ossification process is considered to be an amorphous calcium phosphate. It has long been recognised that mitrochondria can concentrate calcium and phosphate and form electron-dense granules (Lehninger 1970). The mitochondria of the chondrocytes in the growth plate are rich in these mineral granules (Martin and Matthews 1969; Holtrop 1972; Shapiro et al. 1976; see this chapter, Hypertrophic zone), which are thought most likely to contain amorphous calcium phosphate stabilised with phospholipid (Ali et al. 1978; Posner et al. 1978). Matrix vesicles begin to accumulate calcium at the level in the hypertrophic zone where mitochondria begin to lose calcium (Brighton and Hunt 1974, 1976), and it therefore seems possible that the mitochondria of the chondrocytes concentrate calcium and phosphate, then export these ions to give locally high levels for the growth of hydroxyapatite crystals in and near the matrix vesicles. The first apatite crystals in matrix vesicles may be formed in the proliferative zone and the further nucleation and complete mineralisation occur in the lower hypertrophic zone by the rapid release of calcium phosphate from mitochondria of degenerative chondrocytes (Ali 1976).

Bone collagen and its mineralisation

The various possible mechanisms responsible for the mineralisation of collagenous tissues are comprehensively reviewed by Glimcher (1976), and the reader requiring detailed background knowledge is referred to that article. This chapter is also not the place in which to give details of the different types of collagen and their chemistry, and such information is available elsewhere. There are at least five types of collagen (Table 1.1). Bone collagen is a type I collagen and has the same general chemical composition and chemical structure as other type I collagens. It differs, however, in its mechanical and physicochemical properties. Important differences have also been noted in the

Table 1.1. The different types of collagen

Type	Molecular form	Tissue
Type I	$[a1(I)]_2a2(I)$	Bone, dermis, tendon, cornea, dentin
Type II	$[a1(II)]_3$	Cartilage
Type III	$[a1(III)]_3$	Fetal and infant dermis, early scar tissue, granulomas, cardiovascular system
Type IV	$[a1(IV)]_3$ $[a2(IV)]_3$	Basement membranes
Type V	$[a1(V)]_2a_2(V)$ $a1(V), a_2(V)a_3(V)$ $[a1(V)]_3$	Pericellular collagens, exocytoskeleton-like

packing arrangement of collagen molecules in the fibrils of soft tissue and those of bone or dentine (Katz and Li 1973a, b).

A model of the packing of collagen molecules has been presented by Hodge and Petruska (1963) in which molecules are overlapped by about 9% of their length and linear aggregates are staggered laterally to form a fibril in which there are spaces between the ends of the molecules, referred to as holes (Fig. 1.14). The region of the fibril containing both holes and overlapped molecules is referred to as the hole zone, and the region consisting only of overlapped molecules as the overlap zone. The holes may be seen by negative staining techniques using electron microscopy. Three-dimensional models of this two-dimensional concept propose either a cylindrical or hexagonal arrangement (Miller and Wray 1971; Katz and Li 1973a, b; Glimcher 1976). Katz and Li suggested the presence of spaces within the fibrils described as 'pores'.

Although the exact three-dimensional array of collagen molecules in the collagen fibrils of any of the connective tissues is not known with certainty, it is likely that there is considerable space within them which can accommodate other substances, for example calcium and phosphate. The gap between adjacent molecules in a bone collagen fibril is greater than in certain soft tissue collagens, so that the rate of diffusion of ions into the interstices of the fibril will be correspondingly greater in bone collagen fibrils.

Almost all the mineral present in normal lamellar bone is located within the collagen fibrils (Glimcher 1976). The volume present outside the collagen fibrils is only 5%–10% (Boyde 1972). The mineral phase is initially deposited within the fibrils, and mineral is subsequently deposited between the fibrils.

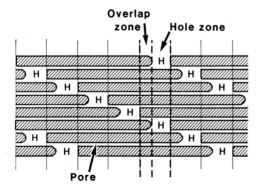

Fig. 1.14. Diagram to show overlapping of collagen molecules, hole zones (*H*), and pores in proposed model of the packing arrangement of collagen in bone

At all stages of mineralisation, the predominant ultrastructural organisation shows more of the mineral phase located in certain specific regions of collagen fibrils, and when an axial periodicity of the mineral phase has been observed, its period has been approximately the same as that of collagen fibrils themselves (viz. ~ 700 Å).

Collagen molecules or polymers of these molecules secreted into the extracellular space by the osteoblasts are assembled into fibrils prior to impregnation with mineral. There is therefore a stage in the calcification of bone in which the collagen fibrils in the extracellular tissue space are free of solid-phase calcium and phosphate. The deposition of a mineral phase within and on the surface of the fibrils occurs preferentially in the hole zone of the fibril, and there continues to be a preferential distribution of the mass of the mineral phase at this site as against the overlap zone, at least until full mineralisation of the fibril occurs (Glimcher 1976).

Although more of the mineral phase is located within the hole zone region, solid-phase calcium and phosphate particles are deposited in the pores of both the hole zone and the overlap region. The mass of mineral phase and number and size of particles increase with time so that eventually a great number of larger particles completely fill the holes and pores. After initiation of calcification of collagen fibrils, there are several rate-dependent processes which occur concurrently within the fibrils. These include heterogeneous nucleation (see p. 15) of new amorphous calcium phosphate, growth of amorphous calcium phosphate particles and transition of these to poorly crystalline hydroxyapatite with nucleation onto the surfaces of amorphous calcium phosphate.

Once the initial solid phase has been formed, most of the additional material is deposited by secondary nucleation (Glimcher 1976). The internal geometry of the spaces within the collagen fibril permits the particles of the mineral phase to 'overlap' one another and thus provide the continuity necessary to provide structural rigidity throughout the fibril.

The presence of calcium and phosphate granules in intracellular organelles and extracellular matrix vesicles is described elsewhere in this chapter (see p. 13). The relationship between such calcium deposits and mineralisation of collagen is not yet clearly defined.

A relationship seems to exist between the disappearance of calcium-phosphate particles from mitochondria and the onset of calcification, while the concentration of these ions within matrix vesicles appears to precede extracellular deposition, at least in the case of the calcification of cartilage. Whether such mechanisms also apply to the calcification of bone in the postnatal organism has been questioned by Glimcher (1976). Certainly, the method of secretion of collagen by osteoblasts at bone surfaces and the temporal relationships of the calcification of osteoid are not well understood. The relationship between mitochondrial calcification, matrix vesicle formation and the calcification of collagen fibrils in endochondral ossification is highly theoretical. It seems likely that mitochondria and matrix vesicles play a role in calcification by altering local conditions in the extracellular fluid space in such a way that heterogeneous nucleation of calcium-phosphate particles occurs within collagen fibrils. In addition, calcification may be regulated by cellular means, such as the presence of soluble inhibitors and the synthesis of enzymes which degrade such inhibitors. Proteoglycans, for example, act as inhibitors of calcification since they are able to bind calcium, exclude phosphate ions and decrease the diffusion of ions into tissue.

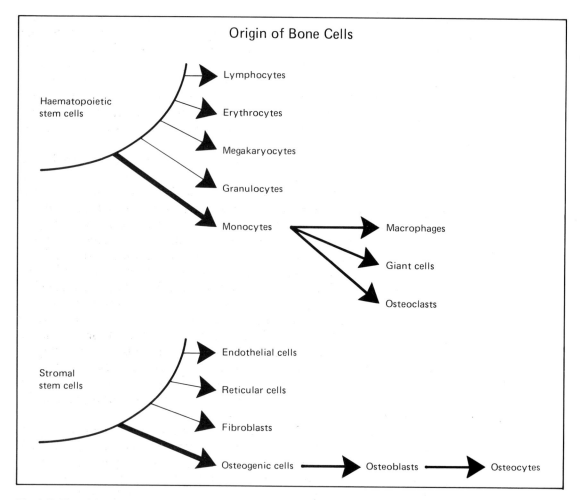

Fig. 1.15. The origin of bone cells

Origin of bone cells

The question of the origin of cells present in bone has been much discussed in the past. The possibility of a common precursor for osteoclasts and osteoblasts and for interchange between these two types was, until fairly recently, favoured by some (for example Rasmussen and Bordier 1974). It is now becoming increasingly apparent that the two main cell types in bone, the osteoclast and osteoblast, are derived from different cell lineages, namely the haematopoietic and stromal cell systems respectively (Fig. 1.15). The subject has been reviewed by Owen (1983).

Osteoblast

Osteoblasts originate from connective tissue cells (Friedenstein 1976) and have as their immediate precursors cells termed 'preosteoblasts', which are fibroblast-like cells located near osteoblastic and bone surfaces (Owen 1980).

Alkaline phosphatase activity provides a means of differentiating these osteo-genic cells (Pritchard 1952). Studies of the regeneration of bone marrow after its depletion and of the transplantation of bone marrow have provided evidence that marrow stroma and osteogenic soft tissue are each capable of giving rise to both osseous tissue and bone marrow stroma. A series of references to this work is provided in the reviews by Owen (1980, 1983). Friedenstein (1976) has shown that cultured marrow fibroblasts or marrow cells placed in diffusion chambers and implanted in vivo are capable of forming calcified tissue.

Fibroblasts derived from the stroma of other tissues (thymus, spleen, lymph node) form only soft fibrous tissue unless an inducing agent is present, in which case calcified tissue is formed (Friedenstein et al. 1970). Cartilage and bone formation in skin and muscle may be induced by agents such as transitional (bladder) epithelium, decalcified bone matrix, or a bone morphogenetic protein (Urist et al. 1978). There are therefore 'determined' and 'inducible' osteo-genic precursor cells (Friedenstein 1976), the former requiring no additional stimulus, while the latter do not show osteogenic potential unless subjected to the action of local inducers. Various experiments have been performed to identify osteogenic and haematopoietic tissue after transplantation of different cell types between animals; for example the use of chromosome markers (Friedenstein et al. 1968). The results of these studies lead to the conclusion that stromal tissue is derived from a separate cell line from that which gives rise to haematopoietic tissue (Friedenstein 1976). Nevertheless, a close relationship exists between bone and bone marrow formation, and it seems likely that bone and bone marrow stromal tissue influence haematopoiesis (see, for example, Friedenstein 1976; Owen 1980).

The various factors which affect bone morphogenesis in the postnatal organism have been most recently reviewed by Nogemi and Oohira (1984). Pluripotential cells arise by proliferation and migration from periosteum, bone marrow stroma and other connective tissues, and their subsequent differentiation is much dependent on local conditions. An osteogenic factor called bone morphogenetic protein (BMP) has been isolated from bone, dentin and osteosarcomatous tissue. It is believed to influence mesenchymal cells to differentiate into chondrocytes or osteoblasts. Further information is available elsewhere (Urist and Mikulski 1979; Urist 1981; Urist et al. 1982; Nogemi and Oohira 1984).

Osteoblasts synthesise bone collagen but also secrete several other components into bone matrix. Extracellular protein which binds calcium by the presence of γ-carboxyglutamic acid is known as osteocalcin. Its formation is vitamin K dependent and stimulated by $1,25(OH)_2$ vitamin D (Price et al. 1980; Price and Baukol 1981). Another group comprising proteins analogous to fibronectin are known as osteonectin and bind both to collagen and calcium (Lee and Glimcher 1981; Termine et al. 1981).

Osteoclast

There is a large body of indirect evidence for the origin of the osteoclast from circulating mononuclear cells and hence ultimately from a haematopoietic stem cell. References to this work are available in the review by Owen (1980). Studies of the pathology and treatment of osteopetrosis in rodents have also thrown important light on this question (see, for example, Walker 1975; Loutit and Nisbet 1979), and these are mentioned in a little more detail in Chapter 2. Granulocytes, monocytes and osteoclasts of beige mice have giant lysosomes, but these are absent from fibroblasts and osteoblasts, suggesting two different cell lines. Intravenous infusion of bone marrow from beige mice into lethally irradiated osteopetrotic microphthalmic mice results in the population of bone by osteoclasts with giant lysosomes (Ash et al. 1980). Although the granulocyte series may in theory provide the osteoclast precursor on the evidence of this work, a lineage from monocytes and macrophages is much more likely. Resorptive activity by monocytes and macrophages incubated with bone in vitro and the fact that resorbing bone is chemotactic for these cells provides further evidence (Mundy et al. 1977, 1978; Kahn et al. 1978; Teitelbaum et al. 1979). Radiolabelling experiments suggest that cells local to bone surfaces are the immediate precursors of both osteoblasts and osteoclasts (Young 1962; Owen 1970). Further information about the origin of osteoclasts is available in Chambers (1980), Bonucci (1981) and Marks (1983).

In summary, the haematopoietic stem cell is the precursor of the osteoclast, though the exact cell line to which this cell belongs has not been conclusively established. The stromal stem cell in the marrow gives rise to osteogenic cells, and fibroblast-like cells in osseous tissues are determined osteogenetic precursor cells. Connective tissue precursor cells in other tissues require an inductive factor before becoming capable of osteogenic activity.

Cells in bone

Three types of cells are distinguishable within bone, namely the osteoblasts, osteocytes and osteoclasts. Under normal conditions osteoblasts may be incorporated in bone matrix to become osteocytes. There is a close relationship between the bone-forming cells and the cell lines which form fibrous tissue or cartilage. Conversion of cells from one type to another is encountered under pathological conditions, for example in the formation of chondroid tissue by periosteal cells in fracture callus under certain circumstances.

Osteoblasts

Osteoblasts are seen as a layer of plump polyhedral cells covering the bone surfaces (Fig. 1.16). They show marked cytoplasmic basophilia and have nuclei rich in ribonucleic acid. Differentiating osteoblasts contain glycogen, which is absent, however, from those cells which are actively forming bone. Alkaline phosphatase is present in osteoblasts which are actively forming bone and in the tissue immediately adjacent. Surfaces of osseous tissue on which there is active deposition of bone show a narrow zone of osteoid tissue, or preosseous matrix, which differs from bone matrix in that it is not calcified (Fig. 1.17). Ultrastructurally, osteoid consists of coarse collagen fibres containing foci of initial calcification. The interface between osteoid and calcified bone is referred to as the 'calcification front'. It may be demonstrated with

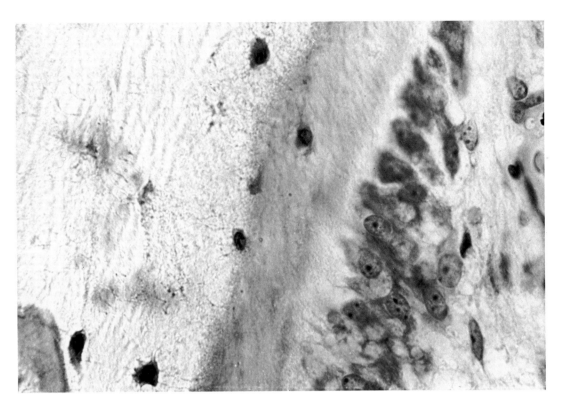

Fig. 1.16. Osteoblasts forming a layer at the surface of osteoid (*right*) bone. Note also incorporation of cells to become osteocytes. (Methylmethacrylate, thionin × 1000)

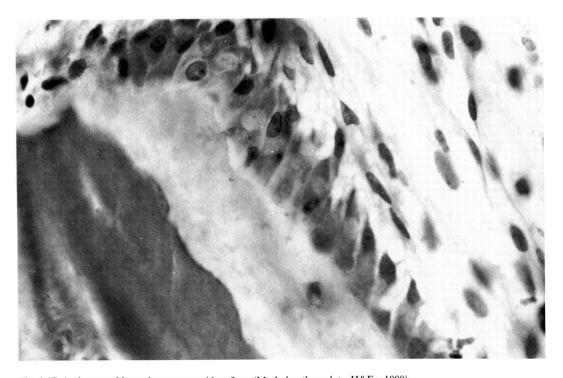

Fig. 1.17. Active osteoblasts along an osteoid surface. (Methylmethacrylate, H&E × 1000)

lipid strains (Irving 1963), or by ultraviolet (UV) light microscopy after the administration of tetracycline, which is fluorescent and becomes incorporated at sites of calcification (Milch et al. 1958). The dynamics of mineralisation and osteoid formation may be studied using labels which fluoresce with different colours, as well as tetracycline (Bordier et al. 1976; Parfitt et al. 1976; Teitelbaum and Nichols 1976).

Resting osteoblasts are usually flattened, with less basophilic cytoplasm, and are closely applied to the bone surface. The surfaces of the trabecular bone and Haversian systems are covered by a thin layer of osteoprogenitor (preosteoblast) cells and osteoblasts, which are together termed the endostium. Such cells cover most of the inner bone surfaces, apart from those areas where there is osteoclastic activity or where they are interspersed with early haematopoietic cells.

Electron microscopy shows that the osteoblast has abundant rough endoplasmic reticulum and plentiful free ribosomes and polyribosomes (Fig. 1.18). The Golgi zone is well developed and mitochondria are numerous. The large ovoid nucleus is eccentrically placed. Accumulations of particulate glycogen are often present and there are lysosomes and coated vesicles, the latter frequently fusing with the cell membrane. The cell surface has a small number of short microvilli. The appearances are those of a cell which is actively involved in protein synthesis, namely collagen fibrils and ground substance of the bone matrix.

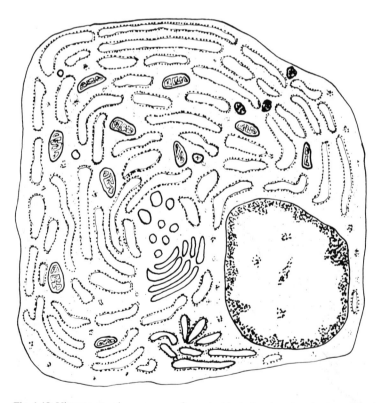

Fig. 1.18. Ultrastructural appearance of an osteoblast, showing abundant rough endoplasmic reticulum, free ribosomes, well-developed Golgi zone and numerous mitochondria, together with eccentrically placed nucleus

Osteocytes

Osteocytes are small darkly staining cells completely surrounded by mineralised bone matrix with the exception of a 1–2 μm wide space which forms the osteocyte lacuna. This zone is occupied by collagen fibrils having a different configuration (see below). Each osteocyte possesses several long cytoplasmic processes which pass through the bone matrix in narrow tunnels, the canaliculi (Fig. 1.19). The narrow space between matrix and the cytoplasmic process is thought to contain interstitial fluid in which metabolites are able to pass to the cells.

Ultrastructural examination shows the osteocytes to have small nuclei and sparse cytoplasm with few mitochondria and a small Golgi zone (Fig. 1.20). The amount of endoplasmic reticulum varies with the activity of the cell, those cells nearer to the bone surface generally containing more rough endoplasmic reticulum. Osteocytes are formed by the incorporation of osteoblasts at bone surfaces when transformation occurs, with the development of long cellular processes (Fig. 1.21) and loss of the organelles associated with protein synthesis, as the cells become surrounded by mineralised bone matrix.

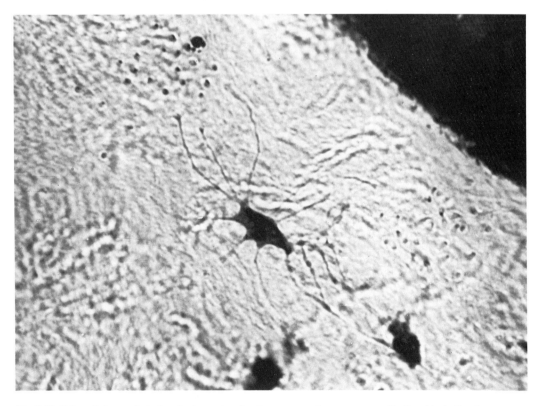

Fig. 1.19. Osteocyte lacuna in trabecular bone showing the presence of numerous canaliculi and including those seen in cross-section (*top left*). (Methylmethacrylate, thionin × 1000)

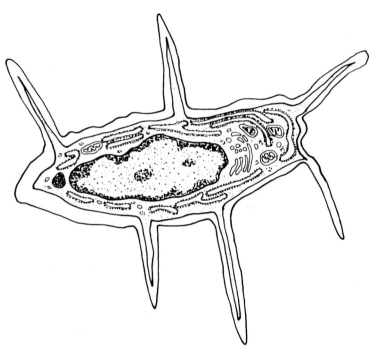

Fig. 1.20. Ultrastructural appearance of an osteocyte, showing sparse organelles with few mitochondria, small Golgi zone and little rough endoplasmic reticulum

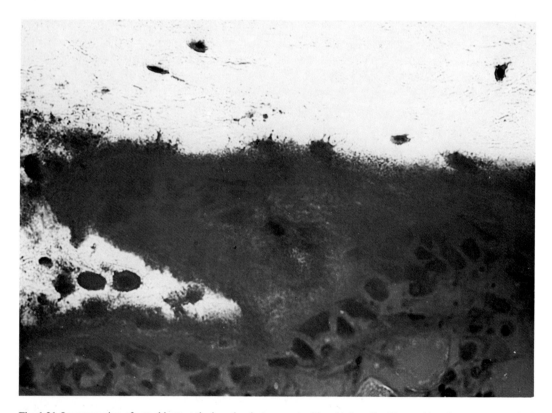

Fig. 1.21. Incorporation of osteoblasts at the junction between osteoid and mineralised bone. Also shows osteocyte (*top*) and surface osteoblasts (*bottom*). (Methylmethacrylate, thionin × 500)

It has been suggested that osteocytes play a role in degradation of the bone matrix surrounding them in the process of osteocytic osteolysis (Belanger 1969). These cells also appear capable of forming small amounts of bone after they have become embedded in bone (Rasmussen and Bordier 1974; Baud 1976). There is certainly a large variation in the size of osteocyte lacunae even in normal bone. Baud and Auil (1971) have classified osteocyte lacunae into four different types, namely:

1. Inactive—small lacuna with a smooth border
2. Osteolytic—large lacuna with an irregular border and plentiful lysosomes in the osteocyte
3. Osteoplastic—large lacuna with recently formed matrix of radially arranged collagen and abundant endoplasmic reticulum in the osteocyte
4. Empty lacuna containing cellular debris

Permanent enlargement of lacunae is said to occur in relation to the death of osteocytes and in relation to endosteal resorption in growing bone (Jande and Belanger 1973; Parfitt 1976). There is some confusion about the term 'osteocytic osteolysis' and there are problems in its use with respect to enlarged osteocyte lacunae. These are also seen in woven bone, fracture callus and other sites of rapidly forming bone and are in no way associated with resorptive activity under these circumstances. The appropriateness of methods used to assess osteocyte lacunar size has also been called into question, since microradiography and von Kossa-stained sections prepared for light microscopy as well as many electron microscopic methods delineate only the mineralised phase of bone. It is thus not possible to differentiate 'true' from 'apparent' enlargement of lacunae, the latter being due to the presence of a halo of unmineralised matrix in the presence of, for example, a mineralisation defect. Such considerations as these are discussed in more detail by Boyde (1981), who has presented the case against the existence of osteocytic osteolysis. The reader wishing to have more detailed information about the subject and the arguments against osteocytic resorption is referred to this review, which also provides a useful bibliography on the whole subject.

Apart from the resorption of bone by osteocytes, the question also arises as to whether these cells are capable of bone formation by the process of 'osteoplasis', in which bone is deposited on the walls of the lacunae (Vittali 1968; Baud and Auil 1971; Baylink and Wergedal 1971). The thin layer of bone immediately adjacent to the osteocyte which contains minimal amounts of collagen and which may be mineralised to a high degree, is referred to as perilacunar bone. It is suggested that this bone plays a role in calcium homeostasis.

The relative significance of osteocytic resorption and osteoplasis, if they occur, must be small in proportion to the activity of osteoclasts and osteoblasts (Baylink and Wergedal 1971; Parfitt 1976). Proponents of osteocytic osteolysis suggest that calcium must be mobilised in this way in order to explain how plasma calcium levels rise so rapidly after administration of parathyroid hormone. However, parathyroid hormone has effects on the kidney and intestine which must also be taken into account, and a rapid response of osteoclasts to parathyroid hormone in the rat has been demonstrated (Holtrop 1976), with a significant increase in ruffled borders and clear zones demonstrable as soon as 30 min after hormone administration. Boyde (1981) has calculated that 1 mg of calcium could be removed by normal osteoclastic activity from the skeleton in 1 min under normal circumstances. If the action of parathyroid hormone on osteoclasts is further taken into account, there would seem to be little need to postulate an osteocytic mechanism to account for the release of calcium from bone.

Osteoclasts

Osteoclasts are multinucleate giant cells occurring singly or in small groups on the inner surfaces of trabecular and compact bones (Fig. 1.22). In routinely stained sections, the cytoplasm is moderately acidophilic and the nuclei round or oval, usually with a single prominent nucleolus. Osteoclasts are easily picked out in sections stained with thionin or toluidine blue, when they show purple-red metachromasia of the cytoplasm. Active bone resorption may be identified by the presence of osteoclasts in resorption lacunae (Howship's lacunae) at the bone surface. Such resorbing surfaces have a crenated irregular appearance and do not contain osteoid. This has led to the idea that osteoclasts are active only at sites where there is mineralised bone matrix. A striated border to the cell cytoplasm is sometimes visible by light microscopy at the contact surface (Hancox 1972). The mechanism by which osteoclasts resorb bone remains a matter for debate. Apatite crystals or collagen fibres may be removed first (Scott and Pease 1956; Dudley and Spiro 1961; Gonzales and Karnovsky 1961), or both organic and inorganic components may be removed simultaneously (Cameron and Robinson 1958). Another alternative is that

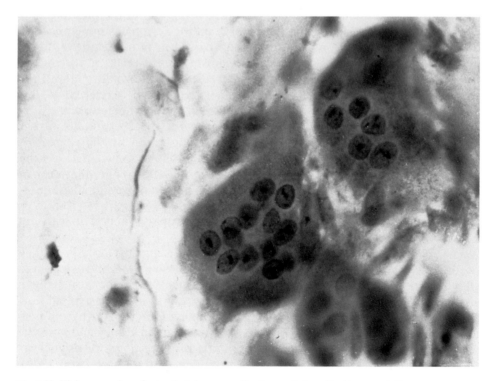

Fig. 1.22. High-power view of osteoclasts in a resorption lacuna (mineralised bone on *left*). (Methylmethacrylate, thionin × 1000)

osteoclasts are responsible for demineralisation of the bone and that exposed collagen fibrils are subsequently phagocytosed by mononuclear cells (Heersche 1978).

Ultrastructural studies have shown that osteoclasts contain plentiful mitochondria, which are concentrated in the cytoplasm between the nucleus and the cell border furthest from the bone. There are several well-developed Golgi zones in the region of the nuclei and moderate amounts of loosely arranged rough endoplasmic reticulum are present. The surface of the osteoclast immediately adjacent to bone matrix is differentiated into a clear zone and a ruffled border (Fig. 1.23). The clear zone lacks organelles and is characterised by moderately dense granular cytoplasm. The ruffled border shows deep invaginations of the cell membrane with numerous microvilli. The cytoplasm deep to the ruffled border contains smooth and coated vesicles, phagosomes and residual bodies. The ruffled zone is considered to be the area of active resorption and is surrounded by the clear zone. The matrix adjacent to the ruffled border shows loss of mineral deposits, and small masses of apparently detached crystals are distinguishable (Hancox 1972).

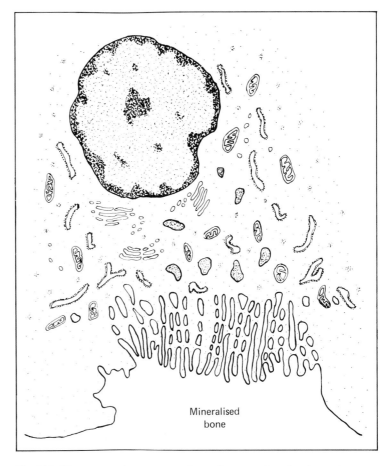

Mineralised
bone

Fig. 1.23. Ultrastructural appearance of part of an osteoclast, showing nucleus, mitochondria, Golgi zone and rough endoplasmic reticulum. There are deep invaginations of the cell membrane at the ruffled border of the cell which is immediately adjacent to bone. The clear zone on either side of the ruffled border is lacking in organelles

Bone resorption

'Resorption' is the term used to indicate removal of both mineral and organic matrix from bone. It is a process necessary for the remodelling of bone and probably for the long-term maintenance of serum calcium levels. Removal of mineral and organic matrix are apparently linked, since large amounts of decalcified matrix are never present at resorbing surfaces and unmineralised matrix is not resorbed. Although some bone resorption may occur in relation to osteocytes (see p. 25), the principal cell responsible is the osteoclast. Resorption of calcified and uncalcified cartilage also occurs and this is mediated by cells morphologically similar to osteoclasts, usually referred to as chondroclasts. The maintenance of calcium levels is not brought about by a simple physicochemical process, and cellular activity is required (Borle 1967; Raisz 1976). Understanding the precise mechanisms of bone resorption in relation to calcium homeostasis is made all the more difficult by the limitations of the methods applicable to its study. These methods include the use of tracers which will become incorporated into bone, measurement of hydroxyproline in blood and urine and quantitative morphological studies. All have drawbacks, and these are discussed briefly elsewhere (Raisz 1976). Morphological methods depend on the use of radiography or histology. Marked increases in resorption rate can produce radiographic changes such as subperiosteal resorption in the small bones of the hand distinguishable in clinical X-ray films. Direct quantitation of changes in tissue includes the use of microradiography or undecalcified sections (Jowsey et al. 1965), or examination of histological sections to include the counting of osteoclasts (Schenk et al. 1969) or measurements on bone surfaces with or without tetracycline labelling (Frost 1964). Sequential labelling with tetracyclines can be used to identify growing and resorbing surfaces (Harris et al. 1968).

The regulation of bone resorption under physiological conditions has to subserve two functions, namely the maintenance of the skeleton as a structural support system which is constantly being remodelled and the fulfilment of a metabolic role in mineral homeostasis. It is clear that maintenance of calcium homeostasis is partly dependent on bone resorption and cellular events. However, when bone turnover is low and an adequate supply of calcium is available, alterations in calcium level in the blood and extracellular fluid space can be rapidly restored by events in the renal tubule and intestinal mucosa.

Remodelling with changes in overall bone structure occurring during growth and development consists largely in the removal of bone from one site and its deposition in another (e.g. the inner and outer aspects of the cortex of long bones, the resorption of calcified cartilage and the deposition of bone in endochondral ossification; see this chapter, Metaphysis). Net gains and losses of osseous tissue must be closely controlled during the period of growth of the skeleton to prevent imbalance between the two processes. It is clear that when such an imbalance occurs, pathological conditions result, as, for example, in the development of osteosclerosis in the condition of osteopetrosis, in which there is a defect in osteoclast function (see Chap. 2, Osteopetrosis).

Tension and compression of bone have an effect on its formation and resorption, and, although the mechanism is not clearly understood, piezoelectric effects have been suggested as one way in which bone cell activity is modified under these circumstances (Bassett 1968; see Chap. 9, Bone response to exogenous electrical stimuli). Local effects which stimulate resorption of bone include increased oxygen tension, heparin and prostaglandins. Studies of radiolabelled explants of rodent bone in vitro show links between prosta-glandin production by macrophages and that of a soluble factor, osteoclast activating factor (OAF), produced by lymphocytes (Yoneda and Mundy 1979a, b). Such a local mechanism may be responsible for bone resorption in relation to chronic inflammation or near tumours.

The major physiological control of bone resorption in calcium homeostasis is mediated through the action of parathyroid hormone. Maintenance of nor-mal ionised calcium concentrations in the serum and of normal rates of bone turnover are dependent on the continuous secretion of this hormone. The effect of vitamin D and parathyroid hormone are closely linked in the regula-tion of bone resorption, while calcitonin is a specific hormonal inhibitor. Thyroid hormones, glucocorticoids and sex hormones also have important effects on bone metabolism. Other factors have been summarised recently by Russell et al. (1983) and include OAF, prostaglandins, interleukin 1 and the retinoids.

There is yet much to know about osteoclast function. It is possible that production of acid conditions locally is responsible for resorption of bone, through hydrogen ion production from carbonic anhydrase or lactate, and that citrate plays a role as a calcium-chelating agent. Unmineralised bone matrix seems likely to be degraded by extracellular proteinases, such as colla-genase and metalloproteinases, and by lysosomal acid hydrolases. Various

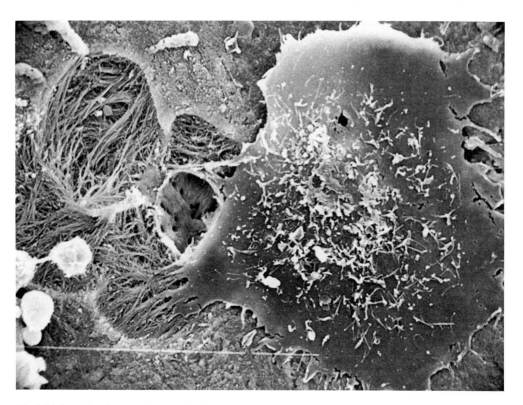

Fig. 1.24. Scanning electron micrograph of an osteoclast (*right*) cultured on a bone slice, to show resorption pits in which collagen fibres are clearly seen (*left*). (Bar = 10 μm)

techniques have been used to study osteoclast function indirectly, such as the release of calcium from fetal or newborn mouse calvariae. Recently, it has been possible to study the effect of isolated osteoclasts in vitro on bone slices (Athanasou et al. 1984; Chambers et al. 1984; Fig. 1.24), and such techniques present the possibility of further understanding osteoclasts and bone resorption.

Control of bone cell function

Some of the factors affecting osteoblasts and osteoclasts in their formation and removal of bone have already been mentioned, as has the requirement for coordination of both processes so that there are no net gains or losses (see this chapter, Osteoblast; Bone resorption). There is a close relationship between the rate of bone formation and resorption under normal conditions and this is seen in various pathological states as well. Observations of cell populations in cortical and trabecular bone have led to the development of the concept that they act together in a unit, and the 'basic multicellular unit' (BMU), 'bone remodelling unit' (BRU) and 'bone structural unit' (BSU) are all terms which have been used (see, for example, Frost 1976; Courpron et al. 1980; Ellis 1981; Parfitt 1982). The relationship between osteoblasts and osteoclasts may be termed 'coupling' (Parfitt 1982) and is as yet poorly understood, but possibilities include the activity of soluble mediators produced by one cell type and influencing the other, the effects of bone matrix components such as osteocalcin and osteonectin, and the influence of cellular interaction by direct contact.

Other aspects, particularly the effects of hormones and vitamin D on bone, are described elsewhere in this book. The regulation of bone formation has recently been reviewed by Raisz and Kream (1983a, b).

References

Ali SY (1976) Analysis of matrix vesicles and their role in the calcification of epiphyseal cartilage. Fed Proc 35: 135–142

Ali SY, Sajdera SW, Anderson HC (1970) Isolation and characterization of calcifying matrix vesicles from epiphyseal cartilage. Proc Natl Acad Sci USA 67: 1513–1520

Ali SY, Wisby A, Gray JC (1978) Electron probe analysis of cryosections of epiphyseal cartilage. Metab Bone Dis Relat Res 1: 97–103

Amstutz HC, Sissons HA (1969) The structure of the vertebral spongiosa. J Bone Joint Surg [Br] 51: 540–550

Anderson HC (1967) Electron microscopic studies of induced cartilage development and calcification. J Cell Biol 35: 81–101

Anderson HC (1969) Vesicles associated with calcification in the matrix of epiphyseal cartilage. J Cell Biol 41: 59–72

Anderson HC (1976) Matrix vesicle calcification. Introduction. Fed Proc 35: 105–108

Ash P, Loutit JF, Townsend KMS (1980) Osteoclasts derived from haemopoietic stem cells. Nature 283: 669–670

Athanasou NA, Gray A, Revell PA, Fuller K, Cochrane T, Chambers TJ (1984) Steriophotogrammetric observations on bone resorption by isolated rabbit osteoclasts. Micron Microscopia Acta 15: 47–53

Bachra BN (1970) Calcification of connective tissue. Int Rev Connect Tissue Res 5: 165–208

Bassett CAL (1968) Biologic significance of piezoelectricity. Calcif Tissue Res 1: 252–272

Baud CA (1976) Osteocyte, osteocytic functions and morphometry of periosteocytic lacunae. In: Meunier PJ (ed) Bone histomorphometry. 2nd international workshop. Armour Montagu, Paris, pp 429–432.

Baud CA, Auil E (1971) Osteocyte differential count in normal human alveolar bone. Acta Anat 78: 321–327

Baylink DJ, Wergedal JE (1971) Bone formation by osteocytes. Am J Physiol 221: 669–678

Belanger LF (1969) Osteocytic osteolysis. Calcif Tissue Res 4: 1–12

Betts F, Blumenthal NC, Posner AS, Becker GL, Lehringer AL (1975) The atomic structure of intercellular amorphous calcium phosphate deposits. Proc Natl Acad Sci USA 72: 2088–2090

Bonucci E (1967) Fine structure of early cartilage calcification. J Ultrastruct Res 20: 33–50

Bonucci E (1981) New knowledge on the origin, function and fate of osteoclasts. Clin Orthop 158: 252–269

Bordier Ph J, Marie P, Miravet L, Ryckewaert A, Rasmussen H (1976) Morphological and morphometrical characteristics of the mineralisation front. A vitamin D regulated sequence of the bone remodeling. In: Meunier PJ (ed) Bone histomorphometry. 2nd international workshop. Armour Montagu, Paris, pp 335–354

Borle AB (1967) Membrane transfer of calcium. Clin Orthop Relat Res 52: 267–291

Boskey AL (1978) The role of calcium-phospholipid-phosphate complexes in tissue mineralisation. Metab Bone Dis Relat Res 1: 137–142

Boskey AL, Posner AS (1977) The role of synthetic and bone extracted Ca-phospholipid-PO$_4$ complexes in hydroxyapatite formation. Calcif Tissue Res 23: 251–258

Boyde A (1972) Scanning electron microscope studies of bone. In: Bourne GH (ed) The biochemistry and physiology of bone, 2nd edn, vol 1. Academic, New York, pp 259–310

Boyde A (1981) Evidence against 'osteocytic osteolysis'. In: Jee WSS, Parfitt AM (eds) Bone histomorphometry. 3rd international workshop. Metab Bone Dis Relat Res 2 (Suppl): 239–255

Brighton CT (1978) Structure and function of the growth plate. Clin Orthop 136: 22–32

Brighton CT, Hunt RM (1974) Mitochondrial calcium and its role in calcification. Histochemical localisation of calcium in electron micrographs of the epiphyseal growth plate with K-pyroantimonate. Clin Orthop 100: 406–416

Brighton CT, Hunt RM (1976) Histochemical localization of calcium in growth plate mitochondria and matrix vesicles. Fed Proc 35: 143–147

Brighton CT, Ray RD, Soble LW, Kuettner KE (1969) In vitro epiphyseal-plate growth in various oxygen tensions. J Bone Joint Surg [Am] 51: 1383–1396

Brighton CT, Sugioka Y, Hunt RM (1973) Cytoplasmic structures of the epiphyseal-plate chondrocytes. Quantitative evaluation using electron micrographs of rat costochondral junctions with special reference to the fate of hypertrophic cells. J Bone Joint Surg [Am] 55: 771–784

Cameron DA, Robinson RA (1958) The presence of crystals in the cytoplasm of large cells adjacent to sites of bone resorption. J Bone Joint Surg [Am] 40: 414–418

Cecil RNA, Anderson HC (1978) Freeze-fracture studies of matrix vesicle calcification in epiphyseal growth plate. Metab Bone Dis Relat Res 1: 89–95

Chambers TJ (1980) The cellular basis of bone resorption. Clin Orthop 151: 283–293

Chambers TJ, Revell PA, Fuller K, Athanasou NA (1984) Resorption of bone by isolated rabbit osteoclasts. J Cell Sci 66: 383–399

Chung SMK, Batterman SC, Brighton CT (1976) Shear strength of the human femoral capital epiphyseal plate. J Bone Joint Surg [Am] 58: 94–103

Courpron P, Lepine P, Arlet M, Lips P, Meunier PJ (1980) Mechanisms underlying the reduction in age of the mean wall thickness of trabecular basic structure unit (BSU) of human iliac bone. In: Jee WSS, Parfitt AM (eds) Bone histomorphometry. 3rd international workshop. Metab Bone Dis Relat Res 2 (Suppl): 323–329

Dudley RH, Spiro D (1961) The fine structure of bone cells. J Biophys Biochem Cytol 11: 627–671

Ellis HA (1981) Metabolic bone disease. In: Anthony PP, MacSween RNM (eds) Recent advances in histopathology, vol 11. Churchill Livingstone, Edinburgh, pp 185–202

Enlow DH, Conklin JL (1964) A study of lipid distribution in compact bone. Anat Res 148: 279

Fleisch H, Bisaz S (1962) Mechanism of calcification: Inhibitory role of pyrophosphate. Nature 195: 911

Friedenstein AJ (1976) Precursors of mechanocytes. Int Rev Cytol 47: 327–359

Friedenstein AJ, Petrakova KU, Kurolesova AI, Frolova GP (1968) Heterotopic transplants of bone marrow—analysis of precursor cells of osteogenic and hematopoietic tissues. Transplantation 6: 230–246

Friedenstein AJ, Chailakhjan RK, Lalykina KS (1970) The development of fibroblast colonies in monolayer cultures of guinea pig bone marrow and spleen cells. Cell Tissue Kinet 3: 393–402

Frost HM (1964) Dynamics of bone remodelling. In: Frost HM (ed) Bone biodynamics. Little, Brown, Boston, pp 315–333

Frost HM (1976) A method of analysis of trabecular bone dynamics. In: Meunier PJ (ed) Bone histomorphometry. 2nd international workshop. Armour Montague, Paris, pp 445–476

Glauert A, Mayo CR (1973) The study of three dimensional structure relationships in connective tissues by high voltage electron microscopy. J Microsc 97: 83–94

Glimcher MJ (1976) Composition, structure, and organization of bone and other mineralized tissues and the mechanism of calcification. In: Aurbach GD (ed) Handbook of physiology—Endocrinology VII. Williams and Wilkins, Baltimore, pp 25–116

Gonzales F, Karnovsky MJ (1961) Electron microscopy of osteoclasts in healing fractures of rat bone. J Biophys Biochem Cytol 9: 299–316

Hancox NM (1972) Biological structure and function. No. 1. In: Harrison RJ, McMinn RMH (eds) Biology of bone. Cambridge University Press, Cambridge

Harris WH, Haywood EA, Lavorgna J, Hamblen DL (1968) Spatial and temporal variations in cortical bone formation in dogs. J Bone Joint Surg [Am] 50: 1118–1128

Heersche JNM (1978) Mechanism of osteoclastic bone resorption: a new hypothesis. Calcif Tissue Res 26: 81–84

Hodge AJ, Petruska JA (1963) Recent studies with the electron microscope on ordered aggregates of the tropocollagen macromolecule. In: Ramachandran GN (ed) Aspects of protein structure. Academic, New York, pp 289–300

Holtrop ME (1972) The ultrastructure of the epiphyseal plate. II The hypertrophic chondrocyte. Calcif Tissue Res 9: 140–151

Holtrop ME (1976) Quantitation of the ultrastructure of the osteoclast for the evaluation of cell function. In: Meunier PJ (ed) Bone histomorphometry. 2nd international workshop. Armour Montagu, Paris, pp 133–145

Irving JT (1963) The sudanophilic material in the early stages of calcification. Arch Oral Biol 8: 735–745

Irving JT, Wuthier RE (1968) Histochemistry and biochemistry of calcification with special reference to the role of lipids. Clin Orthop 56: 237—260

Jande SS, Belanger LF (1973) The life cycle of the osteocyte. Clin Orthop 94: 281–305

Jowsey J, Kelley PJ, Riggs BL, Bianco AJ, Scholz DA, Gershon-Cohen J (1965) Quantitative microradiographic studies of normal and osteoporotic bone. J Bone Joint Surg [Am] 47: 785–806

Kahn AJ, Stewart CC, Teitelbaum SL (1978) Contact-mediated bone resorption by human monocytes in vitro. Science 199: 988–990

Kashiwa HK, Homorous J (1971) Mineralised spherules in the cells and matrix of calcifying cartilage from developing bone. Anat Res 170: 119–128

Katchburian E (1973) Membrane-bound bodies as initiators of mineralization of dentine. J Anat 116: 285–302

Katz EP, Li S-T (1973a) The intermolecular space of reconstituted collagen fibrils. J Mol Biol 73: 351–369

Katz EP, Li S-T (1973b) Structure and function of bone collagen fibrils. J Mol Biol 80: 1–15

Kember NF (1960) Cell division in endochondral ossification; a study of cell proliferation in rat bones by the method of tritiated thymidine autoradiography. J Bone Joint Surg [Br] 42: 824–839

Kuhlman RE (1960) A microchemical study of the developing epiphyseal plate. J Bone Joint Surg [Am] 42: 457–466

Kuhlman RE (1965) Phosphatases in epiphyseal cartilage—their possible role in tissue synthesis. J Bone Joint Surg [Am] 47: 545–550

Lee SL, Glimcher MJ (1981) Purification, composition and ^{31}P NMR spectroscopic properties of a noncollagenous phosphoprotein isolated from chicken bone matrix. Calcif Tissue Int 33: 385–394

Lehninger AL (1970) Mitochondria and calcium transport. Biochem J 119: 129–138

Loutit JF, Nisbet NW (1979) Resorption of bone. Lancet II: 26–29

Marks SC (1983) The origin of osteoclasts: evidence, clinical implications and investigative challenges of an extra-skeletal source. J Pathol 12: 226–256

Martin JH, Matthews JL (1969) Mitochondrial granules in chondrocytes. Calcif Tissue Res 3: 184–193

Martin JH, Matthews JL (1970) Mitochondrial granules in chondrocytes, osteoblasts and osteocytes. Clin Orthop 68: 273–278

Matsuzawa T, Anderson HC (1971) Phosphatases of epiphyseal cartilage studied by electron microscopic cytochemical methods. J Histochem Cytochem 19: 801–808

Milch RA, Hall DP, Tobie JE (1958) Fluorescence of tetracycline antibiotics in bone. J Bone Joint Surg [Am] 40: 897–910

Miller A, Wray TS (1971) Molecular packing in collagen. Nature 230: 437–439

Mundy CR, Altman AJ, Gondek MD, Bandelin JG (1977) Direct resorption of bone by human monocytes. Science 196: 1109–1111

Mundy CR, Varani J, Orr W, Gondek MD, Ward PA (1978) Resorbing bone is chemotactic for monocytes. Nature 275: 132–135

Nogemi H, Oohira A (1984) Postnatal new bone formation. Clin Orthop 184: 106–113

Odutaga AA, Prout RES (1974) Lipid analysis of human enamel and dentine. Arch Oral Biol 19: 729–731

Owen M (1970) The origin of bone cells. Int Rev Cytol 28: 215–238

Owen M (1980) The origin of bone cells in the postnatal organism. Arthritis Rheum 23: 1073–1079

Owen M (1983) Bone cell differentiation. In: Dixon AStJ, Russell RGG, Stamp TCB (eds) Osteoporosis. A multidisciplinary problem. Royal Society of Medicine International Congress and Symposium Series, No 55. Academic Press and Royal Society of Medicine, London, 25–29

Parfitt AM (1976) The actions of parathyroid hormone on bone: relation to bone remodelling and turnover, calcium homeostasis and metabolic bone disease. Metabolism 25: 809–844

Parfitt AM (1982) The coupling of bone formation to bone resorption: a critical analysis of the concept and of its relevance to the pathogenesis of osteoporosis. Metab Bone Dis Relat Res 4: 1–6

Parfitt AM, Villanueva AR, Crouch MM, Mathews CHE, Duncan M (1976) Classification of osteoid seams by combined use of cell morphology and tetracycline labelling. Evidence for intermittency of mineralization. In: Meunier PJ (ed) Bone histomorphometry. 2nd international workshop. Armour Montagu, Paris, pp 299–310

Peress NS, Anderson HC, Sajdera SW (1974) The lipids of matrix vesicles from bovine fetal epiphyseal cartilage. Calcif Tissue Res 14: 275–282

Posner AS, Betts F, Blumenthal NC (1978) Properties of nucleating systems. Metab Bone Dis Relat Res 1: 179–183

Price PA, Baukol SA (1981) 1,25 dihydroxyvitamin D₃ increases serum levels of the vitamin-K dependant bone protein. Biochem Biophys Res Commun 99: 928–935

Price PA, Parthemore JG, Deftos LJ (1980) New biochemical marker for bone metabolism: measurement by radioimmunoassay of bone GLA protein in the plasma of normal subjects and patients with bone disease. J Clin Invest 66: 878–883

Pritchard JJ (1952) A cytological and histochemical study of bone and cartilage formation in the rat. J Anat 86: 259–277

Rabinowitch AL, Anderson HC (1976) Biogenesis of matrix vesicles in cartilage growth plates. Fed Proc 35: 112–116

Raisz LG (1976) Mechanisms of bone resorption. In: Aurbach GD (ed) Handbook of physiology— Endocrinology VII. Parathyroid gland. Williams and Wilkins, Baltimore, pp 117–136

Raisz LG, Kream BE (1983a) Regulation of bone formation. N Engl J Med 309: 29–35

Raisz LG, Kream BE (1983b) Regulation of bone formation. N Engl J Med 309: 83–89

Rasmussen J, Bordier P (1974) Bone cells—morphology and physiology. In: The physiology and cellular basis of metabolic bone disease. Williams and Wilkins, Baltimore, pp 9–69

Russell RGG, Kanis JA, Gowen M, Gallagher JA, Beresford J, Guilland-Cumming D, Coulton LA, Preston CJ, Brown BL, Sharrard M, Beard DJ (1983) Cellular control of bone formation and repair. In: Dixon AStJ, Russell RGG, Stamp TCB (eds) Osteoporosis. A multidisciplinary problem. Royal Society Medicine International Congress and Symposium Series No 55. Academic Press and Royal Society of Medicine, London, pp 31–42

Sayegh FS, Solomon GC, Davis RW (1974) Ultrastructure of intracellular mineralization in the deer's antler. Clin Orthop 99: 267–284

Schenk RK, Merz WA, Muller J (1969) A quantitative histological study on bone resorption in human cancellous bone. Acta Anat 74: 44–53

Scott BL, Pease DC (1956) Electron microscopy of the epiphyseal apparatus. Anat Rec 126: 465–495

Shapiro F, Holtrop ME, Glimcher MJ (1977) Organisation and cellular biology of the perichondrial ossification groove of Ranvier. J Bone Joint Surg [Am] 59: 703–723

Shapiro IM (1970) The association of phospholipids with anorganic bone. Calcif Tissue Res 5: 13–20

Shapiro IM, Burke A, Lee NH (1976) Heterogeneity of chondrocyte mitochondria. A study of the Ca^{2+} concentration and density banding characteristics of normal and rachitic cartilage. Biochim Biophys Acta 451: 583–591

Silberman M, Frommer J (1974) Initial locus of calcification in chondrocytes. Clin Orthop 98: 288–293

Spycher MA, Moore H, Ruettner JR (1969) Electron microscopic investigations on aging and osteoarthritic human articular cartilage. Z Mikrosk Anat Forsch 98: 512–524

Sutfin LV, Holtrop ME, Ogilvie RE (1971) Microanalysis of individual mitochondrial granules with diameters less than 1,000 angstroms. Science 174: 947–949

Teitelbaum SL, Nichols SH (1976) Tetracycline-based morphometric analysis of trabecular bone kinetics. In: Meunier PJ (ed) Bone histomorphometry. 2nd international workshop. Armour Montagu, Paris, pp 311–319

Teitelbaum SL, Stewart CC, Kahn AJ (1979) Rodent peritoneal macrophages as bone resorbing cells. Calcif Tissue Int 27: 255–261

Termine JD, Conn KM (1976) Inhibition of apatite formation by phosphorylated metabolites and macromolecules. Calcif Tissue Res 22: 149–157

Termine JD, Kleinmann HK, Whitson SW, Conn KM, McGarvey ML, Martin GR (1981) Osteonectin, a bone-specific protein linking mineral to collagen. Cell 26: 99–105

Thyberg J, Friberg U (1972) Electron microscopic enzyme histochemical studies on the cellular genesis of matrix vesicles in epiphyseal plate. J Ultrastruct Res 41: 43–59

Tonna EA (1961) The cellular complement of the skeletal system studied autoradiographically with tritiated thymidine (H³TDR) during growth and aging. J Biophys Biomed Cytol 9: 813–824

Urist MR (1981) New bone formation induced in post fetal life by bone morphogenetic protein. In: Becker RA (ed) Mechanisms of growth control. Thomas, Springfield, Ill, pp 406–434

Urist MR, Mikulski AJ (1979) A soluble morphogenetic protein extracted from bone matrix with a mixed aqueous and nonaqueous solvent. Proc Soc Exp Biol Med 162: 48–53

Urist MR, Nakagawa M, Nakata N, Nogemi H (1978) Experimental myositis ossificans: cartilage and bone formation in muscle in response to a diffusible bone matrix-derived morphogen. Arch Pathol Lab Med 102: 312–316

Urist MR, Lietze A, Mizutani H, Takagi K, Triffitt JT, Amstatz J, De Lange R, Termine J, Finerman GAM (1982) A bovine low molecular weight bone morphogenetic protein (BMP) fraction. Clin Orthop 162: 219–232

Vittali P (1968) Osteocytic activity. Clin Orthop 56: 213–226

Vogel JJ, Boyan-Salyers BD (1976) Acidic lipids associated with the local mechanism of calcification, a review. Clin Orthop 118: 230–241

Vogel JJ, Boyan-Salyers B, Campbell MM (1978) Protein-phospholipid interactions in biologic calcification. Metab Bone Dis Relat Res 1: 149–153

Walker DG (1975) Bone resorption restored in osteopetrotic mice by transplants of normal bone marrow and spleen cells. Science 190: 784–785

Wuthier RE (1968) Lipids of mineralizing epiphyseal tissues in the bovine fetus. J Lipid Res 9: 68–78

Wuthier RE (1976) Lipids of matrix vesicles. Fed Proc 35: 117–121

Yoneda T, Mundy GR (1979a) Prostaglandins are necessary for osteoclast activating factor production by activated peripheral blood leukocytes. J Exp Med 149: 279–283

Yoneda T, Mundy GR (1979b) Monocytes regulate osteoclast activating factor production by releasing prostaglandins. J Exp Med 150: 338–350

Young RW (1962) Cell proliferation and specialization during endochondral osteogenesis in the rat. J Cell Biol 14: 357–370

Chapter 2

Abnormal Development of the Skeletal System

The classification of constitutional disorders of bone includes a vast number of different conditions. In many of them only a few cases have been described. It is not therefore proposed to attempt a comprehensive account of abnormalities of skeletal development, details of which are available elsewhere. This chapter concerns itself with dwarfism and some of the chondrodystrophies, osteogenesis imperfecta, osteopetrosis and a few other miscellaneous conditions.

The chondrodysplasias

General considerations

The chondrodysplasias are a heterogeneous group of disorders which are associated with abnormalities in the size and shape of the limbs, trunk and skull. Frequently there is disproportionate shortness of stature. Classification is based on the clinical, genetic and radiographic features of each disorder. The names used for many of the chondrodysplasias denote the part of the bone affected, namely epiphyseal, metaphyseal, diaphyseal dysplasias. Where the spine is involved, the prefix 'spondylo-' is added and where the skull is affected the prefix 'cranio-' is used, for example spondyloepiphyseal dysplasia, craniometaphyseal dysplasia. Other disorders have descriptive names derived from Greek, such as diastrophic (twisted), thanatophoric (death-bearing) and metatropic (changing) dysplasia.

Broad distinctions between groups of patients may be made on the basis of clinical characteristics, i.e. age of presentation, whether the condition is lethal in the newborn period, occurrence of associated non-skeletal features and natural history of the skeletal and non-skeletal manifestations. The family history is obligatory. Certain conditions may be defined by their inheritance pattern, e.g. X-linked recessive spondyloepiphyseal dysplasia tarda.

Knowledge of the radiographic changes in a particular individual plays an important part in diagnosis, and it is therefore important to perform a full skeletal survey of any case suspected of having a chondrodysplasia. Anteroposterior and lateral views of the skull, spine and chest, anteroposterior views of the upper limbs including the hands, the lower limbs and the pelvis and a lateral view of at least one ankle are essential. Interpretation of radiographs is best performed by someone with a special interest in these disorders. In general, the field of chondrodysplasias is a little like that of bone tumours in that the pathologist should not attempt to tackle the question of diagnosis alone but as part of a team in which all the available clinical, genetic and radiological information, as well as the histopathology, is brought to bear on the problem. Referral to an expert in the field is also made more reasonable if all appropriate information, radiographs and biopsy samples are available.

Methods for the histological processing of growth plate specimens are described by Sillence et al. (1979). Biopsies of the costochondral junction and the iliac crest provide a source of tissue for examination of endochondral ossification and show appearances similar to those in the growth plate of long bones.

In the few cases seen at autopsy by the present author, several ribs, limb bones and vertebral bodies have also been examined. After formalin fixation tissue may be decalcified and sectioned, or better, undecalcified sections may be prepared in glycol or methyl methacrylate, both methods enabling assessment of the degree of calcification. Glycol methacrylate has the advantage of water miscibility so that more histochemical studies may be performed with water-soluble stains, enzymes and their substrates. Electron microscopic methods are described by Sillence et al. (1979) and Stanescu et al. (1984). (See also this chapter, Ultrastructural studies.)

Recently, several groups of workers have examined the chondro-osseous pathology of well-documented cases of chondrodysplasia. In some of these disorders, the histological appearances seem to be characteristic, in others the appearances are non-specific, while in yet others no abnormalities are demonstrable. Thus, on a pathological basis, the chondrodysplasias may be divided into those with normal chondro-osseous morphology (e.g. achondroplasia, hypochondroplasia), those with a generalised defect in resting cartilage which secondarily affects the growth plate (e.g. achondrogenesis, Kniest syndrome, diastrophic dwarfism) and those with a defect in the growth plate itself (e.g. thanatophoric dysplasia, metaphyseal chondrodysplasias) (Rimoin et al. 1976). Some of these have recently been subdivided further by Stanescu et al. (1984) into those with a proteoglycan defect (pseudoachondroplasia, Kniest syndrome, spondylometaphyseal dysplasia, Koslowski type) and those with collagen abnormalities (diastrophic dysplasia, fibrochondrogenesis).

Should the morbid anatomist be faced with the problem of a stillborn baby or death in an infant suspected of having one of the chondrodysplasias, it is essential that a thorough autopsy examination be performed with respect to all systems, not just the bones, since the coexistent features are of considerable importance in deciding to which group an affected individual belongs.

The principal clinical and radiological features of many of the chondrodysplasias are outlined below, together with details of the pathological changes so far available. Although the number of disorders may appear large, it is hoped that the non-specialist pathologist will be provided with sufficient information to make a start in his investigation of an affected individual. The age at which different disorders are first identifiable, spinal involvement, lethality and mode of inheritance are summarised in Table 2.1. Those conditions in which cleft palate, contractures, polydactyly or cardiovascular anomalies occur are shown in Table 2.2. Details of those conditions identifiable at birth are given in pp. 38–47 and those which become apparent later in pp. 48–49.

Table 2.1. The chondrodysplasias. Summary of age at presentation, spinal involvement, lethality and genetic information

Name of disorder	Spinal involvement	Lethality	Inheritance
Identifiable at birth			
Achondroplasia	−	Lethal in homozygous form; otherwise not lethal	Dominant/sporadic
Achondrogenesis	−	Lethal	? some types recessive
Thanatophoric dysplasia	−	Lethal	Sporadic
Asphyxiating thoracic dysplasia	−	Lethal	Recessive
Short-rib-polydactyly syndrome	−	Lethal	Recessive
Campomelic dysplasia	−	Lethal	Sporadic
Diastrophic dysplasia	+	Sometimes lethal	Recessive
Metatropic dysplasia	+	Sometimes lethal	Recessive
Chondrodysplasia punctata	−	Sometimes lethal	Dominant/sporadic
Chondroectodermal dysplasia	−	Sometimes lethal	Recessive
Spondyloepiphyseal dysplasia congenita	+		Dominant
Kniest dysplasia	+		Sporadic
Identifiable later in life			
Hypochondroplasia	−		Dominant
Metaphyseal dysplasia	−		Recessive
Spondylometaphyseal dysplasias	+		?
Multiple epiphyseal dysplasias	−		Dominant
Pseudoachondroplasia	+		Dominant and recessive types
Spondyloepiphyseal dysplasia tarda	+		X-linked recessive

−, absent or minimal; +, significant

Table 2.2. Chondrodysplasias in which other easily recognisable abnormalities occur

Cleft palate	Diastrophic dysplasia
	Campomelic dysplasia
	Spondyloepiphyseal dysplasia congenita
	Kniest dysplasia
Contractures (club foot, flexed digits etc.)	Diastrophic dysplasia
	Chondrodysplasia punctata
	Metatropic dysplasia
	Campomelic dysplasia
	Kniest dysplasia
Supernumerary digits (polydactyly)	Short-rib-polydactyly syndrome
	Asphyxiating thoracic dysplasias
	Chondroectodermal dysplasia
Abnormalities of heart and great vessels	Achondrogenesis I
	Thanatophoric dysplasia
	Short-rib-polydactyly syndromes
	Chondroectodermal dysplasia

Achondroplasia

Achondroplasia is the most common form of short-limbed dwarfism. Affected infants are rhizomelic, that is they have shortening of the proximal part of the limbs (Fig. 2.1). The large head has a protuberant frontal region and depressed nasal bridge, resulting from shortness of the base of the skull. Lordosis and dorsolumbar kyphosis are often present and there is anteroposterior flattening of the pelvic inlet, which gives rise to obstetric problems in adult life. Although achondroplasia has an autosomal dominant inheritance, over 80% of cases have no family history and are sporadic (Sillence et al. 1979).

Radiological changes in the long bones, pelvis and lumbar spine at birth are diagnostic (Langer et al. 1967; Rimoin 1976; Sillence et al. 1978). The features are short, broad limb bones, progressive narrowing of the interpedicular distance in the spine, flattening of the acetabulum and small sacroiliac notches.

Some confusion has existed over the histological appearances in achondroplasia, mainly because of the widespread misdiagnosis of short-limbed dwarfs as suffering from this condition in the past. The growth plate, contrary to earlier descriptions, is well organised with normal columns of chondrocytes containing normal numbers of cells (Fig. 2.2; Rimoin et al. 1970; Silberberg 1976; Rimoin et al. 1976; Sillence et al. 1979). Minor abnormalities have been described in some areas of the growth plate with clumps of proliferating chondrocytes separated by fibrous septa (Ponseti 1970; Stanescu et al. 1970). The

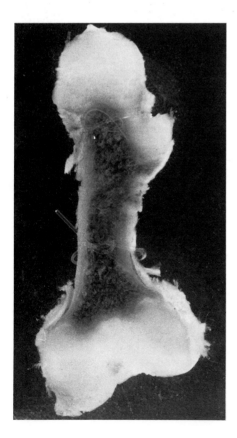

Fig. 2.1. Femur from a stillborn achondroplastic infant, showing shortening of the bone with broadening at either end

cartilage shows relatively normal chondrocytes and matrix by electron microscopy (Rimoin et al. 1976; Silberberg 1976), but some increase in the number of dead cells surrounded by micro-scars containing focal aggregations of collagen fibrils. The cells show the presence of membrane-bound intracellular inclusions which contain electron-dense granules and thread-like material (Sillence et al. 1979).

Homozygous achondroplasia is a more severe form of the disorder, which should be suspected in the affected offspring of two achondroplastic parents. Although some of these infants may survive for several years, most die of respiratory disease during the first few months of life (see Table 2.1; Sillence et al. 1979). Differentiation from thanatophoric dysplasia, other neonatal skeletal dysplasias and the heterozygous form of achondroplasia is on clinical, radiological and histological grounds. The histological appearances show normal (Fig. 2.3) and abnormal areas of endochondral ossification with absence of regular column formation, a short growth zone and a wide zone of randomly arranged hypertrophic chondrocytes (Sillence et al. 1979). Periosteal overgrowth gives rise to cupping of the epiphyseal region in both hetero- and homozygous forms of achondroplasia (Fig. 2.4).

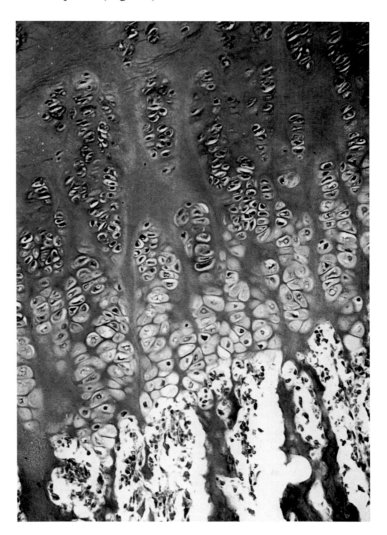

Fig. 2.2. Achondroplasia.
Costochondral junction growth plate showing relatively normal endochondral ossification with cartilage column formation. (H&E × 500)

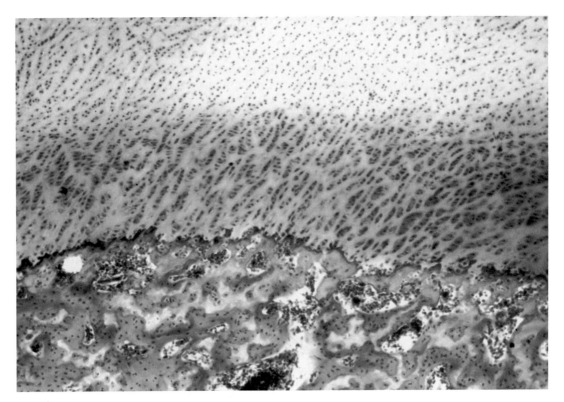

Fig. 2.3. Achondroplasia. Junction of vertebral body and intervertebral disc from a stillborn infant showing regular cartilage column formation. (H&E × 250)

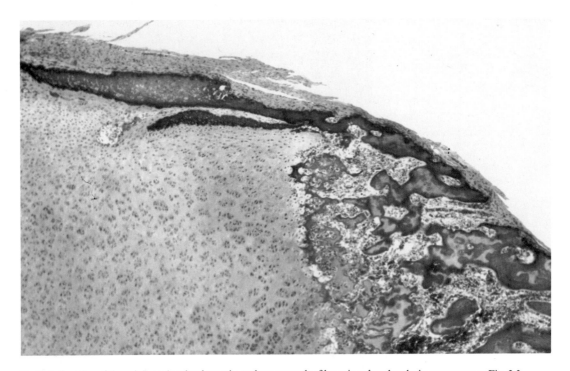

Fig. 2.4. Cupping of the epiphyseal region by periosteal overgrowth of bone in achondroplasia, same case as Fig. 2.3. (H&E × 150)

Achondrogenesis

Two autosomally recessive syndromes in which there is severe failure of growth are classified as achondrogenesis. The affected infants are either stillborn or die in the neonatal period. The two syndromes are known as *achondrogenesis I (Parenti–Fraccaro)* and *achondrogenesis II (Langer–Saldino)*. The former may have associated congenital heart defects, namely patent ductus arteriosus, ventricular septal defect and patent foramen ovale (Sillence et al. 1979).

Achondrogenesis I shows no disproportion of the skull, which is soft, being made up of islands of bone in a membranous calvaria. Radiologically the skull and vertebral bodies show total absence of ossification. The long bones are short and square and the ribs frequently fractured (Spranger et al. 1974; Maroteaux et al. 1976; Sillence et al. 1978). Histopathological examination shows marked abnormalities of endochondral ossification, with hypercellularity throughout the growth plate (Yang et al. 1974). The cells have an irregular distribution so that there is little chondrocyte column formation. Irregular vascular penetration and disorderly calcification of the cartilage occur.

Achondrogenesis II is clinically different in that the head is disproportionately large. The limbs are shortened and the trunk has a squared appearance (Langer et al. 1969; Saldino 1971; Yang et al. 1974). The diagnostic radiological features are underdeveloped ossification centres in the vertebral bodies and pelvis. There is severe shortening of the limb bones with widening of the metaphyses and cupping of the ends of the bones. The cranial vault shows well-developed ossification (Beighton 1978). The histopathological appearances differ markedly from those of any other chondrodysplasia (Sillence et al. 1979). Macroscopically the epiphyseal cartilage is lobulated and shows increased vascularity. There is hypercellularity of the reserve cartilage on microscopy, and hypertrophic chondrocytes are separated by only small amounts of matrix (Maroteaux et al. 1976; Sillence et al. 1979). Complete disorganisation of endochondral ossification is seen at the growth plate, with lack of column formation. Irregular vascular invasion results in the formation of groups of degenerate chondrocytes surrounded by calcified cartilage. Primary trabeculae are sometimes horizontally arranged. They are irregular and decreased in number (Sillence et al. 1979). Overgrowth of membranous bone is responsible for the cupping at the ends of the long bones, seen radiologically.

Thanatophoric dysplasia

Thanatophoric dysplasia has received its name from the Greek *thanatos* (death) and *phoros* (bearing), since affected infants are either stillborn or die of respiratory distress in the neonatal period. The mode of inheritance is unknown and the great majority of cases are sporadic. The trunk is relatively normal in length but the head is large and shows craniofacial disproportion. There is marked shortening of the limbs and narrowing of the thorax. Anomalies in the cardiovascular and central nervous systems include patent ductus arteriosus, atrial septal defect, coarctation of the aorta, absence of the corpus callosum, and other abnormalities of the cerebrum and cerebellum. The diagnostic radiological features are marked platyspondyly of the lumbar vertebrae, which have an inverted 'U' appearance, curvature of the femora

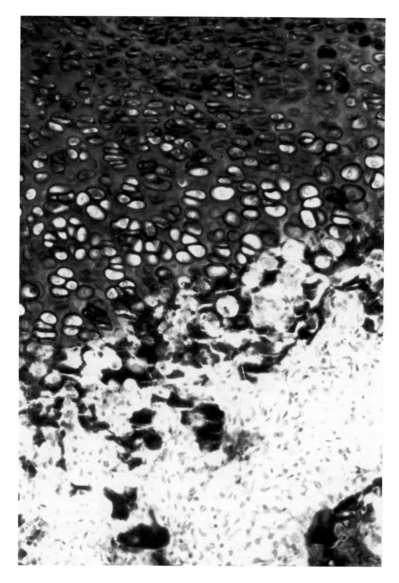

Fig. 2.5. Thanatophoric dysplasia. Costochondral junction growth plate showing disorganised endochondral ossification with lack of cartilage column formation and ballooning of chondrocytes. (H&E × 500)

with medial and lateral spikes at their low ends, and short flared ribs (Beighton 1978). Histological examination shows fairly normal resting cartilage with round or spindle-shaped cells in a homogeneous matrix (Rimoin 1974; Maroteaux et al. 1976; Rimoin et al. 1976). There is disruption of endochondral ossification at the growth plate with no regular column formation (Fig. 2.5). Small areas of regularly orientated hypertrophic cells may be present, but irregular arrangement of short spicules of calcified cartilage is due to abnormal vascular invasion.

Short-rib-polydactyly syndromes

Two different syndromes are included in the category of lethal neonatal skeletal dysplasia known as short-rib-polydactyly syndrome. There is severe narrowing of the thorax, and the limbs are short with polydactyly. The inheritance is autosomally recessive in type. The chief problems in diagnosis are differentiation from asphyxiating thoracic dysplasia and from chondroectodermal dysplasia (see below).

A wide variety of congenital anomalies is present in *short-rib-polydactyly dysplasia I (Saldino–Noonan)*, including abnormalities of the great vessels, polycystic kidneys, hypoplastic lungs, atresia of the oesophagus and urogenital anomalies. Radiological examination shows extremely short, horizontally orientated ribs. The vertebral bodies are distorted and the pelvis has small iliac bones and flattened roofs to the acetabula. An unusual radiological feature is the presence of pointed ends to the femora (Lowry and Wignall 1975; Beighton 1978).

Histological abnormalities of chondro-osseous development have been reported (Sillence et al. 1979). The cartilage shows reduced numbers of chondrocytes with disorganised column formation. Primary trabeculae are broad and there is extension of bone into the cartilage, giving rise to irregularity of the region of chondro-osseous transformation. Cartilage extends into the metaphysis.

Short-rib-polydactyly dysplasia II (Majewski) is extremely rare. There is severe reduction in the development of the ribs with polydactyly. Facial clefts, low-set ears, and other associated malformations may be present. Radiological examination shows horizontally arranged short ribs, very short limbs and polydactyly of the hands and feet. Histology shows irregularity of chondrocyte column formation at the growth plate.

Chondroectodermal dysplasia (Ellis–van Creveld syndrome)

Chondroectodermal dysplasia is characterised by short-limbed dwarfism. It was first described by Ellis and van Creveld (1940), and a large number of subsequent cases have occurred in the Amish community in the USA, where consanguinity is an important factor (McKusick et al. 1964). Other features include postaxial polydactyly, narrowing of the rib cage, congenital heart disease and ectodermal anomalies affecting the hair, teeth and nails (Ellis and van Creveld 1940). The form of inheritance is autosomally recessive. Confusion with asphyxiating thoracic dysplasia (see below) may occur, partly as the result of the similarity in the radiographic features of the two disorders. In Ellis–van Creveld syndrome the limbs show acromelic micromelia (shortening of the distal segment of the limb). The changes in the pelvis and limbs are virtually the same as in asphyxiating thoracic dysplasia. Accurate differentiation on radiological grounds may be difficult and this is reviewed by Cremin and Beighton (1978).

There are inconsistencies in the histological appearances described by different authors. Smith and Hand (1958) described nuclear abnormalities of chondrocytes and islands of bone in the metaphyseal cartilage. Other reports describe the presence of bone in the epiphyseal cartilage, irregular vascularisation and column formation with extension of cartilage along the periosteum and into the metaphyseal bone, and abnormalities in chondrocyte size and number (Figs. 2.6, 2.7; Sillence et al. 1979).

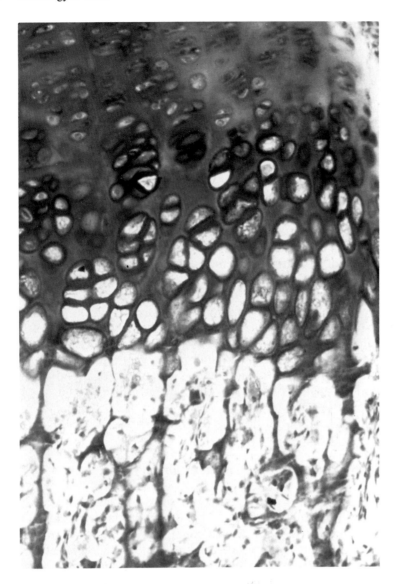

Fig. 2.6. Chondroectodermal dysplasia. Lower femoral growth plate showing irregular column formation and abnormally large chondrocytes. (H&E × 650)

Asphyxiating thoracic dysplasia (Jeune syndrome)

The main clinical feature of asphyxiating thoracic dysplasia is severe narrowing of the chest with immobility. Confusion with chondroectodermal dysplasia may occur when there is polydactyly. The severe thoracic involvement results in early death with respiratory distress and infection, but milder forms are compatible with life, and in later childhood the shape of the thorax tends to revert to normal (Herdman and Langer 1968). Friedman et al. (1975) have reported the case of an adult patient who developed renal and hepatic complications. Renal failure usually occurs in those children surviving initial respiratory problems (Langer 1968; Oberklaid et al. 1977).

Radiological examination shows limb bones which are neither markedly shortened or bowed, but the epiphysis of the femoral head, which is not normally visible until about 4 months of life, is present in the affected neonate

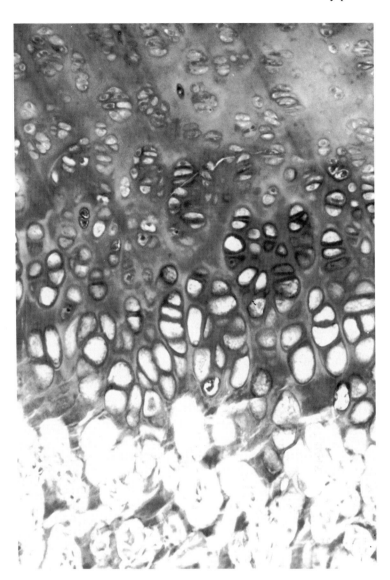

Fig. 2.7. Chondroectodermal dysplasia. Costochondral junction growth plate, showing irregular column formation and large chondrocytes. Same case as Fig. 2.6. (H&E × 650)

or early in infancy (Cremin 1970). The short ribs are horizontal in position and have flared anterior ends. Ossification of the sternum may be incomplete in the affected neonate. There is some doubt about the homogeneity of asphyxiating thoracic dysplasia when milder forms are included. The histological abnormalities described have varied considerably (Sillence et al. 1979). They include reduction in the numbers of proliferating chondrocytes, irregular vascularisation during endochondral ossification and the presence of islands of cartilage in the metaphyses. Lipid inclusions in chondrocytes have been reported in an ultrastructural study (Phillips et al. 1974).

Stippled epiphyses and chondrodysplasia punctata

The presence of multiple spotty foci of calcification in the cartilaginous parts of the neonatal and infantile skeleton, often called 'stippled epiphyses', is a striking feature on radiological examination. However, this is a radiological sign and not a diagnosis. The appearances are present in a number of different disorders, including multiple epiphyseal dysplasia, several of the mucolipidoses, the mucopolysaccharidoses, trisomy 18, trisomy 21, anencephaly, cretinism and peripheral resistance to thyroxine. Similar radiological appearances may also be seen in the fetal warfarin syndrome (Becker et al. 1975; Shaul et al. 1975), fetal hydantoin syndrome and congenital cytomegalovirus and rubella infections (Sheffield et al. 1976).

Apart from all these conditions, there are three congenital dysplasias in which stippling of the epiphyses occurs. All show hypoplasia of the nasal cartilage and may be associated with erythroderma. The three separate entities are called chondrodysplasia punctata of autosomal dominant type (Conradi–Hunerman chondrodysplasia punctata), autosomal recessive type (rhizomelic chondrodysplasia punctata) and the X-linked variant.

Neonates with rhizomelic chondrodysplasia punctata have symmetrical rhizomelic shortening of the limbs. The face is flattened and the bridge of the nose is depressed. The fingers are short and fixed in flexion. Contractures of the limb joints may be present. Cataracts and skin manifestations are sometimes seen. Most patients die in infancy with neonatal respiratory distress (Sillence et al. 1979). The main radiological features are in the spine and limbs. There are multiple well-defined radiodense areas at the proximal ends of the long bones. Large irregular opacities surround or occupy the ossification centres. Stippling is usually absent or mild in the spine.

Clinically, the facial and dermal changes of Conradi–Hunerman chondrodysplasia punctata are like those of the rhizomelic form. The shortening of the limbs is less severe and may be asymmetrical. There may be spinal deformity. Early death occurs in severe forms, but milder forms are compatible with survival. There is widespread stippling of the feet, ankles, patellae, hands and wrists in severe forms. There may also be marked stippling in the spine, pelvis, sternum, ribs and mandible (Cremin and Beighton 1978). No consistent histopathological abnormalities have been described so far in the cases studied (Raap 1943; Coughlin et al. 1950; Ford et al. 1951; Briggs et al. 1953; Sugarman 1974; Visekzul et al. 1974). Areas of myxoid fibrous tissue, microcystic degeneration and dysplastic calcification in the proliferative cartilage have been described in both conditions.

No histopathological studies have been performed in sex-linked chondrodysplasia punctata, which shares some clinical features with the Conradi–Hunerman type (Sillence et al. 1979).

Other types of chondrodysplasia identifiable at birth

There are numerous other types of chondrodysplasia which are identifiable at birth. The main clinical, radiological and histological features of some of them are summarised in Table 2.3. Only brief comments about these disorders need be given here.

Bent limbs (campomelia) are the most prominent feature of campomelic dysplasia. Increased curvature of the limbs may also occur in thanatophoric dysplasia, osteogenesis imperfecta and hypophosphatasia. In diastrophic dwarfism there is a distinctive 'hitch-hiker' thumb (and great toe) appearance, caused by shortening of the abnormally shaped first metacarpal bone, which

Table 2.3. Summary of the clinical, radiological and histological features of other chondrodysplasias identifiable at birth

Name of disorder	Clinical features	Radiological features	Histological appearances at the growth plate
Campomelic dysplasia	1. Short-limbed dwarfism 2. Anterolateral bowing of legs 3. Talipes equinovarus 4. Altered facies (flat nose, cleft palate, micrognathia) 5. Low-set ears 6. Hypotonia	1. Cortices of limb bones thickened at angle of bowing 2. Hypoplastic fibulae 3. Talipes equinovarus 4. Platyspondyly with undermineralised bone 5. Hypoplastic facial bones 6. Short skull base with flattened sella turcica	Normal or mild changes in endochondral ossification
Diastrophic dysplasia	1. Short-limbed dwarfism with short trunk 2. Talipes equinovarus 3. Progressive scoliosis 4. 'Hitch-hiker' thumb 5. Cleft palate 6. Contractures of joints 7. Pinnae of ears distorted	1. Shortened, broadened limb bones 2. Delayed appearance of epiphyses 3. Flared metaphyses 4. Severe talipes equinovarus 5. Joint dislocation, including hip dysplasia 6. Thoracolumbar scoliosis 7. Hypoplasia of cervical vertebral bodies $\pm$ subluxation	1. Three or four chondrocytes in irregularly distributed lacunae in resting cartilage, contain large amounts of collagen, surrounded by proteoglycan and cellular debris, outside which is circumferentially arranged collagen 2. Fibrous cystic areas in resting cartilage 3. Growth plate shorter than normal
Metatropic dysplasia	1. Changing body proportions 2. Progressive kyphoscoliosis 3. Short extremities with enlarged bone ends	1. Short limb bones with enlarged metaphyses and epiphyseal dyplasia 2. Narrow rib cage, short ribs, in newborn 3. Severe platyspondyly— later wedge-shaped vertebrae	1. Vacuolated chondrocytes containing metachromatic granules in resting cartilage 2. Normal cell proliferation and maturation of growth plate 3. Irregular vascular invasion 4. Unossified cartilage in metaphysis
Spondyloepiphyseal dysplasia congenita	1. Short-limbed dwarfism 2. Severe kyphoscoliosis and thoracic deformity in childhood 3. Dislocation of hips 4. Talipes equinovarus 5. Cleft palate 6. Myopia, retinal detachment	1. Severe platyspondyly 2. Shortening of all long bones 3. Severe epiphyseal dysplasia 4. Coxa vara deformity 5. Instability of cervical spine with hypoplasia of odontoid process 6. Kyphoscoliosis developed	1. Regular chondrocyte proliferation and maturation 2. Parts of cartilage may be hypocellular 3. Irregular vascular invasion
Kniest dysplasia	1. Short-limbed dwarfism with short trunk 2. Kyphoscoliosis 3. Talipes equinovarus 4. Cleft palate 5. Myopia, retinal detachment 6. Deafness 7. Inguinal hernia	1. Playtyspondyly 2. Underminetalised skeleton with irregular expansion of epiphyses 3. Dysplastic femoral heads with wide acetabular margins	1. Resting and growth cartilige show large amounts of vacuolated matrix and degenerating chondrocytes 2. Columns widely separated by vacuolated matrix 3. Irregular vascular invasion

results in an abduction deformity. The diagnosis of diastrophic dysplasia is suggested in the neonatal period by the presence of limb shortening, club feet and dislocation of joints.

Spondyloepiphyseal dysplasias have been divided into 'congenita' and 'tarda' types, depending upon whether the features of the condition are present at birth. Abnormalities of the spine and epiphyses predominate, as is readily apparent from the name.

Hypochondroplasia

Hypochondroplasia is not usually apparent at birth. Skeletal disproportion and mild lumbar lordosis become apparent only in early childhood. Affected individuals may come to have shortening of the limbs and features resembling achondroplasia, although the appearance of the face is usually normal (Walker et al. 1971; Beighton 1978; Sillence et al. 1979). Mildly affected individuals may be very little different from normal. The radiological appearances of the skeleton are reminiscent of achondroplasia. Lengthening of the distal end of the fibula in relation to the tibia is a useful diagnostic sign (Frydman et al. 1974). Histological examination shows essentially normal endochondral ossification at the growth plates (Sillence et al. 1979).

Metaphyseal dysplasias

The metaphyseal dysplasias are a heterogeneous group of disorders recognisable later in life. Epiphyseal and spinal development are usually relatively normal. Details of the various types will not be given here and the reader is referred to the book by Beighton (1978) and the review by Sillence et al. (1979). Immunological incompetence and endocrine abnormalities are features of some of these conditions.

The histological features of all types have been found to be similar by Rimoin and his colleagues (Rimoin et al. 1976; Sillence et al. 1979). There is disorganisation of the growth plate, with clusters of abnormally large cells being formed instead of orderly columns. The cells are surrounded by large amounts of dense fibrous material. Vascular invasion of the cell clusters is irregular or absent. Continued growth of a tongue of hypertrophic cartilage into the metaphysis is the result where vascular invasion is absent, as might be expected.

Multiple epiphyseal dysplasias

The multiple epiphyseal dysplasias are a group of disorders in which changes are maximal in the epiphyses. Metaphyseal and axial skeletal involvement is minimal. Several different types have been described. The group is heterogeneous and the classification problematic (Lie et al. 1974; Spranger 1976; Sillence et al. 1979). The height of some patients is normal while others show a mild degree of shortening of stature, which becomes apparent during childhood. There are no consistent extraskeletal manifestations and general health is good. Early onset of degenerative joint disease in adult life is common.

The epiphyses may have a stippled appearance on radiological examination in infancy. Fragmentation of the epiphyses of the long bones becomes more obvious with increasing age, and this applies especially to the femoral heads.

Histological examination of sites of endochondral ossification shows essentially normal appearances (Fairbank 1947; Rimoin 1975), although histochemical and electron microscopic changes have been described (Sillence et al. 1979).

Other types of chondrodysplasia not identifiable at birth

The main features of some other types of chondrodysplasia which do not become apparent until childhood are shown in Table 2.4. They represent a varied collection of disorders, all of which show predisposition to the early development of degenerative joint disease. Descriptions of the histochemical, ultrastructural and possible biochemical defects in some of these disorders are available in Stanescu et al. (1984).

Table 2.4. Summary of the main features of other chondrodysplasias not identifiable at birth

Name of disorder	Clinical features	Radiological features	Histological appearances at the growth plate
Pseudoachondroplasia (heterogeneous group)	1. Short stature, shortening of limbs 2. Normal craniofacial proportions 3. Resembles achondroplasia 4. Sometimes spinal deformity with scoliosis and lumbar lordosis 5. Secondary osteoarthrosis in early adulthood	1. Irregularity of epiphyses of long bones 2. Cupping and widening of metaphyses 3. Shortened metacarpals and phalanges	1. Various degrees of disruption of the growth plate 2. Two to six larger chondrocytes than normal accumulated in single lacuna
Spondylometaphyseal dysplasias	1. Dwarfism with short trunk 2. Growth retardation not apparent in first 2 years of life 3. Kyphoscoliosis 4. Pectus carinatum 5. Coxa vara, knee deformities 6. Secondary osteoarthrosis of early onset	1. Skeleton normal at birth 2. Platyspondyly in early childhood 3. Progressively more irregular metaphyses, multiple radiolucent areas 4. Epiphyses not involved	Non-specific, irregular column formation and vascular invasion of growth plate
Spondyloepiphyseal dysplasia tarda (heterogeneous group)	1. Variable 2. Dorsal kyphoscoliosis develops between ages 5 and 10 years 3. Progressive shortening of trunk 4. Severe disability in middle age with degenerative changes in spine and hips 5. Some have X-linked inheritance	1. Skeleton more or less normal in early life 2. Progressive platyspondyly and kyphoscoliosis	1. Essentially normal maturation of chondrocytes 2. Larger clusters of proliferating cells than normal

Ultrastructural studies

The electron microscopic appearances of cells in growing cartilage in the chondrodysplasias have been described in recent papers. Some of the findings are briefly summarised here.

In achondroplasia and hypochondroplasia, the chondrocytes and matrix of the growth plate are ultrastructurally normal, except that in achondroplasia there is a relative increase in the numbers of dead cells and there are focal scars. Intracytoplasmic inclusions have been described in the chondrocytes in achondroplasia and diastrophic, metatropic, asphyxiating thoracic and spondylometaphyseal dysplasia. The inclusions contain glycogen in diastrophic dysplasia and lipid in asphyxiating thoracic dysplasia. Granular and thread-like material is present in the inclusions seen in achondroplasia and spondylometaphyseal dysplasia. String-like material is associated with glycogen in the inclusions present in metatropic dysplasia. Abnormalities in the matrix are present in several conditions. Disorganised collagen fibrils with tapered ends and the presence of abnormal amounts of mature collagen have been described in short-rib-polydactyly I.

Ultrastructural studies may prove a useful means of further differentiating the chondrodysplasias. The reader is referred to the articles by Silberberg (1976), Rimoin et al. (1976), Hwang et al. (1979), Sillence et al. (1979) and Stanescu et al. (1984), where further details may be obtained.

Osteogenesis imperfecta

Osteogenesis imperfecta is a disorder, or rather a group of disorders, characterised by a marked tendency for the bones to fracture on slight provocation.

Classification

Severely affected infants having 'osteogenesis imperfecta congenita' are stillborn with shortened deformed limbs and numerous fractures which have occurred during intrauterine life. A less severe form, 'osteogenesis imperfecta tarda', may present for the first time in childhood and carries a more favourable prognosis. Although cases usually have been placed in these two broad categories, other methods of classification have also been suggested; for example, division of osteogenesis imperfecta into four different types has been suggested by Sillence and Rimoin (1978).

Osteogenesis imperfecta I

Osteogenesis imperfecta I is the largest group in this classification and shows a dominant inheritance. There is increased bone fragility and the sclerae are blue. Presenile deafness develops and there is sometimes a family history of deafness. Scoliosis may be moderately severe but marked long bone deformity is uncommon. Affected infants are of normal birth weight and rarely have numerous fractures.

Osteogenesis imperfecta II

Osteogenesis imperfecta II is recessive and is the most frequent form to affect the newborn, who are usually stillborn or die during the neonatal period. Affected individuals are small for gestational age, have short, bowed limbs

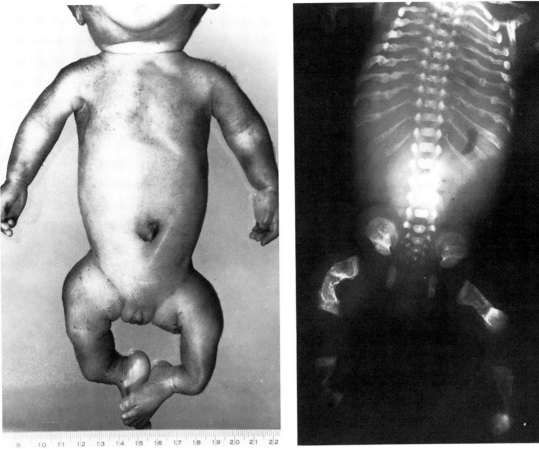

Fig. 2.8.   **Fig. 2.9.**

Fig. 2.8. Stillborn infant with osteogenesis imperfecta, showing shortened deformed limbs

Fig. 2.9. Fractured ribs and right femur in infant shown in Fig. 2.8

and numerous fractures (Fig. 2.8). Radiological examination shows beaded fractured ribs, concertina-like femora, platyspondyly and poor ossification of the cranial vault (Fig. 2.9).

Osteogenesis imperfecta III

Fractures are present at birth in two-thirds of affected infants or appear during the first year of life of babies with osteogenesis imperfecta type III. Blue sclerae are present during infancy but tend to become paler or appear normal in adolescence. Inheritance is recessive.

Osteogenesis imperfecta IV

Patients with type IV osteogenesis imperfecta show dominant inheritance and do not have blue sclerae, dentigenesis imperfecta or impairment of hearing (Sillence and Rimoin 1978).

Biochemical abnormalities

It will be appreciated from the above description that osteogenesis imperfecta represents a heterogeneous group of related disorders, but that there are often abnormalities of the sclerae and teeth as well as increased bone fragility. These features prompted the search for a generalised biochemical abnormality. Bauze et al. (1975) showed instability of polymeric structural collagen from the skin of patients with severe osteogenesis imperfecta, and this was interpreted as being the result of a decrease in the number of types of cross-links in the collagen (Smith et al. 1975). Cells from the skin of infants with severe osteogenesis imperfecta synthesised type III and type I collagen in culture, whereas cells from normal skin synthesised predominantly type I collagen (Penttinen et al. 1975; Sykes et al. 1977). The rate of synthesis of collagen was increased in the skin of patients with osteogenesis imperfecta, according to Kovac et al. (1974).

Studies of bone collagen yielded conflicting results. Dickson et al. (1975) demonstrated abnormalities in the non-collagenous protein of bone matrix in children with osteogenesis imperfecta, but no pronounced changes in the collagen of bone were detected by Eastoe et al. (1973), Brickley et al. (1974) and Fujii and Tanzer (1977). Increased amounts of hydroxylysine were demonstrated in bone collagen from an infant with osteogenesis imperfecta congenita compared with age-matched controls by Trelstad et al. (1977). Other results presented by Fujii and Tanzer (1977) suggested delayed maturation of cross-linking of bone collagen in osteogenesis imperfecta. Nicholls and Pope (1979) described a collagen defect in a severely affected infant with osteogenesis imperfecta. It will be appreciated from the above that osteogenesis imperfecta may be a biochemically heterogeneous group of disorders.

Recent findings from different laboratories confirm the idea that there may be a collagen synthesis deficit in osteogenesis imperfecta and show this to involve type I collagen. The review by Shapiro and Rowe (1983) gives further information and references. Current knowledge is summarised in Table 2.5. The clinical features of the various types have already been described. Type I osteogenesis imperfecta shows decreased production of $(\alpha 1)$I procollagen. Clinical separation from type IV disease may be difficult, yet patients with this form have a quite different type of biochemical abnormality. Little is known at present of the defect in type III osteogenesis imperfecta, while type II disease shows failure of secretion of type I collagen into extracellular matrix. It is likely that further developments in the understanding and classification of osteogenesis imperfecta will be along the lines of the precise recognition of biochemical defects rather than clinical or pathological description.

Histological appearances

There are considerable differences to be found among the reports of the histological appearances seen in osteogenesis imperfecta. These may reflect the differences in the clinical and radiological types of disease already mentioned above. The main points relating to the findings of various workers have been reviewed by Falvo and Bullough (1973).

Most reports of osteogenesis imperfecta congenita describe the bone as having a woven bone pattern, whereas in osteogenesis imperfecta tarda the bone

Table 2.5. Classification of osteogenesis imperfecta according to biochemical data, inheritance and other features (after Shapiro and Rowe 1983)

Type	Biochemical abnormality	Inheritance	Frequency	Sclerae	Dentinogenesis imperfecta
I	Marked decrease in type I collagen synthesis $a1:a2(I)$ ratio normal	Dominant (sporadic)	50%	Blue	25%
II	Failure to secrete type I collagen $a1(I)$ and $a2(I)$ deletions and insertions	Recessive	5%	Blue	Unknown, but occurs
III	Normal type I collagen synthesis $a1:a2$ ratio normal Defect unknown	Recessive (genetic compound)	20%	White, sometimes blue	25%
IV	Variable decrease in type I collagen synthesis $a1:a2$ ratio elevated $a2$ chain deletions Failure to process $a2(I)$ chains	Dominant (sporadic and genetic compound)	25%	Blue, may lighten with age	25%

is lamellar in type. There is no agreement as to the cellular characteristics of the bone. The numbers of osteoblasts are decreased in osteogenesis imperfecta according to some authors, but increased according to others. A majority of descriptions of osteogenesis imperfecta congenita show osteoblasts to be decreased in number. Similar discrepancies exist over the number of osteoclasts present (Falvo and Bullough 1973). There appears to be general agreement that there are normal or increased numbers of osteocytes in the bone. Increased numbers of osteocytes, the large size of osteoblasts and the increase in the number of bone surfaces with osteoid seams found by Falvo and Bullough (1973) were considered suggestive of increased bone production. Abundant osteoid formation and increased numbers of osteocytes were also observed by Doty and Matthews (1971).

Tetracycline labelling has shown an increase in the rate of bone turnover in osteogenesis imperfecta (Ramser et al. 1966; Albright and Albright 1971), but assessment of bone mineral turnover in a severely affected child given fluoride treatment by Forbes et al. (1968) showed no difference in bone mineral turnover from normal.

Many healing fractures in osteogenesis imperfecta show differences from normal callus in that there is often metaplastic cartilage present (Figs. 2.10, 2.11; Spencer 1962). The hyperplastic callus which forms in some patients with osteogenesis imperfecta comprises fibromucoid cartilage-like tissue (King and Bobechko 1971), and such areas may occasionally appear tumour-like. True osteosarcoma occurring in osteogenesis imperfecta has been reported occasionally (Jewell and Lofstrom 1940; Klenerman et al. 1967; Rutkowski et al. 1979).

The epiphyseal cartilage of the long bones is normal in all respects in osteogenesis imperfecta according to Knaggs (1924), Key (1926) and Follis (1953), although Engfeldt et al. (1954) found the epiphyseal plate to be irregular and broader than normal in their cases.

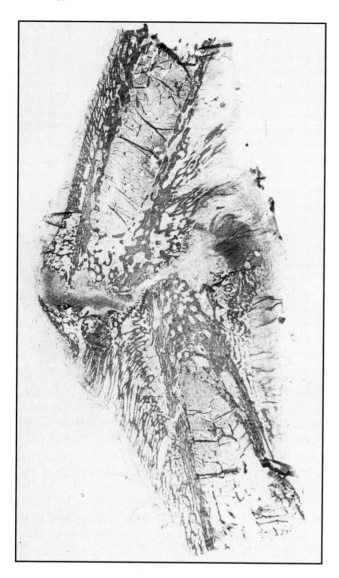

Fig. 2.10. Healing fracture of the shaft of the femur in an infant with osteogenesis imperfecta who died aged 6 days. (H&E × 75)

Follis (1953) failed to demonstrate any histochemical differences from normal, but Spencer (1962) showed an increase in the 'acid mucopolysaccharide' content of the cartilage matrix and cells. Doty and Matthews (1971) showed the fine structure of the osteoclasts and osteocytes to be not different from normal, and no abnormalities were revealed in these cells by enzyme histochemical methods. There were qualitative differences in the phosphatase staining of the osteoblasts, and these cells contained large accumulations of glycogen. The results suggested to Doty and Matthews that the defect in osteogenesis imperfecta was confined to the osteoblasts.

No alteration in collagen fibre diameter or periodicity was found by Doty and Matthews (1971) or Riley and Brown (1971), who used transmission electron microscopy. Teitelbaum et al. (1974) examined bone collagen in osteogenesis imperfecta congenita by scanning electron microscopy and showed aggregation of thin collagen fibres into the large collagen bundles of normal

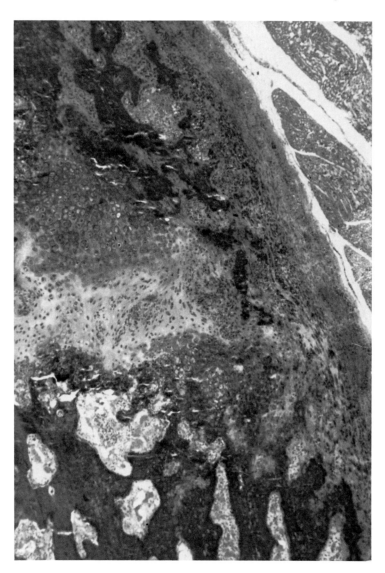

Fig. 2.11. Higher power view of a fractured rib from the same case as Fig. 2.10, showing a large amount of metaplastic cartilage in the callus. (H&E × 550)

bone. This finding is of some interest in view of the biochemical evidence for abnormalities of collagen in osteogenesis imperfecta (Trelstad et al. 1977; Fujii and Tanzer 1977).

Osteopetrosis

'Osteopetrosis' is the term often used to describe the condition first described by Albers-Schönberg (1904), which is also known as 'marble bone disease' or even 'osteosclerosis fragilis generalisata'. Several different entities are now recognisable within a group of conditions characterised by varying combinations of bony sclerosis and defects of bone modelling. All might be termed 'osteopetroses' or 'osteoscleroses'. There are considerable differences over the classification of these disorders in the literature, and that used here is the Paris nomenclature for constitutional disorders of bone (McKusick and Scott 1971). Briefly, they are divisible into osteoscleroses, craniotubular dysplasias, craniotubular hyperostoses, and other sclerosing and hyperostotic disorders. It is proposed to discuss only the osteoscleroses. The reader is referred to the review by Beighton et al. (1977) and the book by Beighton (1978) for details of the other conditions.

In the osteoscleroses it is the sclerosis that predominates, and changes in overall bone modelling are relatively minor. Three conditions are included, namely osteopetrosis of autosomal recessive and dominant types and pycnodysostosis.

Osteopetrosis of autosomal dominant type (syns. osteopetrosis tarda, benign osteopetrosis)

The benign or tarda form of osteopetrosis is inherited as an autosomal dominant condition and corresponds to the disease originally described by Albers-Schönberg (1904). The mother of the original patient was also affected. Osteopetrosis of this type is relatively common. While presenting features may be facial palsy, deafness or pathological fractures in a small proportion of patients, individuals may only be diagnosed incidentally when radiological examination is performed. Problems with dental extraction sometimes occur, and osteomyelitis of the mandible may develop. There may be mild anaemia.

The skeleton is usually radiologically normal at birth, but sclerotic foci develop within the bones during childhood giving the appearances of striations and endobones (or 'bones within bones'). These changes usually disappear by about the age of 20 years. Although skeletal involvement is widespread, the extremities are sometimes spared. Thickening of the vertebral end plates gives rise to the 'rugger jersey' spine appearance, and the calvaria is denser than normal, often with obliteration of the sinuses. The skull changes are most marked in the basal region and result in distortion of the cranial foramina.

Osteopetrosis of autosomal recessive type (syns. precocious osteopetrosis, malignant osteopetrosis, osteopetrosis congenita)

The malignant or congenita form of osteopetrosis is evident during infancy, when bony overgrowth is associated with failure to thrive, bruising, abnormal bleeding and anaemia with bone marrow depression. The haematological manifestations have been considered by some workers to be due to the encroachment of persistent endochondral tissue upon the bone marrow (McCune and Bradley 1934; Solcia et al. 1968), while others have thought haemolysis and hypersplenism contributed to the anaemia (Engfeldt et al. 1955; Sjolin 1959; Gamsu et al. 1961). A basic disturbance in the development of both haematopoietic and osseous tissue has been suggested by McCune and Bradley (1934) and Solcia et al. (1968). The question of the role of bone marrow cells in osteopetrosis will be returned to later (see p. 60). Hepatosplenomegaly is a feature. There is decreased resistance to infection and there may be osteomyelitis of the jaw bone. Increased bone fragility occurs and is associated with pathological fractures.

Death takes place in the first decade from overwhelming infection or haemorrhage. Survival into adulthood is extremely rare, though there are occasional atypical individuals, for example two brothers described by Funderburk (1975).

The predominant radiological feature is generalised osteosclerosis. There are transverse bands in the metaphyseal regions and longitudinal striations in the shafts of tubular bones in penetrated radiographs. Endobones (see under Osteopetrosis of autosomal dominant type) are present in the axial skeleton and the spine shows the typical 'rugger jersey' appearance. Progressive thickening of the skull and narrowing of cranial foramina occur, as they do in the dominant form of osteopetrosis. The ends of long bones, particularly the distal femur and proximal humerus, develop into a flask shape.

Macroscopic and histological appearances

The histological appearances of the bones in osteopetrosis have been described by Zawisch (1947), Pines and Lederer (1947), Cohen (1951), Engfeldt et al. (1960) and Shapiro et al. (1980). The findings are consistent with the conclusion that the principal defect in this disease is a failure of resorption of bone and calcified cartilage. The abnormality in resorption of calcified cartilage formed during endochondral ossification results in the filling of the metaphyseal and diaphyseal regions with calcified cartilage surrounded by new bone. Similarly, failure of osteoclastic resorption at the periphery of the metaphyseal–diaphyseal junction leads to the widening of the metaphysis. It is upon examination of the bones of severely affected patients that pathological descriptions are mainly based.

Macroscopically, the metaphyses and diaphyses of long bones are increased in diameter and the epiphyses normal in shape, size and position (Fig. 2.12). The increase in diameter of the diaphysis is due to thickening of the bone cortex and accumulation of subperiosteal new bone. A bone marrow cavity is not usually seen in the long bones. The vertebrae show similar changes. The skull is thickened and contains little bone marrow, and the nerve foramina are smaller than normal with rounded elevated and smooth edges. There may be beading of the costochondral junctions.

Histological examination of the epiphyses shows normal appearances apart from occasional clumped chondrocytes and widening of cell columns near the growth plate. The matrix of the articular and epiphyseal growth cartilage is normal. Vascular penetration of the hypertrophic cartilage cells in the growth plates appears normal. The characteristic features of osteopetrosis are seen in the metaphysis and diaphysis. In the metaphysis large amounts of calcified cartilage persist and are surrounded by both woven and lamellar bone (Fig. 2.13). These appearances represent thickened primary trabeculae. They are present throughout the metaphysis and fill the medullary cavity of the diaphysis. Virtually no bone marrow may be present between these dense trabeculae (Fig. 2.14), especially in the diaphyseal region. The persisting remnant of the original cortical bone of the primary centre of ossification could still be recognised at the periphery of the metaphysis and diaphysis in the case described by Shapiro et al. (1980). Adjacent to this primary centre true Haversian bone was present and woven bone was transforming peripherally into true lamellar bone. Secondary epiphyseal centres of ossification show similar

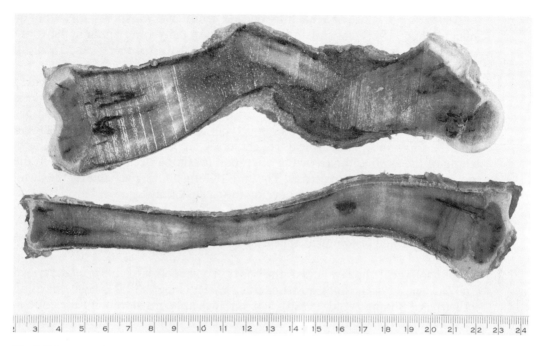

Fig. 2.12. Femur and tibia from a child aged 7½ years with osteopetrosis, showing epiphyses which are normal in shape, size and position and metaphyses which are increased in diameter. There is a fracture of the femur. No bone marrow cavity is present in either bone

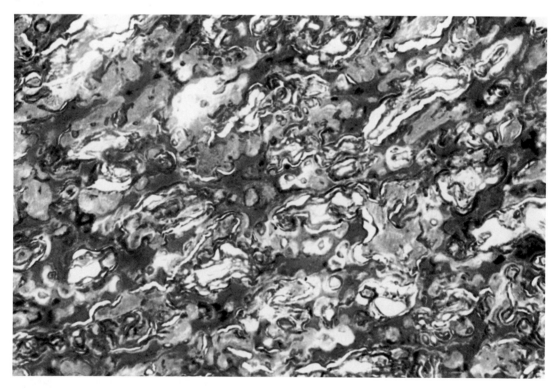

Fig. 2.13. Histological appearances of metaphyseal bone in osteopetrosis in a child aged 7½ years, showing almost complete obliteration of the bone marrow spaces. The bone is made up of persistent calcified cartilage surrounded by abundant woven and lamellar bone. The patient had hepatosplenomegaly, severe anaemia, blindness and bilateral femoral fractures. (H&E × 250)

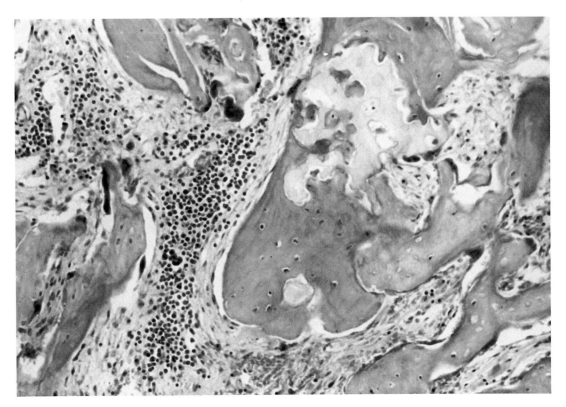

Fig. 2.14. Higher power view of bone in osteopetrosis, showing the presence of numerous osteoclasts. Note small collection of bone marrow cells. (H&E × 500)

appearances to those seen at the site of endochondral ossification at the growth plate (Cohen 1951; Shapiro et al. 1980). Central cores of calcified cartilage persist and are surrounded by woven bone. Membranous bone of the skull and mandible shows narrow intertrabecular spaces containing fibrous or haematopoietic tissue. The bone of the tables of the skull shows variability in appearance with immature bone, characterised by increased cellularity and arrangement of cells into columns near the sutures (Cohen 1951). Normally cancellous bone between the two tables of the skull is resorbed and replaced by haematopoietic tissue in the first 2 years of life, but this cancellous bone persists in osteopetrosis.

Attention has been paid to the appearances of the osteoclasts at the light and electron microscopic levels by Bonucci et al. (1975) and Shapiro et al. (1980). Numerous osteoclasts are present close to both calcified cartilage and woven bone. Large osteoclasts with very numerous nuclei have been seen. Shapiro et al. (1980) studied a large number of osteoclasts ultrastructurally. These cells were found adjacent to cartilage or bone in about the same percentage as in control normal bone of a child, but the osteoclasts were more numerous in osteopetrotic bone. The most striking feature was the lack of ruffled borders and clear zones, even in osteoclasts adjacent to the surface of bone. By contrast, around 30% of osteoclasts in normal bone showed ruffled borders and even more had a surrounding clear zone in the portion of the cell adjacent to the bone surface.

Osteopetrosis in animals

Although osteopetrosis is a rare condition in man, several animal models of the disease have become available over recent years, and the study of these has led to important advances in understanding of the pathogenesis of the disease.

In mice, there are four different mutations which have osteopetrosis, namely the grey-lethal (*gl*), microphthalmic (*mi*), osteosclerotic (*oc*) and osteopetrotic (*op*) strains. Three forms in the rat are known as incisor absent (*ia*), osteopetrotic (*op*) and toothless (*tl*), and osteopetrosis is also present in rabbits, dogs and cows (Milhaud and Labat 1978). Morphologically and radiologically these osteopetrotic strains of rodents show increased bone mass with shorter, broader bones and lack of development of bone marrow cavities in tubular bones. Histological examination of the bone shows features like those of human disease, with columns of calcified cartilage extending from the region of endochondral ossification into the shaft of the tubular bones.

The basic defect in osteopetrotic rodents appears to be a failure of resorption of endosteal bone. Osteopetrotic *gl* and *mi* mice were cured after a period of parabiosis with uninvolved littermates by Walker (1973), who proposed that blood-borne stem cells from the uninvolved parabiont were responsible for the restoration of bone resorptive activity. It is now believed that the fundamental abnormality in osteopetrosis is one of differentiation of osteoclast precursor cells or a functional defect of osteoclasts. The ultrastructure of the osteoclasts in five different osteopetrotic animal mutants has been described (Milhaud and Labat 1978). In the *ia* rat the ruffled borders to the cells were poorly developed and lacking in acid phosphatase activity, but with the onset of bone resorption these features of the osteoclasts were restored to normal (Marks 1973; Schofield et al. 1974). Spontaneous cure of osteopetrosis occurs in this strain of rat. The injection of bone marrow cells from normal littermates into osteopetrotic *op* rats (Milhaud et al. 1975) and *mi* mice (Walker 1975) has proved an effective way of restoring resorptive activity. Bone marrow cells from normal littermates failed, however, to restore *tl* rats to normal (Marks 1977). It therefore seems that there may be different mechanisms at work in different strains of osteopetrotic rodents. The work of Milhaud and his colleagues suggests that the position may be more complicated (Milhaud and Labat 1978). Thus, the *op* rat, as well as developing osteopetrosis, also loses weight and develops signs of 'runt disease' with evidence of thymic deficiency. Bone marrow cells correct the osteopetrosis and cure the thymic deficiency. Thymectomised *op* rats fail to respond to injection of bone marrow cells, both with respect to the 'runt disease' and the osteopetrosis, whereas similar animals receiving grafts of thymus from normal littermates show restoration of bone and bone marrow to normal as well as recovery of thymic function. In other words, normal thymus is able to cure the wasting and bone disease in the *op* rat.

Bone marrow transplantation has recently been applied, with some success, for the treatment of the lethal autosomal recessive form of osteopetrosis in human infants (Ballet et al. 1977; Coccia et al. 1980). Further advances in this field are awaited.

Pycnodysostosis

The characteristics of pycnodysostosis (Greek *pycnos*, thick or dense; *dys-* + *-osteon* + *-osis*, defective bone) were defined by Maroteaux and Lamy (1962). Short stature becomes evident in early childhood. Affected individuals have small faces with a receding chin. The teeth are misplaced and carious. The cranium bulges and the anterior fontanelle remains patent. There are defects of the terminal phalanges, which are shortened, and the fingernails are dysplastic. Osteosclerosis with increased bone fragility predisposes to spontaneous fracture (Roth 1976). Maroteaux and Lamy (1965) have suggested that Henri de Toulouse-Lautrec suffered from this condition, and the appearance of the painter certainly serves as a useful *aide-memoire* to the features of the condition. He was short in stature and carried a stick, suffering two femoral fractures in childhood as a result of minor trauma. It is suggested that his stovepipe hat was worn to cover a patent anterior fontanelle and the beard to cover a receding chin. His parents were first cousins.

Pycnodysostosis is inherited as an autosomal recessive disorder and first appears during childhood. The large brachycephalic skull has an open anterior fontanelle and the sutures are separated even in adults. The mandibular angle is commonly obtuse. The outer ends of the clavicles may be underdeveloped. Abnormalities of segmentation may occur in both the cervical and the lumbar regions of the spine. Further details of the specific features of pycnodysostosis may be found in the review by Elmore (1967). The differential diagnosis of pycnodysostosis is clearly presented by Roth (1976) and by Elmore (1967). The primary differentiation is from osteopetrosis, and the main points are set out in Table 2.6.

Table 2.6. Differential diagnosis between osteopetrosis and pycnodysostosis (after Elmore 1967; Roth 1976)

Feature	Osteopetrosis	Pycnodysostosis
Base of skull	Dense	Dense
Cranial sutures	Closed	Usually open
Paranasal sinuses	Unaerated	Unaerated or dysplastic
Mandible	Normal	Obtuse angle
Clavicle	Normal	Sometimes abnormal
Hands and feet	Normal	Tapered distal phalanges Short phalanges
Pelvis	Coxa vara	Coxa plana or coxa valga
Cranial nerve involvement	Facial palsy, deafness, optic and trigeminal nerves	Absent
Bone density	Increased	Increased
Spontaneous fractures	Present	Present
Medullary cavity	Obliterated	Present
Blood picture	Anaemia, bleeding tendancy (AR)	Normal
Hepatosplenomegaly	Present (AR)	Absent
Development of infections	Present	Absent
Genetics	AD and AR	AR
Stature	Normal, no consistent abnormality	Short

AD, autosomal dominant; AR, autosomal recessive

Histological appearances

There are few reports of the histological appearances of the bones in pycnodysostosis. They are stated simply to be similar to those of osteopetrosis by Shuler (1963), Elmore (1967) and Taylor et al. (1978). They confirm the radiological findings of an imperfect medullary cavity, but there is microscopic evidence of haematopoiesis (Elmore 1967). The histochemistry and electron microscopy of the growth plate of a case has recently been described (Stanescu et al. 1984). The growth plate was narrowed, contained small islands of cells and had short, thick primary trabeculae.

Some other forms of abnormal skeletal development

Cleidocranial dysplasia (cleidocranial dysostosis)

Cleidocranial dysplasia is a condition in which there is abnormal development of the clavicles associated with mild shortness of stature. There is increased mobility of the shoulder, resulting from hypoplasia of the clavicle, and there may be recurrent dislocation of the shoulder, elbows or hip joints. Radiologically the clavicles are totally absent or present only in their medial parts. The clavicles are composed of fragments which articulate normally with the sternum but have no articulation at their lateral ends, where they are either freely mobile or joined by fibrous bands to the choracoid process, acromion, first rib or glenoid cavity. Hypoplasia of the pubic and iliac bones may also occur. The facies are characteristic with a broad forehead and wide parietal region, and radiology shows patent fontanelles and widening of the sutures. These are gradually closed in later life by irregular islands of bone, but a large frontal defect often persists. The unformed ossification centres of the calvaria form a mosaic of small bones.

Congenital dislocation of the hip

Almost all examples of so-called congenital dislocation of the hip are not present at birth and are not therefore strictly congenital. Truly congenital dislocation of the hip with bilateral displacement is rare and is often known as 'atypical' congenital dislocation of the hip. The acetabular socket is diminished in size and flattened by the presence of accumulated cartilaginous tissue. There is shortening of the neck of the femur and associated anomalies may include torticollis, spina bifida, agenesis of the sacrum, contractures of the knee joint, hypoplasia of the fibula or femur and club foot.

The more common form of congenital dislocation of the hip occurs more frequently in some families than in the general population. The cartilaginous parts of the hip joint are almost intact in the predisposed neonate, but hypoplasia of the osseous nuclei occurs. The roof of the acetabulum is more oblique than normal with the socket flattened, and there is increased anteversion of the femoral head in the stage before luxation. The ossification centre for the head of the femur appears later on the affected side. The femoral head may remain in contact with the original articular surface of the acetabulum after subluxation has occurred, but it protrudes from the socket. The flattened elongated acetabular roof shows a depression at the site where the femoral head rests. At a later stage, the flattened femoral head moves over the rim of the acetabulum and there is no longer contact with the original socket. A secondary socket is formed opposite the dislocated femoral head. Fibro-cartilage is formed in the fat pad around the ligamentum teres and fuses with the hyaline cartilage of the flattened original socket. Displacement is always upwards but additionally may be anterior, posterior or lateral. Coxa vara or coxa valga deformities result when the direction of the femoral neck is altered. Information on the growth of the acetabulum in the normal child and the changes in congenital hip dysplasia is available in the publications of Ponseti (1978a, b).

Slipped femoral capital epiphysis

Slipping of the epiphysis of the femoral head occurs slightly more often in males than females and presents at the age of 10–16 years in the former, a year or so earlier in the latter. The condition may be unilateral or bilateral. It is rarely synchronously bilateral, although subsequent involvement of the opposite side is more likely with unilateral disease.

The epiphysis is not altered in an uncomplicated case. There is fragmentation, reduplication and folding of the epiphyseal cartilage into the epiphysis. Thus, slipping of the epiphysis follows disruption of the epiphyseal cartilage plate (Sutro 1935; Ponseti and McClintock 1956). The region of the epiphyseal plate shows increased vascularity with fibrous tissue and new bone formation. The femoral head and neck eventually become reunited to form a synostosis and there is frequently malalignment. Ischaemic necrosis of the slipped epiphysis is one complication. More rarely there is necrosis of the femoral and acetabular articular cartilages. Secondary osteoarthrosis may develop.

References

Albers-Schönberg H (1904) Röntgenbilder einer seltenen Knockenerkrankung, Munch Med Wochenschr 51: 365 (Cited by Beighton 1978)

Albright JP, Albright JA (1971) Osteogenesis imperfecta: serial rib biopsies in three patients treated with low doses of fluoride. J Bone Joint Surg [Am] 53: 801 (abstr)

Ballet JP, Griscelli C, Coutris G, Milhaud G, Maroteaux P (1977) Bone marrow transplantation in osteopetrosis. Lancet II: 1137 (letter)

Bauze RJ, Smith R, Francis MJO (1975) A new look at osteogenesis imperfecta. J Bone Joint Surg [Br] 57: 2–12

Becker MH, Genieser NB, Finegold M, Miranda D, Spackman T (1975) Chondrodysplasia punctata. Is maternal warfarin therapy a factor? Am J Dis Child 129: 356–359

Beighton P (1978) Inherited disorders of the skeleton. Genetics in medicine and surgery series. Churchill Livingstone, Edinburgh

Beighton P, Horan F, Hammersma H (1977) A review of the osteopetroses. Postgrad Med J 53: 507–516

Bonucci E, Sartori E, Spina M (1975) Osteopetrosis fetalis. Report on a case, with special reference to ultrastructure. Virchows Arch Pathol Anat 368: 109–121

Brickley DM, Eyre DR, Glimcher MJ (1974) Studies on the chemical composition, structure, reducible crosslinks and solubility properties of the collagen from patients with osteogenesis imperfecta. J Bone Joint Surg [Am] 56: 859 (abstr)

Briggs JN, Emery JL, Illingworth RS (1953) Congenital stippled epiphyses. Arch Dis Child 28: 209–212

Coccia PF, Krivit W, Cervenka J, Clawson C, Kersey JH, Kim TH, Nesbit ME, Ramsay NKC, Warkentin PI, Teitelbaum SL, Kahn AJ, Brown DM (1980) Successful bone-marrow transplantation for infantile malignant osteopetrosis. N Engl J Med 302: 701–708

Cohen J (1951) Osteopetrosis. Case report, autopsy findings and pathological interpretation: failure of treatment with vitamin A. J Bone Joint Surg [Am] 33: 923–937

Coughlin EJ, Guare HT, Moskowitz AJ (1950) Chondrodystrophia calcificans congenita. J Bone Joint Surg [Am] 32: 938–942

Cremin BJ (1970) Infantile thoracic dystrophy. Br J Radiol 43: 199–204

Cremin BJ, Beighton P (1978) Bone dysplasias of infancy. A radiological atlas. Springer, Berlin Heidelberg New York

Dickson IR, Millar EA, Veis A (1975) Evidence for abnormality of bone matrix proteins in osteogenesis imperfecta. Lancet II: 586–587

Doty SB, Matthews RS (1971) Electron microscopic and histochemical investigation of osteogenesis imperfecta tarda. Clin Orthop 80: 191–201

Eastoe JE, Martens P, Thomas NR (1973) The amino-acids composition of human hard tissue collagens in osteogenesis imperfecta and dentinogenesis imperfecta. Calcif Tissue Res 12: 91–100

Ellis RW, van Creveld S (1940) A syndrome characterized by ectodermal dysplasia; polydactyly, chondroplasia and congenital morbus cordis. Arch Dis Child 15: 65–84

Elmore SM (1967) Pycnodysostosis: a review. J Bone Joint Surg [Am] 49: 153–162

Engfeldt B, Engström A, Zetterström R (1954) Biophysical studies of the bone tissue in osteogenesis imperfecta. J Bone Joint Surg [Br] 36: 654–661

Engfeldt B, Karlberg P, Zetterström R (1955) Studies on the skeletal changes and on the etiology of the anaemia in osteopetrosis. Acta Pathol Microbiol Scand 36: 10–20

Engfeldt B, Fajers C-M, Lodin H, Pehrson M (1960) Studies on osteopetrosis. III Roentgenological and pathologic-anatomical investigations on some of the bone changes. Acta Paediatr 49: 391–408

Fairbank T (1947) Dysplasia epiphysialis multiplex. Br J Surg 34: 225–232

Falvo KA, Bullough PG (1973) Osteogenesis imperfecta: a histometric analysis. J Bone Joint Surg [Am] 55: 275–286

Follis RH (1953) Histochemical studies on cartilage and bone. III Osteogenesis imperfecta. Bull Johns Hopkins Hosp 93: 386–399

Forbes GB, Taves DR, Smith FA, Kilpper RW (1968) Bone mineral turnover in a patient with osteogenesis imperfecta estimated by fluoride excretion. Calcif Tissue Res 25: 283–287

Ford GD, Schneider M, Brandon JR (1951) Congenital stippled epiphyses. Paediatrics 8: 380–392

Friedman JM, Kaplan HG, Hall JG (1975) The Jeune syndrome (asphyxiating thoracic dystrophy) in an adult. Am J Med 59: 857–862

Frydman M, Hertz M, Goodman RM (1974) The genetic entity of hypochondroplasia. Clin Genet 5: 223–229

Fujii K, Tanzer ML (1977) Osteogenesis imperfecta: biochemical studies of bone collagen. Clin Orthop 124: 271–277

Funderburk SJ (1975) Osteopetrosis in two brothers with severe mental retardation. Birth Defects 11: 91–98

Gamsu H, Lorber J, Rendle-Short J (1961) Haemolytic anaemia in osteopetrosis. A report of two cases. Arch Dis Child 36: 494–499

Herdman RC, Langer LO (1968) The thoracic asphyxiant dystrophy and renal disease. Am J Dis Child 116: 192–201

Hwang WS, Tock EPC, Tan KL, Tan LKA (1979) The pathology of cartilage in chondrodysplasias. J Pathol 127: 11–18

Jewell FC, Lofstrom JE (1940) Osteogenic sarcoma occurring in fragilitas ossium. Radiology 34: 741–745

Key JA (1926) Brittle bones and blue sclera. Hereditary hypoplasia of the mesenchyme. Arch Surg 13: 523–567

King JD, Bobechko WP (1971) An orthopaedic description and surgical review. J Bone Joint Surg [Br] 53: 72–89

Klenerman L, Ockenden BG, Townsend AC (1967) Osteosarcoma occurring in osteogenesis imperfecta. Report of two cases. J Bone Joint Surg [Br] 49: 314–323

Knaggs RL (1924) Osteogenesis imperfecta. Br J Surg 11: 737–759

Kovac MJ, Wolf JW, Thompson RC, Schwartz ER (1974) The biosynthetic rate and hydroxylysine content of collagen in osteogenesis imperfecta. J Bone Joint Surg [Am] 56: 859–860

Langer LO (1968) Thoracic-pelvic-phalangeal dystrophy: asphyxiating thoracic dystrophy of the newborn; infantile thoracic dystrophy. Radiology 91: 447–456

Langer LO Jr, Baumann PA, Gorlin RJ (1967) Achondroplasia. Am J Roentgenol Radium Ther Nucl Med 100: 12–26

Langer LO Jr, Spranger JW, Greinacher I, Herdman RC (1969) Thanotophoric dwarfism: a condition confused with achondroplasia in the neonate, with brief comments on achondrogenesis and homozygous achondroplasia. Radiology 92: 285–294

Lie SO, Siggers DC, Dorst JP, Kopits DE (1974) Unusual multiple epiphyseal dysplasias. Birth Defects 12: 165–185

Lowry RW, Wignall N (1975) Saldino–Noonan short rib-polydactyly dwarfism syndrome. Paediatrics 56: 121–123

Marks SC (1973) Pathogenesis of osteopetrosis in the *ia* rat: reduced bone resorption due to reduced osteoclastic function. Am J Anat 138: 165–190

Marks SC (1977) Osteopetrosis in the toothless (*tl*) rat: presence of osteoclasts but failure to respond to parathyroid extract or to be cured by infusion of spleen or bone marrow cells from normal litter mates. Am J Anat 149: 289–297

Maroteaux P, Lamy M (1962) La pycnodysostose. Presse Med 70: 999–1002

Maroteaux P, Lamy M (1965) The malady of Toulouse-Lautrec. JAMA 191: 715–717

Maroteaux P, Stanescu V, Stanescu R (1976)The lethal chondrodysplasias. Clin Orthop 114: 31–45

McCune DJ, Bradley C (1934) Osteopetrosis (marble bones) in an infant. Review of the literature and report of a case. Am J Dis Child 48: 949–1000

McKusick VA, Scott CI (1971) A nomenclature for constitutional disorders of bone. J Bone Joint Surg [Am] 53: 978–986

McKusick VA, Egeland JA, Eldridge R, Krusen DE (1964) Dwarfism in the Amish. The Ellis–van Creveld Syndrome. Bull Johns Hopkins Hosp 115: 306–336

Milhaud G, Labat M-L (1978) Thymus and osteopetrosis. Clin Orthop 135: 260–271

Milhaud G, Labat M-L, Graf B, Juster M, Balmain N, Moutier R, Toyana K (1975) Démonstration cinétique, radiographique et histologique de le guèrison de l'ostéopétrose congénitale du rat. CR Seances Acad Sci 280: 2485–2488

Nicholls AC, Pope FM (1979) Biochemical heterogeneity of osteogenesis imperfecta: new variant. Lancet I: 1193 (letter)

Oberklaid F, Danks DM, Mayne V, Campbell P (1977) Asphyxiating thoracic dysplasia: clinical, radiological and pathological information on 10 patients. Arch Dis Child 52: 758–765

Penttinen RP, Lichtenstein JR, Martin GR, McKusick VA (1975) Abnormal collagen metabolism in cultured cells in osteogenesis imperfecta. Proc Natl Acad Sci USA 72: 586–589

Phillips SJ, Magsamen BF, Punnett HH, Kisternmacher ML, Campo RD (1974) Fine structure of skeletal dysplasia as seen in pseudo-achondroplastic spondylo-epiphyseal dysplasia and asphyxiating thoracic dystrophy. Birth Defects 10: 314–326

Pines B, Lederer M (1947) Osteopetrosis: Albers–Schönberg Disease (marble bones). Report of a case and morphologic study. Am J Pathol 23: 755–775

Ponseti IV (1970) Skeletal growth in achondroplasia. J Bone Joint Surg [Am] 52: 701–716

Ponseti IV (1978a) Growth and development of the acetabulum in the normal child. J Bone Joint Surg [Am] 60: 575–585

Ponseti IV (1978b) Morphology of the acetabulum in congenital dislocation of the hip. J Bone Joint Surg [Am] 60: 586–599

Ponseti IV, McClintock R (1956) The pathology of slipping of the upper femoral epiphysis. J Bone Joint Surg [Am] 38: 71–83

Raap G (1943) Chondrodystrophia calcificans congenita. Am J Roentgenol Radium Ther Nucl Med 49: 77–82

Ramser JR, Villanueva AR, Pirok D, Frost HM (1966) Tetracycline based measurements of bone dynamics in 3 women with osteogenesis imperfecta. Clin Orthop 49: 151–162

Riley FC, Brown DM (1971) Morphological and biochemical studies in osteogenesis imperfecta. J Lab Clin Med 78: 1000 (abst)

Rimoin DL (1974) Histopathology and ultrastructure of cartilage in the chondrodystrophies. Birth Defects 10: 1–18

Rimoin DL (1975) The chondrodystrophies. Adv Hum Gen 5: 10–118

Rimoin DL (ed) (1976) Skeletal dysplasias. Clin Orthop 114: 2–179

Rimoin DL, Hughes GN, Kaufman RL, Rosenthal RE, McAlister WH, Silberberg R (1970) Endochondral ossification in achondroplastic dwarfism. N Engl J Med 283: 728–735

Rimoin DL, Silberberg R, Hollister DW (1976) Chondro-osseous pathology in the chondrodystrophies. Clin Orthop 114: 137–152

Roth VG (1976) Pycnodysostosis presenting with bilateral subtrochanteric fractures. A case report. Clin Orthop 117: 247–253

Rutkowski R, Resnick P, McMaster JH (1979) Osteosarcoma occurring in osteogenesis imperfecta. J Bone Joint Surg [Am] 61: 606–608

Saldino RM (1971) Lethal short-limbed dwarfism: achondrogenesis and thanatophoric dwarfism. Am J Roentgenol Radium Ther Nucl Med 112: 185–197

Schofield BH, Levin LS, Doty SB (1974) Ultrastructure and lysosomal histochemistry of *ia* rat osteoclasts. Calcif Tissue Res 14: 153–160

Shapiro R, Rowe DW (1983) Collagen genes and brittle bones. Ann Intern Med 99: 700–704

Shapiro R, Glimcher MJ, Holtrop ME, Tashjian AH, Brickley-Parsons D, Kenzora JE (1980) Human osteopetrosis. J Bone Joint Surg [Am] 62: 384–399

Shaul WI, Emery H, Hall JG (1975) Chondrodysplasia punctata and material warfarin use during pregnancy. Am J Dis Child 129: 360–362

Sheffield LJ, Danks DM, Mayne VM, Hutchinson LA (1976) Chondrodysplasia punctata: 23 cases of a mild and relatively common variety. J Pediatr 89: 916–923

Shuler SE (1963) Pychodysostosis. Arch Dis Child 38: 620–625

Silberberg R (1976) Ultrastructure of cartilage in chondrodystrophies. Birth Defects 10: 306–313

Sillence DO, Rimoin DL (1978) Classification of osteogenesis imperfecta. Lancet I: 1041–1042

Sillence DO, Rimoin DL, Lachman R (1978) Neonatal dwarfism. Pediatr Clin North Am 25: 453–483

Sillence DO, Horton WA, Rimoin DL (1979) Morphologic studies in the skeletal dysplasias. Am J Pathol 96: 813–859

Sjolin S (1959) Studies on osteopetrosis. II. Investigations concerning the nature of the anaemia. Acta Paediatr Scand 48: 529–544

Solcia E, Rondini G, Copella C (1968) Clinical and pathological observations on a case of newborn osteopetrosis. Helv Paediatr Acta 23: 650–658

Smith HL, Hand AM (1958) Chondro-ectodermal dysplasia (Ellis–van Creveld syndrome): report of two cases. Paediatrics 21: 298–307

Smith R, Francis MJO, Bauze RJ (1975) Osteogenesis imperfecta. Q J Med 44: 550–573

Spencer AT (1962) A histochemical study of long bones in osteogenesis imperfecta congenita. J Pathol Bacteriol 83: 423–427

Spranger J (1976) The epiphyseal dysplasias. Clin Orthop 114: 46–60

Spranger JW, Langer LO, Wiedemann HR (1974) Bone dysplasias: an atlas of constitutional disorders of skeletal development. Saunders, Philadelphia

Stanescu V, Bona C, Ionescu V (1970) The tibial growing cartilage biopsy in the study of growth disturbances. Acta Endocrinol (Copenh) 64: 577–601

Stanescu V, Stanescu R, Maroteaux P (1984) Pathogenic mechanisms in osteochondrodysplasias. J Bone Joint Surg [Am] 66: 817–836

Sugarman GI (1974) Chondrodysplasia punctata (rhizomelic type): case report and pathologic findings. Birth Defects 10: 334–340

Sutro CJ (1935) Slipping of the capital epiphysis of the femur in adolescence. Arch Surg 31: 345–360

Sykes B, Francis MJO, Smith R (1977) Altered relation of two collagen types in osteogenesis imperfecta. N Engl J Med 296: 1200–1203

Taylor MM, Moore TM, Harvey JP (1978) Pycnodysostosis. A case report. J Bone Joint Surg [Am] 60: 1128–1130

Teitelbaum SL, Kraft WJ, Lang R, Avioli LV (1974) Bone collagen aggregation abnormalities in osteogenesis imperfecta. Calcif Tissue Res 17: 75–79

Trelstad RL, Rubin D, Gross J (1977) Osteogenesis imperfecta congenita. Evidence for a generalised molecular disorder of collagen. Lab Invest 36: 501–508

Visekzul C, Opitz JM, Spranger JW, Hartman HA, Gilbert FF (1974) Pathology of chondrodysplasia punctata rhizomelic type. Birth Defects 10: 327–333

Walker BA, Murdoch JL, McKusick VA, Langer LO, Beals RK (1971) Hypochondroplasia. Am J Dis Child 122: 95–104

Walker DG (1973) Osteopetrosis—cured by temporary parabiosis. Science 180: 874–875

Walker DG (1975) Bone resorption in osteopetrotic mice by transplants of normal bone marrow and spleen cells. Science 190: 784–785

Yang S-S, Brough AJ, Garewal GS, Bernstein J (1974) Two types of heritable lethal achondrogenesis. J Pediatr 85: 796–801

Zawisch Carla (1949) Marble bone disease. Arch Pathol 43: 55–75

Chapter 3

Inborn Biochemical Disorders of Metabolism

Introduction

An increasing number of disorders in which there is a biochemical abnormality in the form of an enzyme deficiency have been identified over recent years. Some of these disorders are classified together as the lysosomal storage diseases, some of which affect the skeletal system. The mucopolysaccharidoses, mucolipidoses and sphingolipidoses all fall within this category and these are described in this chapter. Although hypophosphatasia has effects on bone which are the same as those of rickets and osteomalacia, this has also been included, since an enzyme deficiency is responsible ultimately for the changes. Oxalosis may be primary and is then due to an enzyme defect, though oxalate crystal deposition in bones is much more often secondary to other disease processes.

The mucopolysaccharidoses

The mucopolysaccharidoses are a recessively inherited group of lysosomal storage diseases. Deficiency of specific degradative enzymes results in accumulation of glycosaminoglycans (mucopolysaccharides) in connective tissue cells. Glycosaminoglycans are polysaccharide chains consisting of disaccharide repeating units of alternating uronic acid and hexosamine molecules. They are linked, as side chains, by a characteristic terminal sequence through xylose to serine molecules on a core protein, itself a polypeptide, to form a proteoglycan. All the classified mucopolysaccharidoses, with the exception of Morquio's syndrome, involve a disturbance in dermatan sulphate and heparan sulphate metabolism, either singly or together.

The main degradative pathways for these glycosaminoglycans involve lysosomal glycosidases and sulphatases, a distinct enzyme being required to remove each chemical group. Several enzymes are required to break down each chain. If any one enzyme is missing, the degradative sequence is interrupted and the only available method of catabolism is by hyaluronidase, resulting in the breaking of the glycosaminoglycan into large fragments. It is the storage of these large fragments in cells which is responsible for the pathological changes of the mucopolysaccharidoses. Details of the biochemical disorders in the mucopolysaccharidoses are available in the articles by Neufeld (Neufeld 1974, Neufeld et al. 1975).

The enzyme defects in the separate mucopolysaccharidoses (MPS) are summarised in Table 3.1. The individual disorders are known either by eponymous names or by the designation of Roman numerals (MPS I to VII; McKusick 1969). The Scheie's syndrome was classified as MPS V because it had a distinctive phenotype (Schie et al. 1962) but has been found to be biochemically similar to Hurler's syndrome (Weissmann and Neufeld 1970) and is placed within the Hurler group as MPS I–S.

The severity of clinical features differs, but as a group these disorders are characterised by variable degrees of skeletal dysplasia and the excretion of excessive amounts of glycosaminoglycans in the urine. Details of the biochemical and clinical features of the different disorders are summarised in Tables 3.1 and 3.2.

Table 3.1. The mucopolysaccharidoses. Details of designation and biochemical features

MPS	Eponym	Enzyme defect	Metabolite affected	Inheritance
I–H	Hurler	a-L-iduronidase	Dermatan sulphate, heparan sulphate	Autosomal recessive
I–S	Scheie	a-L-iduronidase	Dermatan sulphate, heparan sulphate	Autosomal recessive
I–H/S	H/S compound	a-L-iduronidase	Dermatan sulphate, heparan sulphate	Autosomal recessive
II severe	Hunter	Sulpho-iduronide sulphatase	Dermatan sulphate, heparan sulphate	X-linked recessive
II mild	Hunter	Sulpho-iduronide sulphatase	Dermatan sulphate, heparan sulphate	X-linked recessive
III A	Sanfilippo	Sulpho-glucosamine sulphatase	Heparan sulphate	Autosomal recessive
III B	Sanfilippo	N-acetyl-B-D-glucosaminidase	Heparan sulphate	Autosomal recessive
IV	Morquio	Sulpho-hexosamine sulphatase	Keratan sulphate	Autosomal recessive
VI severe	Maroteaux–Lamy	Sulpho-galactosamine sulphatase	Dermatan sulphate	Autosomal recessive
VI mild	Maroteaux–Lamy	Sulpho-galactosamine sulphatase	Dermatan sulphate	Autosomal recessive
VII	Sly	β-glucuronidase	Dermatan sulphate	Autosomal recessive

Table 3.2. The mucopolysaccharidoses. Clinical features, intelligence and life expectancy

MPS	Features	Intelligence	Life expectancy

Hurler	Dwarfism
	Hepatosplenomegaly
	Corneal opacities
	Altered facies
	Skeletal changes,
	  including bowed limbs
	  and kyphosis
		Mental retardation	6–10 years

Scheie	Normal stature Corneal opacities Hepatosplenomegaly Claw hands	Normal	Normal

Hunter	Dwarfism
	Hepatosplenomegaly
	Altered facies
	Cardiac abnormalities
	Deafness
	No corneal changes
		Severe form—mental
		  retardation
		Mild form—normal
			Severe form—
			  10–15 years
			Mild form—
			  adulthood or
			  normal

Sanfilippo	Deafness
	Altered facies
	Some skeletal changes
		Severe mental
		  retardation
			Teens to early
			  adulthood

Morquio	Dwarfism
	Kyphoscoliosis and
	  platyspondyly
		Not usually mentally
		  retarded
			Third and
			  fourth decades

Maroteaux–Lamy	Dwarfism
	Corneal opacity
	Platyspondyly and
	  other abnormalities
	  of the hips and spine
		Normal	Second and
			  third decades,
			  or normal

Hurler's syndrome

The features of Hurler's syndrome become manifest during the early years of life. Affected infants appear normal after birth, and presenting symptoms are stiffness of joints, persistent rhinorrhoea, dorsolumbar kyphosis and chest deformity. This disorder becomes fully developed by 1–2 years of age with hepatosplenomegaly, dwarfism, corneal opacities, umbilical hernia and cardiac murmurs. The face becomes altered in appearance with a flattened nasal bridge, wide-set eyes, bulging cheeks and thickening of the lips. There is progressive mental retardation from the age of 2 years. The skeletal features comprise bowing deformities of the limbs, dorsolumbar kyphosis, stubbiness of the fingers and general limitation of joint movement. Dwarfism is due to a combination of growth retardation, bowing of the limbs and spinal changes.

Radiological examination shows generalised rarefaction of tubular bones, delay in the appearance of epiphyseal ossification centres and widening of their metaphyseal ends. Failure of ossification of the anterior half of at least one of the vertebral bodies gives rise to a 'beak-like' appearance to the spine on radiological examination. Macroscopic examination of the tubular bones shows widened irregular epiphyseal plates with gelatinous articular cartilage, which is abnormally thick in places. The lumbar vertebral bodies have oval and irregular outlines in sagittal section and there is cartilage instead of bone in the upper anterior part of each of the 'beaked' dorsolumbar vertebrae

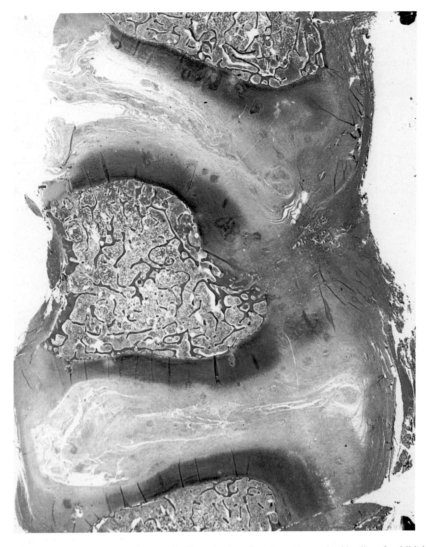

Fig. 3.1. Low-power photomicrograph of a sagittal section through vertebral bodies of a child dying with Hurler's syndrome, showing anterosuperior defect in a vertebral body giving rise to a 'beaked' appearance. (H&E × 4)

(Fig. 3.1). The thickened skull has osteophyte-like protrusions on the floor of the middle and posterior fossae with a narrowed foramen magnum. The sutures are closed earlier than normal.

Hunter's syndrome

All of the mucopolysaccharidoses are autosomally recessively inherited except for Hunter's syndrome, which is an X-linked recessive. The onset of symptoms is delayed, in comparison with Hurler's syndrome. Abnormal behaviour, problems with feeding and mental retardation are usually present by the age of 3 years. Affected males show growth retardation, coarse facial features, head enlargement, hepatosplenomegaly, stiffness and contractures of the joints, deafness and cardiac abnormalities. Corneal changes are not present. The patients survive to age 10–15 years. A milder form of the disease with normal intelligence and survival into adult life is recognised, as reported, for example, by DiFerranti and Nichols (1972).

Maroteaux–Lamy syndrome

Lack of growth between the ages of 2 and 3 years, development of facial features like those of Hurler's syndrome and joint stiffness are present in the Maroteaux–Lamy syndrome. Dwarfism is severe, with the development of a wedge-shaped lumbar kyphosis similar to that seen in Hurler's syndrome and shortening of the limbs and trunk. Corneal opacity is variable but frequently marked. The patients are of normal intelligence.

Morquio's syndrome

All of the mucopolysaccharidoses are due to abnormalities in dermatan and/or heparan sulphate breakdown with the exception of Morquio's syndrome, in which the affected metabolite is keratan sulphate (see Table 3.1). Morquio's syndrome becomes clinically apparent at the age of 1–2 years, when there is disturbance of gait with knock knees, flat feet and hip abnormalities associated with the development of flexion contractures and dislocation. There is dwarfism resulting from growth retardation and kyphoscoliotic deformity of the vertebral column, which is most marked in the dorsolumbar region. Platyspondyly in the dorsal region is also a significant feature. The face shows a wide mouth with broadly spaced teeth and a broad maxilla. Corneal opacity becomes clinically apparent at age 8–10 years. Aortic regurgitation is frequent. Early death is often due to respiratory disease, which may be contributed to by the platyspondyly, kyphoscoliosis and cervical myelopathy resulting from atlantoaxial subluxation.

Examination of the spine shows that the flattened vertebral bodies are increased in diameter anteroposteriorly and have upper and lower borders which slope towards each other anteriorly. Ossification centres are delayed in appearance and development and may resemble multiple epiphyseal dysplasia on radiological examination.

Histological appearances

Histological examination of the bones in Hurler's syndrome shows marked abnormalities of endochondral ossification with diminished thickness of the proliferation zone of the long bones and reduction in the amount of cartilage related to epiphyseal ossification centres. Glycosaminoglycan-containing macrophages fill the bone marrow space and may produce cortical defects when similar collections are present in the periosteal connective tissue cells. Chondro-osseous tissue from patients with the Hurler, Sanfilippo and Morquio syndromes shows similar histological appearances. The chondrocytes in resting cartilage are larger than normal with granular cytoplasm which stains positively for mucopolysaccharides. Areas of loose connective tissue

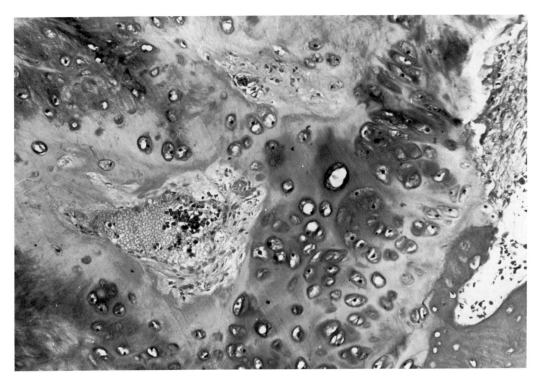

Fig. 3.2. High-power photomicrograph of the costochondral junction of a child with Hurler's syndrome, showing disruption of the growth plate and loose fibrous tissue in the cartilage. (H&E × 500)

are present throughout the resting cartilage and these cause focal disruption of the growth plate and irregularity of the metaphysis in the Hurler and Morquio syndromes (Fig. 3.2). The trabeculae of the iliac crest cartilage in Hurler's syndrome are wider and coarser than normal, contain loose connective tissue and fuse horizontally.

Electron microscopy in Hurler's syndrome shows chondrocytes which are larger than normal and have a granular cytoplasm resulting from the presence of lysosomal vacuoles containing undegraded proteoglycan (Rimoin et al. 1976). Similar appearances are seen in cells in the Sanfilippo and Morquio syndromes (Silberberg et al. 1972). The vacuoles are uniform in appearance in the Hurler and Morquio syndromes, but of two distinct types in the Sanfilippo syndrome (Rimoin et al. 1976).

The mucolipidoses

The mucolipidoses comprise a group of rare disorders which clinically resemble both the mucopolysaccharidoses and the sphingolipidoses in morphological features. The term was introduced by Spranger and Wiedemann (1970) and refers to lysosomal storage diseases in which mucopolysaccharides (glycosaminoglycans) and sphingolipids accumulate in cells. The lymphocytes contain vacuoles, and cultured fibroblasts from affected patients also show the presence of cytoplasmic inclusion bodies. The skeletal changes in all the mucolipidoses, and in the mucopolysaccharidoses, have been termed 'dysostosis multiplex' and are present in varying degrees in the different conditions.

Premature closure of the cranial sutures is fairly common. Widening of the ribs is an early radiological sign of dysostosis multiplex and may occur in the first 3 months of life. The ovoid shape to the vertebral bodies seen in normal infancy may persist beyond the first year, and there may be anterior and superior ossification defects. The iliac bones may be hypoplastic. In the hands, the metacarpals may be short, widened and pointed proximally, with bullet-shaped phalanges (Spranger 1977). Available evidence suggests that all the mucolipidoses are inherited as autosomal recessives (Beighton 1978). The mucolipidoses are classified in the way set out in Table 3.3.

Table 3.3. Classification of the mucolipidoses

1. Mucolipidosis I   (lipomucopolysaccharidosis)
2. Mucolipidosis II (I-cell disease)
3. Mucolipidosis III (pseudo-Hurler polydystrophy)
4. Other mucolipidoses
   a) Generalised gangliosidosis I (GM$_1$ gangliosidosis, pseudo-Hurler disease)
   b) Generalised gangliosidosis II
   c) Juvenile sulphatidosis (mucosulphatidosis—Austin type)
   d) Fucosidosis
   e) Mannosidosis
   f) Others

Mucolipidosis I

Mucolipidoses I is a rare disorder in which retardation of development is apparent by the age of 1 year and the appearance is mildly Hurler-like by 3–4 years. Mild radiographic changes of dysostosis multiplex are seen. The diagnosis may be suspected by the presence of vacuolated cells in the bone marrow, and inclusions are demonstrable in cultured fibroblasts.

Mucolipidosis II

Mucolipidosis II ('I-cell disease') was originally described as a variant of Hurler's syndrome and shows features reminiscent of severe mucopolysaccharidosis. It differs from Hurler's syndrome by virtue of the fact that it is clinically apparent at a younger age and shows faster progression with earlier death. Corneal opacities are less apparent and there is no mucopolysacchariduria.

Affected individuals have gingival hyperplasia, thickening of the skin, mucoid rhinorrhoea, severe joint contractures and claw hand deformity, together with hepatosplenomegaly. Death occurs about the age of 4–5 years. Dense cytoplasmic inclusions are present in cultured fibroblasts and these inclusion cells (I-cells) give the disease its alternative name. The histochemistry and ultrastructure of these I-cells have been described by Hanai et al. (1971). The inclusions are periodic acid-Schiff positive, oil red O positive, metachromatic and osmiophilic. They comprise multivesicular membranous figures, pleomorphic membranous bodies and electron-dense and electron-lucent material, these components being present in varying degrees in most inclusions.

Radiological examination shows irregular periosteal thickening, widening of the diaphyses of the long bones and skeletal changes similar to those of Hurler's syndrome, so that it is only the severity of the changes at a young age which suggests the diagnosis (Kelly 1976).

Mucolipidosis III

Mucolipidosis III is compatible with survival into adult life, though there may be real, but mild, mental retardation and progressive disability, resulting from skeletal dysplasia. The condition is also known as pseudo-Hurler polydystrophy, the term used originally by Maroteaux and Lamy (1966). Onset of symptoms occurs at age 2–4 years with stiffness of the fingers and other joints. Early coarsening of the facial features and radiographic findings of dysostosis multiplex by the age of 6 years suggest a mucopolysaccharidosis. A claw hand deformity is present by 12 years of age. Vertebral involvement comprises spondylolisthesis or kyphosis, and considerable disability may result from progressive destruction of the hip joint (Kelly 1976). The radiological features are described by Nolte and Spranger (1976), and descriptions of a number of cases in which the diagnosis was certain are given by Kelly et al. (1975). Cultured fibroblasts show cytoplasmic vacuoles.

Generalised gangliosidosis I

Generalised gangliosidosis I shows Hurler-like clinical and radiological features, present at birth, and there is widespread periosteal reaction in the long bones (Beighton 1978). This condition is also known as neurovisceral lipidosis, and death occurs by the end of the second year of life with accumulation of gangliosides in the liver and brain. Skeletal changes are relatively minor components of the other mucolipidoses. Further details may be obtained from Kelly (1976) and Beighton (1978).

The sphingolipidoses

The sphinglolipidoses include Gaucher's disease, Tay–Sachs disease, Fabry's disease, Niemann–Pick disease and infantile metachromatic leucodystrophy. Skeletal involvement is a clinically significant feature only of Gaucher's disease. The changes in Niemann–Pick disease are also briefly described below.

Gaucher's disease

Gaucher's disease is a disorder characterised by the presence of cerebroside-laden cells in the lymphoreticular system and bone marrow. Three forms of the disease are now recognised, namely an adult or chronic non-neuropathic type, an infantile cerebral type and a juvenile type. These three categories are sometimes given the numerical designations type I, II and III respectively (Brady 1977). The infantile and juvenile forms are lethal and show no evidence of skeletal involvement, the patients dying because of the accumulation of cerebrosides in the brain. A relatively normal lifespan is common in the adult form of Gaucher's disease, and the author has personally seen a case presenting for the first time at the age of 69 years. Splenomegaly is a frequent presenting feature of this form of Gaucher's disease, though there may be a haemorrhagic diathesis. The skeletal manifestations are bone pain, pathological fractures, degenerative joint disease, osteomyelitis and so-called pseudo-osteomyelitis, aseptic necrosis of the femoral head and spinal deformities, notably kyphoscoliosis (Arkin and Schein 1948; Davies 1952; Seinsheimer and Mankin 1977; Goldblatt et al. 1978). 'Pseudo-osteomyelitis' refers to the clinical picture, in which there is localised tenderness, redness, swelling and warmth over a bone in a patient who is usually pyrexial with a raised erythrocyte sedimentation rate and a polymorphonuclear leucocytosis. Blood culture is consistently negative and the acute attacks settle, usually after a few days (Goldblatt et al. 1978). Adult non-neuropathic Gaucher's disease has a high prevalence among Ashkenazi Jews (Beighton 1978). This type of 'adult' Gaucher's disease presenting in infancy has been described in 11 non-Jewish children under the age of 4 years by Hodson et al. (1979). The skeletal manifestations were pseudo-osteomyelitis, bone pain, fractures and arthritis. In view of this finding, it may be more appropriate to use the term 'non-neuropathic' rather than 'adult-type' Gaucher's disease for this particular disorder.

The changes of skeletal involvement by Gaucher's disease in childhood have been described by Todd and Keidon (1952), Wood (1952) and Amstutz and Carey (1966). The radiological features of the hip often resemble Perthes disease (Reed and Sosman 1942; Todd and Keidon 1952; Amstutz and Carey 1966; Jaffe 1972).

The radiological appearances include areas of radiolucency, which may be circumscribed or diffuse with scalloping of the cortex resulting from the presence of large collections of Gaucher cells. Pathological fractures, sclerotic foci related to ischaemic necrosis and widening of the lower third of the femur to give an 'Erlenmeyer flask' appearance with cortical thinning and patchy sclerosis are also features (Amstutz and Carey 1966; Jaffe 1972; Myers et al. 1975; Goldblatt et al. 1978).

Macroscopic examination of longitudinally sectioned bones shows the presence of greyish nodules which stand out from the surrounding marrow and are partly surrounded by fibrous tissue. Sectioned long bones may show diffuse replacement of the medullary cavity by similar greyish tissue. Thinning of the related cortex may be present. Replacement of the diploic spaces of the calvaria by yellowish or greyish deposits of Gaucher cells results in severe thinning of the tables of the skull. Collapse of the femoral head results where there is necrosis of bone and of the Gaucher cell collections. Vertebral collapse may occur for similar reasons, sometimes resulting in the formation of an angular 'gibbus' deformity (Jaffe 1972). Osteonecrosis under these circumstances is almost certainly related to impairment of the blood supply to bone by massive infiltration with Gaucher cells.

Histological examination shows the presence of numerous Gaucher cells which are typically large and polyhedral with eosinophilic cytoplasm (Fig. 3.3)

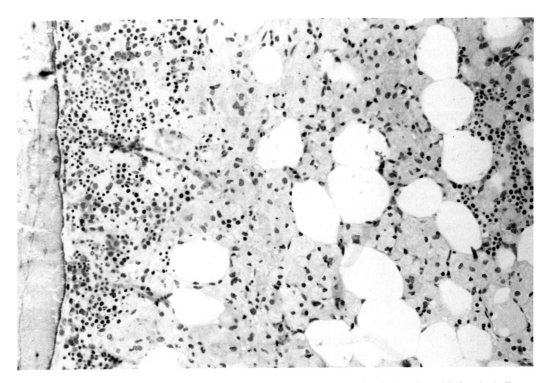

Fig. 3.3. Photomicrograph of bone and bone marrow from a woman presenting for the first time with Gaucher's disease at the age of 69 years. Shows large pale Gaucher cells in the *centre*, bone trabecula with adjacent haematopoietic tissue to the *left*. (H&E × 500)

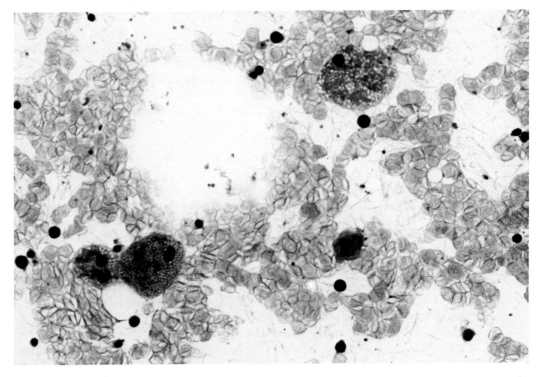

Fig. 3.4. Photomicrograph of bone marrow aspirate from the case shown in Fig. 3.3, showing large Gaucher cells with granular appearance in the cytoplasm. (Azan × 1200)

in which striations may be just discernible. The author has personally found the azan stain to be an effective way of demonstrating the granular or striated appearance of the inclusions (Fig. 3.4), while Weinberg (1978) advocates the use of periodic acid–methenamine silver stain to distinguish Gaucher cells from normal marrow histiocytes. A detailed histochemical study has been performed by Fisher and Reidbord (1962). The cytoplasm shows an intense periodic acid–Schiff reaction which is unaffected by diastase treatment. The oil red O stain for neutral fat is positive but only with frozen sections, and there is intense reaction in stains for acid phosphatase, lipase and non-specific esterase. These findings have been confirmed by Burns et al. (1977), who also carried out studies of the surface markers of Gaucher cells and showed that they possessed many of the characteristics of the monocyte–macrophage series.

The ultrastructural appearances of Gaucher cells have been described by DeMarsh and Kautz (1975), Fisher and Reidbord (1962) and Djaldetti et al. (1979). The cells contained round, ovoid and elongated membrane-bound inclusion bodies containing fine tubular structures. The scanning electron microscopic appearances of the surfaces of Gaucher cells were considered by Djaldetti et al. (1979) to support the view that these cells are derived from the reticuloendothelial system, and evidence of phagocytic activity was occasionally seen.

The metabolic defect in Gaucher's disease leads to accumulation of an excessive quantity of glycolipid known as glucocerebroside. There is insufficiency of an enzyme, glucocerebrosidase, that catalyses the cleavage of glucose from glucocerebroside. Patients with infantile Gaucher's disease have virtually no detectable glucocerebrosidase activity, those with the juvenile form of the disease up to 20% of normal glucocerebrosidase activity, and those with the non-neuropathic adult form 20%–45% of that found in normal individuals (Brady et al. 1965; Brady 1977). It is assumed that the amount of residual glucocerebrosidase activity in the brain in adult-type Gaucher's disease is sufficient to catabolise glucocerebroside derived from ganglioside metabolism so that no pathological accumulation in nerve cells results (Brady 1977).

Niemann–Pick disease

Niemann–Pick disease is a lipid storage disorder which is transmitted as an autosomal recessive trait. Patients with this disorder have been divided into five basic categories on clinical grounds. In none of them is skeletal involvement a significant clinical feature of the illness, which comprises neurological involvement and organomegaly in variable degrees (Brady 1977).

The basic metabolic disorder is one of abnormal storage of sphingomyelin in various tissues. Sphingomyelin is ubiquitous as a component of cell membranes. The enzymatic deficiency in this disorder is that of sphingomyelinase. Lipid-laden cells are present in various tissues, most notably the spleen, lymph nodes, liver and bone marrow. They are large cells of the macrophage series with pale foamy or faintly granular cytoplasm, which is sudanophilic. The skeletal changes are described by Jaffe (1972). The bone marrow may appear yellow if heavy infiltration with lipid-laden cells is present. The cortex of the long bones may be thinned and bone trabeculae reduced in number. Secondary ossification centres may be delayed in their appearance because of the generally poor health of the affected infant or young child. In contrast with Gaucher's disease, collapse of the epiphysis of the femoral head and circumscribed areas of radiolucency of the bones are not features of Niemann–Pick disease, even in those subjects surviving into later childhood or adult life (Jaffe 1972).

Hypophosphatasia

Hypophosphatasia is a familial disorder which probably has an autosomal recessive type of inheritance (see below). It is characterised by low serum and tissue alkaline phosphatase levels, defective bone mineralisation with the formation of excessive amounts of unmineralised bone matrix, and increased urinary levels of phosphoethanolamine and pyrophosphate. The biochemical finding of a subnormal serum alkaline phosphatase level may also occur in inanition, hypothyroidism, scurvy, severe anaemia, poisoning with radioactive heavy metals and clofibrate or aminophylline therapy (Schade et al. 1977; Whyte et al. 1979).

The exact incidence of hypophosphatasia is unknown, though Fraser (1957) estimated it to be 1:100 000 for the infantile form of the disease in Toronto. The severity of clinical involvement varies, decreasing with increasing age at the time of onset. Disorders within the diagnosis 'hypophosphatasia' are sometimes divided into congenita, juvenile, tarda and adult types (Beighton 1978). Arbitrary division into three types—infantile, juvenile and adult—was suggested by Fraser (1957). Infantile or neonatal hypophosphatasia is the most common form of the disorder and can be diagnosed in utero by the examination of amniotic fluid cells (Hoar and Rudd 1976; Rathenbury et al. 1976; Rudd et al. 1976). Defective mineralisation of bone, raised intracranial pressure, convulsions, hypercalcaemia and hypercalciuria are features. Autosomal recessive inheritance is well established, and the disease is common among inbred populations (Mehes et al. 1972; Rubecz et al. 1974; Rasmussen and Barrter 1978). Childhood hypophosphatasia has a more benign course, with clinical onset after the age of 6 months. The bone disease is similar to rickets in which, however, spontaneous healing has been observed (Schlessinger et al. 1955; Pimstone et al. 1966). Premature loss of deciduous teeth is common in children surviving with hypophosphatasia, and heterozygotes lose their permanent teeth at an early age (Pimstone et al. 1966). The inheritance of this form is as an autosomal recessive trait (Pimstone et al. 1966; Rasmussen and Barrter 1978). Parental consanguinity has been a feature of several cases (Svejcar and Walther 1975). Heterozygotes are easily recognisable by the demonstration of diminished serum alkaline phosphatase and increased urinary phosphoethanolamine (Rathbun et al. 1961).

Adult hypophosphatasia is the rarest form of the disease. Osteopenia, long bone deformities, recurrent fractures and early loss of the permanent teeth are the main clinical features, and the biochemical changes are less severe than those of the childhood forms. A study of a large kindred of adult hypophosphatasic patients is presented by Whyte et al. (1979), together with a review of the literature. The pattern of inheritance has not been definitely established in this form of hypophosphatasia and both dominant and recessive inheritance have been suggested.

Radiological examination of the neonate with severe involvement shows changes in the whole skeleton with underdevelopment and poor mineralisation of bone. The head may be globular and the skull boneless, being formed as a caput membranaceum, or show partial ossification, so that, for example, only the parietal bones are visible. Failure of ossification of long bones may give rise to coarse and ragged central portions of the bones. Radiolucent areas in the metaphysis may show as streaky or irregular and spotty areas. The metaphyseal parts of the long bones may show widening with radiolucent bands (Jaffe 1972; Cremin and Beighton 1978). This appearance, which resembles that of rickets, is pathognomonic of hypophosphatasia in the neonate. Streaking of the metaphysis may occur in intrauterine rubella and radiolucent metaphyseal bands in congenital syphylis, but the combination of an unossified skull and limb lesions is seen only in hypophosphatasia (Cremin and Beighton 1978). The radiological appearances are less marked in the childhood form of the disorder, so that the separate bones of the calvaria are fairly well mineralised. There is little widening of the metaphyseal regions of the long bones, and radiolucent bands are not usually present in the metaphyses. In the affected adult, the appearances are non-specific and comprise generalised loss of bone density with pathological fractures which may heal slowly but do so completely. Stress fractures and pseudofractures are also seen. The latter are typically situated in the lateral part of the subtrochanteric femur on both sides. Postrachitic deformity of the long bones and an abnormal 'copper-beaten' appearance to the skull are less frequent features (Whyte et al. 1979).

Macroscopically, in the child, the epiphyseal cartilage plates are widened (Fig. 3.5), with disordered arrangement of cartilage cells in the proliferation zone and no mineralisation of the matrix of the proliferating cartilage by

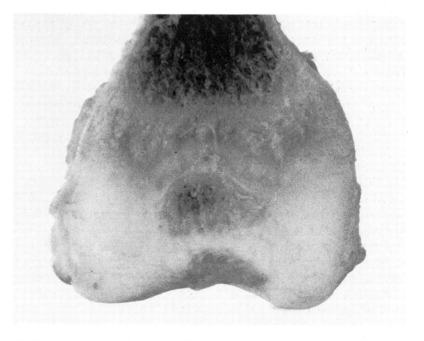

Fig. 3.5. Lower end of the femur of a child with hypophosphatasia, showing widening of the end of the bone and thickening of the growth plate

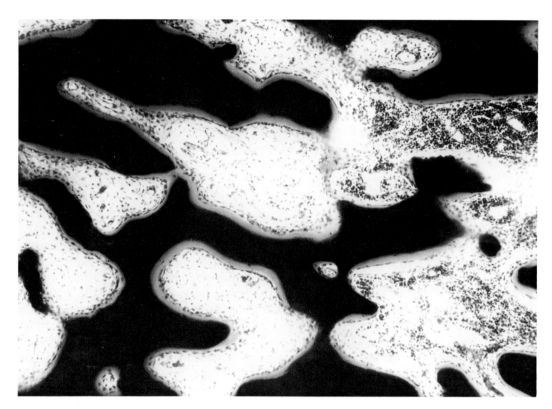

Fig. 3.6. Photomicrograph of bone of a child with hypophosphatasia, showing widened osteoid seams on the bone trabeculae. (Methylmethacrylate, von Kossa × 500)

microscopy. Abundant non-mineralised bone matrix is present in the metaphysis. Enlarged bead-like expansions of the ribs at the costochondral junctions are composed of poorly mineralised osteoid. There may be little widening of growth plates in the older child. The histological features are like those of rickets, with an increase in width of osteoid seams of the bone trabeculae (Fig. 3.6). In the adult, the appearances are those of osteomalacia (Whyte et al. 1979). The defect would seem to be one purely of alkaline phosphatase.

Oxalosis

Raised levels of oxalate may occur in the blood as a result of either endogenous or exogenous processes. When the solubility product of calcium oxalate is exceeded, this salt becomes precipitated in the tissues and gives rise to the condition of oxalosis. The known causes of oxalosis may be divided into 'hereditary' and 'acquired'. The hereditary form of oxalosis, known as primary oxalosis, is a rare autosomally recessive disorder of metabolism, presenting usually in childhood or early adult life with recurrent nephrolithiasis and progressive nephrocalcinosis with high urinary oxalate excretion. Terminal renal failure supervenes usually before the end of the third decade of life. Primary oxalosis and oxaluria results from one of two inborn errors of metabolism

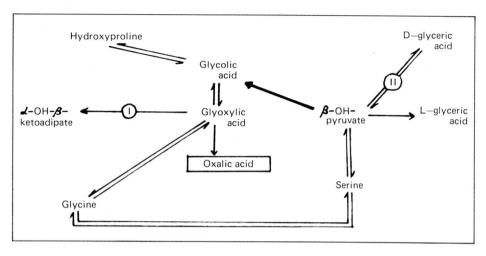

Fig. 3.7. Diagram to represent the sites of the two possible metabolic defects which give rise to primary oxaluria (*I*, 2-oxoglutarate glyoxylate carboligase; *II*, D-glyceric acid dehydrogenase)

(Williams and Smith 1968a). In type I primary oxalosis there is a deficiency of the enzyme 2-oxoglutarate gloxylate carboligase (Koch et al. 1967), while in type II disease the defective enzyme is thought to be D-glyceric acid dehydrogenase (Williams and Smith 1968b; Fig. 3.7). The acquired causes of oxalosis need only be briefly outlined here, but include: (1) excessive dietary intake of oxalate-rich foods, for example rhubarb, spinach; (2) ingestion of ethylene glycol and related glycols (antifreeze); (3) methoxyflurane anaesthesia; (4) so-called enteric oxalosis with increased absorption of normal dietary oxalate in enteric disease; (5) uraemic oxalosis with hyperoxaluria occurring in renal insufficiency from various causes (Chaplin 1977).

Changes in the bones occur in both hereditary (primary) and acquired oxalosis. Descriptions of bone changes in hereditary disease are given by Davis et al. (1950), Dunn (1955), Hughes (1959), Hug and Mihatsch (1975), McKenna and Dehner (1976), Mathews et al. (1979) and Revell et al. (1982). The commonest form of oxalosis is that related to chronic renal failure, and this is certainly the most significant form of acquired disease. The bone changes in oxalosis related to renal failure are described by Milgram and Salyer (1974), Kinnett and Bullough (1976) and Fayemi et al. (1979). Since primary oxalosis may give rise to renal failure and renal failure may cause secondary oxalosis, it is not always possible to be certain whether an individual has primary or secondary oxalosis, especially if the patient is young, there is no family history of renal stone formation and no early clinical presentation with nephrolithiasis and renal calcinosis.

The description below applies mainly to the appearances of bones in primary oxalosis in childhood. The distribution of oxalate crystals in the bones of adults with secondary disease is similar, except that, for example, involvement of growth plates does not occur. Radiological examination in childhood shows the presence of increased density of bones in regions of active bone growth in the end plates of the vertebral bodies (Carsen and Radkowski 1974) and at the epiphysiometaphyseal junction of long bones (Revell et al. 1982). Milgram and Salyer (1974) described similar spinal appearances in secondary oxalosis in children. Further radiodense lines were seen more distal to the plate of the upper humerus by Milgram and Salyer (1974), proximal to the growth plate in the lower femur, in the fingers and in the iliac crests. In addition, there may be a fine radiolucent line in the epiphysis parallel to and situated just deep to the articular cartilage (Carsen and Radkowski 1974; Revell et al. 1982). Macroscopic examination reveals that these radiodense lines correspond to the deposition of calcium oxalate crystals (Fig. 3.8). In addition, there may be periosteal deposition of crystals. Light microscopy shows the presence of birefringent crystals arranged as radiating bundles of needles or as flakes piled one on another. They are situated in the intertrabecular marrow space (McKenna and Dehner 1976; Mathews et al. 1979; Revell et al. 1982), in relation to osteochondral junctions at growth plates, articular cartilage and

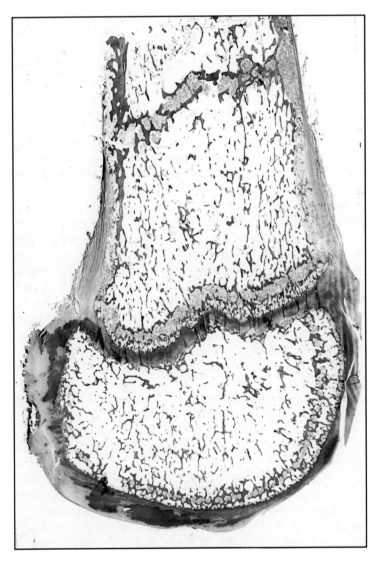

Fig. 3.8. Low-power photomicrograph of the lower end of the femur in a child with primary oxalosis, showing horizontal line of bone and grey material representing oxalate crystals in the upper part of the metaphysis, a second line adjacent to the growth plate and a third arc of bone and crystals parallel with the articular surface. Crystals may also be distinguished at the periosteal surface. (H&E × 3)

in the vertebrae (Hughes 1959; Milgram and Salyer 1974; Revell et al. 1982) and sometimes within bone trabeculae (Hughes 1959; McKenna and Dehner 1976; Revell et al. 1982). The linear deposits of crystals parallel to the growth plate corresponded to horizontally arranged bone trabeculae at a growth arrest line (Harris's line) in the case studied personally by the author (Fig. 3.9). The deposits of oxalate crystals are accompanied by a chronic inflammatory reaction characterised by the presence of histiocytes, foreign body giant cells and fibrosis (Fig. 3.10).

The identification of calcium oxalate deposits in tissue sections has been investigated and reviewed by Chaplin (1974, 1977) and may be carried out on the basis of optical properties, solubility of the crystals, microincineration techniques and tinctorial properties. Briefly, the crystals are of three major forms—rosettes of rods or needles, dipyramids or diamond-shaped crystals and large overlapping plates or flakes. They show positive form birefringence and most are white or have higher first-order polarisation colours. The plates may show second- or third-order colours. The crystals have three refractive indices, and extinction angles are only significant where crystal orientation is known (Peterson and Kuhn 1965). Calcium oxalate is insoluble in water, alkalis, alcohol and other organic solvents, but markedly soluble in mineral acids. Insolubility in acetic acid distinguishes it from other calcium salts.

The von Kossa silver nitrate method which demonstrates anions, such as phosphate, rather than cations, like calcium, fails to give consistent staining of calcium oxalate crystals, according to Chaplin (1977), though in the author's limited experience oxalate deposits stain by this technique even after formic

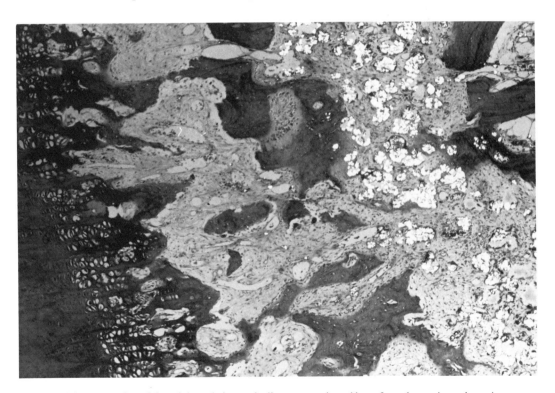

Fig. 3.9. Higher power view of the epiphyseal plate and adjacent metaphyseal bone from the specimen shown in Fig. 3.8, showing endochondral ossification on the *left* and a line of oxalate crystals with related sclerotic trabeculae on the *right*. (Partially crossed polars; H&E × 175)

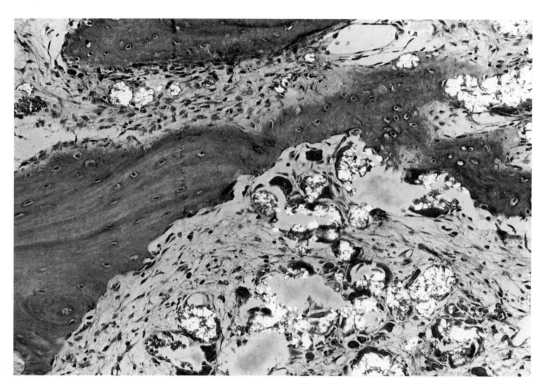

Fig. 3.10. High-power view of the area of crystal deposition showing chronic inflammatory cell reaction with giant cells related to oxalate crystals. There is resorption of the adjacent bone trabecula. (Partially crossed polars; H&E × 500)

acid decalcification of bone. A hydrogen peroxide–silver nitrate method has been developed by Pizzolato (1964) but this has proved capricious in the hands of other workers. The silver nitrate–rubeanic acid method described by Yasue (1969) is a reliable procedure according to Chaplin (1977) and is regarded as selective for calcium oxalate when there has been prior treatment with acetic acid (Chaplin 1974).

Ultimately, proof of the presence of calcium oxalate in tissues depends on the use of analytical methods such as thin layer and gas–liquid chromatography, electron microprobe analysis and X-ray diffraction analysis (Bennett and Rosenblum 1961; Bennington et al. 1964; Evans et al. 1973; Jahn et al. 1980). The crystals have been shown to be whewellite (calcium oxalate monohydrate) by X-ray diffraction analysis (Hughes 1959; Jahn et al. 1980; Revell et al. 1982).

References

Amstutz HC, Carey EJ (1966) Skeletal manifestations and treatment of Gaucher's disease. J Bone Joint Surg [Am] 48:670–701
Arkin AM, Schein AJ (1948) Aseptic necrosis in Gaucher's disease. J Bone Joint Surg [Am] 30:631–641
Beighton P (1978) Inherited disorders of the skeleton. Genetics in medicine and surgery series. Churchill Livingstone, Edinburgh

Bennett B, Rosenblum C (1961) Identification of calcium oxalate crystals in the myocardium of patients with uraemia. Lab Invest 10:947–955

Bennington JL, Haber SL, Smith JV, Warner NE (1964) Crystals of calcium oxalate in the human kidney. Am J Clin Pathol 41:8–14

Brady RO (1977) Heritable catabolic and anabolic disorders of lipid metabolism. Metabolism 26:329–345

Brady RO, Kanfer JO, Shapiro D (1965) Metabolism of glucocerebrosides. II Evidence of an enzymatic deficiency in Gaucher's cells. Biochem Biophys Res Commun 18:221–225

Burns GF, Cawley JC, Flemans RJ, Higgy KE, Worman CP, Barker CR, Roberts BE, Hayhoe FGJ (1977) Surface marker and other characteristics of Gaucher's cells. J Clin Pathol 30:981–988

Carsen G, Radkowski MA (1974) Calcium oxalosis. Pediatr Radiol 113:165–166

Chaplin AJ (1974) Some observations on the demonstration of calcium oxalate in tissue sections. Stain Technol 49:165–173

Chaplin AJ (1977) Histopathological occurrence and characterisation of calcium oxalate: a review. J Clin Pathol 30:800–811

Cremin BJ, Beighton P (1978) Bone dysplasias of infancy. Springer, Berlin Heidelberg New York

Davies FWT (1952) Gaucher's disease in bone. J Bone Joint Surg [Br] 34:454–459

Davis JS, Klingberg WG, Stowell RE (1950) Nephrolithiasis and nephrocalcinosis with calcium oxalate crystals in kidneys and bones. J Pediatr 36:323–334

DeMarsh QB, Kautz J (1957) The submicroscopic morphology of Gaucher cells. Blood 12:324–335

DiFerranti N, Nichols BL (1972) A case of the Hunter syndrome with progeny. John Hopkins Med J 130:325–328

Djaldetti M, Fishman P, Bessler H (1979) The surface ultrastructure of Gaucher cells. Am J Clin Pathol 71:146–150

Dunn HG (1955) Oxalosis: a report of a case with a review of the literature. Am J Dis Child 90:58–80

Evans GW, Phillips G, Mukherjee TM, Snow MR, Lawrence JR, Thomas DW (1973) Identification of crystals deposited in brain and kidney after Xylitol administration by biochemical, histochemical and electron diffraction methods. J Clin Pathol 26:32–36

Fayemi AO, Ali M, Braun EV (1979) Oxalosis in hemodialysis patients. Arch. Pathol Lab Med 103:58–62

Fisher ER, Reidbord H (1962) Gaucher's disease: pathogenetic considerations based on electron microscopic and histochemical observations. Am J Pathol 41:679–692

Fraser D (1957) Hypophosphatasia. Am J Med 22:730

Goldblatt J, Sacks S, Beighton P (1978) The orthopedic aspects of Gaucher disease. Clin Orthop 137:208–214

Goldfischer S, Johnson AB, Morecki R (1976) Hypophosphatasia. A cytochemical study of phosphatase activities. Lab Invest 35:55–62

Hanai J, Leroy J, O'Brien JS (1971) Ultrastructure of cultured fibroblasts in I-cell disease. Am J Dis Child 122:34–38

Hoar DL, Rudd NL (1976) Parental diagnosis of hypophosphatasia. Lancet I:1194 (letter)

Hodson P, Goldblatt J, Beighton P (1979) Non-neuropathic Gaucher disease presenting in infancy. Arch Dis Child 54:707–709

Hug von I, Mihatsch JM (1975) Die primäre oxalose. Fortschr Geb Rontgenstr Nuklearmed 123:153–162

Hughes DTD (1959) The clinical and pathological background of two cases of oxalosis. J. Clin Pathol 12:498–509

Jaffe HL (1972) Metabolic, degenerative and inflammatory disease of bones and joints. Lea and Febiger, Philadelphia

Jahn H, Frank RM, Voegel JC, Schohn D (1980) Scanning electron microscopy and X-ray diffraction studies of human bone oxalosis. Calcif Tissue Res 30:109–119

Kelly TE (1976) The mucopolysaccharidoses and mucolipidoses. Clin Orthop 114:116–136

Kelly TE, Thomas GH, Taylor HA, McKusick VA (1975) Mucolipidoses III: clinical and laboratory findings. Birth Defects 11(6):295–299

Kinnett JG, Bullough PG (1976) Identification of calcium oxalate deposits in bone by electron diffraction. Arch Pathol Lab Med 100:656–658

Koch J, Stockstad ELR, Williams HE, Smith LH (1967) Deficiency of 2,oxo-glutarate: glyoxylate carboligase activity in primary hyperoxaluria. Proc Natl Acad Sci USA 57:1123–1129

Maroteaux P, Lamy M (1966) La pseudopolydystrophie de Hurler. Presse Med 74:2889–2892

Mathews M, Stauffer M, Cameron EC, Maloney N, Sherrard DJ (1979) Bone biopsy to diagnose hyperoxaluria in patients with renal failure. Ann Intern Med 90:777–779

McKenna RW, Dehner LP (1976) Oxalosis. An unusual cause of myelophthisis in childhood. Am J Clin Pathol 66:991–997

McKusick VA (1969) The nosology of the mucopolysaccharidoses. Am J Med 471:730–747

Mehes K, Klujber L, Lassu G, Kajtar P (1972) Hypophosphatasia: Screening and family investigations in an endogamous Hungarian village. Clin Genet 3:60–66

Milgram JW, Salyer WR (1974) Secondary oxalosis of bone in chronic renal failure. J Bone Joint Surg [Am] 56:387–395

Myers HS, Cremin BJ, Beighton P, Sacks S (1975) Chronic Gaucher's disease: radiological findings in 17 South African cases. Br J Radiol 48:465–469

Neufeld EF (1974) The biochemical basis for mucopolysaccharidoses and mucolipidoses. Progr Med Genet 10:81–101

Neufeld EF, Lim TW, Shapiro LJ (1975) Inherited disorders of lysosomal metabolism. Annu Rev Biochem 44:357–376

Nolte K, Spranger J (1976) Early skeletal changes in mucolipidosis III. Ann Radiol (Paris) 19(1):151–159

Peterson BJ, Kuhn RJ (1965) Optical characteristics of crystals in tissue. Cystine and calcium oxalate monohydrate. Am J Clin Pathol 43:401–408

Pimstone B, Eisenberg E, Silverman S (1966) Hypophosphatasia: genetic and dental studies. Ann Intern Med 65:722–729

Pizzolato P (1964) Histochemical recognition of calcium oxalate. J Histochem Cytochem 12:333–336

Rasmussen H, Barrter FC (1978) Hypophosphatasia. In: Stanbury JB, Wyngaarden JB, Frederickson DS (eds) Metabolic basis of inherited disease, 4th edn. McGraw-Hill, New York, p 1340

Rathbun JC, MacDonald JW, Robinson HMC, Wanklin JM (1961) Hypophosphatasia: a genetic study. Arch Dis Child 36:540–542

Rathenbury JM, Blau K, Sandler M, Pryse-Davies J, Clark PJ, Pooley SSF (1976) Prenatal diagnosis of hypophosphatasia. Lancet I:306 (letter)

Reed J, Sosman MC (1942) Gaucher's disease. Radiology 38:579–583

Revell P, Lagier R, Schoenboerner A (1982) Calcium oxalate deposition in growing bone. Anatomical and radiological study in a case of primary oxalosis. Metab Bone Dis Relat Res 4:49–59

Rimoin DL, Silberberg, R, Hollister DW (1976) Chondro-osseous pathology in the chondrodystrophies. Clin Orthop 114:137–152

Rubecz I, Mehes K, Klujber L, Bozzay L, Weisenbach J, Fenyvesi J (1974) Hypophosphatasia: screening and family investigations. Clin Genet 6:155–159

Rudd NL, Miskin M, Hoar DL, Benzie R, Doran TA (1976) Prenatal diagnosis of hypophosphatasia. N Engl J Med 295:146–148

Schade RWB, Demacker PNM, Van't Laar (1977) Clofibrate effect on alkaline phosphatase. N Engl J Med 297:669 (letter)

Scheie HG, Hambrick GW, Barnes S (1962) A newly recognised forme fruste of Hurler's disease (gargoylism). Am J Ophthalmol 53:753–769

Schlessinger B, Luder J, Bodian M (1955) Rickets with alkaline phosphatase deficiency: an osteoblastic dysplasia. Arch Dis Child 30:265–276

Seinsheimer F, Mankin HJ (1977) Acute bilateral symmetrical pathologic fractures of the lateral tibial plateaux in a patient with Gaucher's disease. Arthritis Rheum 20:1550–1555

Silberberg R, Rimoin DL, Rosenthal R, Hasler M (1972) Ultrastructure of cartilage in the Hurler and Sanfilippo syndromes. Arch Pathol 94:500–510

Spranger JW (1977) Catabolic disorders of complex carbohydrates. Postgrad Med J 53:441–448

Spranger J, Wiedemann HR (1970) The genetic mucolipidoses: diagnosis and differential diagnosis. Humangenetika 9:113 (Cited by Beighton 1978)

Svejcar J, Walther A (1975) The diagnosis of the early infantile form of hypophosphatasia tarda. Humangenetika 28(1):49 (Cited by Beighton 1978)

Todd RMcL, Keidan SE (1952) Changes in the head of the femur in children suffering from Gaucher's disease. J Bone Joint Surg [Br] 34:447–453

Weinberg AG (1978) Periodic acid—methenamine silver stain for demonstration of cells in Gaucher's disease. Am J Clin Pathol 69:654 (letter)

Weissmann UN, Neufeld EF (1970) Scheie and Hurler syndromes: apparent identity of the biochemical defect. Science 169:72–74

Whyte MP, Teitelbaum SL, Murphy WA, Bergfeld MA, Avioli LV (1979) Adult hypophosphatasia. Medicine (Baltimore) 58:329–347

Williams HE, Smith LH (1968a) L-glyceric aciduria. A new genetic variant of primary hyperoxaluria. N Engl J Med 278:233–239

Williams HE, Smith LH (1968b) Disorders of oxalate metabolism. Am J Med 45:715–735

Wood HL-C (1952) Gaucher's disease with pseudocoxalgia. J Bone Joint Surg [Br] 34:462–463

Yasue T (1969) Histochemical identification of calcium oxalate. Acta Histochem Cytochem 2:83–95

Chapter 4

Quantitative Methods in Bone Biopsy Examination

Introduction

Although a descriptive approach is normally used in histopathology, there are circumstances in which it is worthwhile to measure the changes seen in tissue sections. Morphometry has a role to play in the study of metabolic bone disease, particularly when groups of patients and methods of treatment are being compared. Whether it is useful or appropriate to apply morphometric methods in routine diagnostic practice is a decision for the individual. Some feel that a pathologist's opinion as to the extent to which particular features are present in a biopsy is sufficient. Undoubtedly care is needed over the reproducibility of techniques and results. The methods are time consuming, but the development of relatively low-cost, semi-automatic computer-linked image analysis systems shows promise of changes in the future. Consideration will be given in this chapter to the measurements which may be made in bone biopsies, the processing and staining methods required and the variables that must be taken into account when assessing the validity of results.

Bone biopsy

Several factors determine the site selected for bone biopsy, apart from ease of clinical availability. The bone specimen should ideally contain cortical and trabecular bone and be from a site where there is representative active bone turnover and in which repeat biopsies are possible with minimal variability. The ribs and iliac crest come nearest to fulfilling these criteria and the iliac crest is usually chosen (Matrajt et al. 1967; Rasmussen and Bordier 1974). Rib biopsy can be performed under local anaesthesia, but among other disadvantages there is the possibility of damage to the pleura. Most bone biopsy techniques involve obtaining a cortex to cortex core from the iliac crest with a wide-bore trephine, for example the Bordier needle (Bordier et al. 1964). Ideally the biopsy should be obtained from a standard site, which by convention is 2 cm below and 2 cm posterior to the anterior superior iliac spine (Melsen et al. 1978a). Alternatively, a vertical core may be taken downwards from the iliac crest. The question of variability at different sites within the iliac crest will be discussed later (see p. 101). The lateral approach to the biopsy of the iliac crest is the method used by most workers now. Wedges of iliac crest obtained at autopsy should include the area normally examined in biopsy specimens.

The complications of bone biopsy have recently been reported by Duncan et al. (1980), who sent a questionnaire to 18 centres and presented data for nearly 15 000 biopsies, three-fifths of which were transiliac, the remainder obtained by a superior approach through the iliac crest. Morbidity was low with both methods of biopsy, the most common problem being haematoma in patients with primary haematological diseases or receiving heparin during haemodialysis. Other complications included neuropathy affecting the lateral cutaneous nerve of the thigh, wound infection, pain, fracture and osteomyelitis. The overall incidence of complications was 0.5%. The same authors also assessed the amount of pain experienced by patients after biopsy. The large majority experienced little, a result similar to that obtained by Johnson et al. (1977), who found that 85% of patients reported the pain as acceptable during and after the procedure.

The experience of the person performing the biopsy determines the suitability of the specimen for histological examination, so that when bone biopsy is performed as an occasional procedure, the specimen is often fragmented. Duncan et al. (1980) have shown that operators with no previous experience produce 16.7% unsatisfactory biopsies, compared with failure on 8.8% of occasions by experienced persons. The same effect was observed when a large number of biopsies were obtained by a single operator in a recent study carried out by the present author and his colleagues: Failure to obtain an adequate sample occurred in the initial stages of the project.

Laboratory processing of the biopsy

Fixation of the biopsy may be in formalin, 70% ethanol or methanol, the alcohols giving better preservation of tetracycline fluorescence (Frost 1969; Parfitt et al. 1976; Melsen and Mosekilde 1980). However, Klein and Jackman (1976) have shown that there is negligible elution of ^{3}H-tetracycline in isotonic saline when bone is taken 3 days after labelling, and the author has experienced no particular difficulty using routine formalin fixation when this interval of time has elapsed between labelling and biopsy. The preparation of undecalcified plastic embedded sections is essential, and the author's own preference is to use methylmethacrylate sectioned at 6–7 μm on a Jung K microtome. Thicker sections (15 μm) may be used for UV microscopy of tetracycline fluorescence.

Staining methods

Bone quantitation is mainly used for the assessment of metabolic bone disease, when changes in the amount of total bone and osteoid together with the activity of the cells at trabecular surfaces are the important features assessed. The histological details are all detectable in haematoxylin and eosin-stained sections, but it is preferable to use other techniques to highlight particular features. Differentiation of osteoid and mineralised bone is readily achieved using von Kossa counterstained with Van Gieson, although almost any other counterstain may be used. The Goldner trichrome method gives good contrast between mineralised and unmineralised bone, as do other trichromes. Solochrome cyanin is used in some centres. A close comparability has been shown between measurements of osteoid volume using solochrome and von Kossa methods (Giroux et al. 1975; Meunier and Edouard 1976), but comparability was less good between solochrome and trichrome, the Goldner process tending to underestimate the amount and extent of the osteoid (Giroux et al. 1975; Meunier et al. 1975). Features at the trabecular surface are reasonably well seen in haematoxylin and eosin and Goldner trichrome methods, although toluidine blue or thionin staining give good definition of cellular details (Fig. 4.1) and both have the advantage of giving an essentially monochromatic staining reaction at the blue end of the spectrum, making them especially suitable for television-linked image analysis systems. Osteoclasts are easily visu-

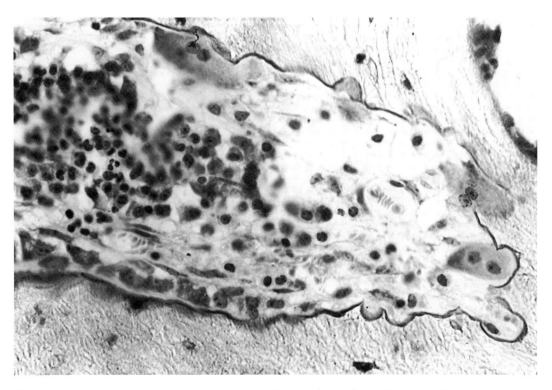

Fig. 4.1. Cellular details at the trabecular bone surface showing osteoclasts and resorption lacunae (*top* and *right*), together with osteoblasts on adjacent bone (*bottom left*). (Methylmethacrylate, thionin × 600)

alised by both of these methods. Some workers fix sections in cold formalin, embed in equal parts methyl/glycol methacrylate and stain for acid phosphatase in order to demonstrate osteoclasts (Evans et al. 1980; Fig. 4.2).

Wide osteoid seams may be difficult to evaluate in the presence of oblique sectioning of trabeculae, and examination of sections by polarisation light microscopy enables the number of bright lamellae present to be counted as a simple aid to assessment (see p. 98). The width of the osteoid seams depends on: (1) the osteoblastic apposition rate, that is the rate of production of osteoid by osteoblasts, and (2) the rate of mineralisation of the osteoid so produced by the osteoblasts (Meunier et al. 1976). An increase in the amount of osteoid present relative to total bone tissue (hyperosteoidosis) need not be due to osteomalacia, and it is necessary to decide whether there is calcification occurring where there are wide osteoid seams. Staining methods for the mineralisation front include solochrome cyanin, Sudan black, cobalt salts and toluidine blue at pH 2.8 (Irving 1958; Irving 1963; Matrajt and Hioco 1972; Rasmussen and Bordier 1974; Meunier et al. 1976). None of these is particularly reliable, and the mineralisation front is best demonstrated by incorporation of a label into the bone before biopsy.

Among the compounds that may be used experimentally in animals are fluorescein derivatives, alazarin red S, procion dyes and haematoporphyrin derivatives (Harris 1960; Goland 1965; Flora 1976). The tetracyclines are used in studies of human bone.

The fluorescence of tetracyclines in bone was described by Milch et al. (1958) and adapted as a means of labelling the mineralisation front by various

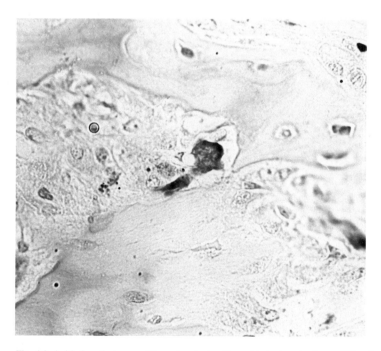

Fig. 4.2. Acid phosphatase positive osteoclasts adjacent to trabecular bone. (Glycol methacrylate, acid phosphatase × 400)

workers (Baud and Dupont 1962; Frost 1962; Harris et al. 1962). The formation of complexes of calcium and magnesium with oxytetracycline has been described by Ibsen and Urist (1962). Tetracyclines are bound at sites of active calcification, there being a close anatomical relationship between tetracycline and ^{45}Ca deposition in bone (Harris et al. 1962; Urist and Ibsen 1963). Further information about the use of tetracycline may be obtained in the articles by Frost (1969), Teitelbaum and Nichols (1976), Flora (1976), Bordier et al. (1976), Frost and Meunier (1976), Treharne and Brighton (1979), Melson and Mosekilde (1980).

Particular points with respect to the histological aspects of using tetracyclines for bone quantitation will be referred to later (see p. 94). Information about the existence of a possible calcification defect can be obtained with a single label, while double-labelling permits measurement of the bone mineralisation rate. Various schedules exist for the performance of both types of labelling. The time required between administration and biopsy before reproducible results are obtained has been found to be 48–72 hours (Bordier et al. 1976). A suitable regimen for single labelling, therefore, is to administer tetracycline for 2–3 days followed by an interval of 3 days before biopsy. Double-labelling is obtained by repeating the doses of tetracycline, separated by an interval of 10 days (i.e. 3 days of tetracycline, 10 days' interval, 3 days of tetracycline, 3 days' interval, biopsy; Fig. 4.3).

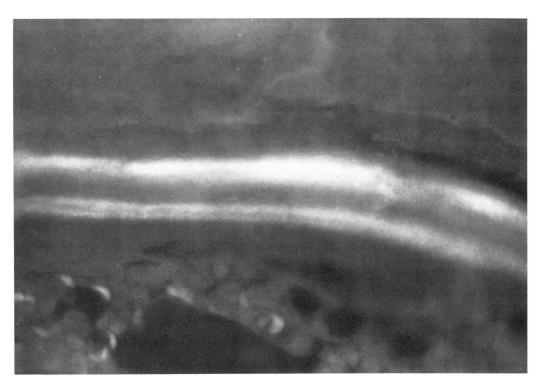

Fig. 4.3. Double-labelling of trabecular bone with tetracycline, which is fluorescent, viewed by UV microscopy. (Methylmethacrylate, unstained section × 800)

Basic principles of measurement

A detailed account of the theory of morphometry is available from other sources (for example, De Hoff and Rhines 1968; Williams 1977; Aherne and Dunnill 1982). The methods involve the application of probability theory to geometry using estimates. Repeated counting is used in order to make these estimates as accurate, that is as near to reality, as possible. The measurements are made on two-dimensional images (allowing for section thickness), but the information derived is normally interpreted in three-dimensional terms (see below).

Bone quantitation may be performed using either (1) inexpensive simple eyepiece graticules and light microscopy, (2) semi-automatic instruments in which a digitising tablet is linked to a desk-top microcomputer or (3) fully automatic computer-linked image analysis equipment.

Point counting with an eyepiece graticule

Point counting is performed by the superimposition of a series of points on the microscope field with an eyepiece graticule and enables the estimation of areas. The points may be randomly arranged or in a regular distribution. Regular arrays of points may be disposed in triangles, squares or hexagons. An arrangement in squares is that most commonly used and is typified by the Zeiss integration plate II. The number of points or hits occurring on a particular feature in a given microscope field is counted and expressed as a percentage of the total number of possible hits (Fig. 4.4). Adjacent fields are

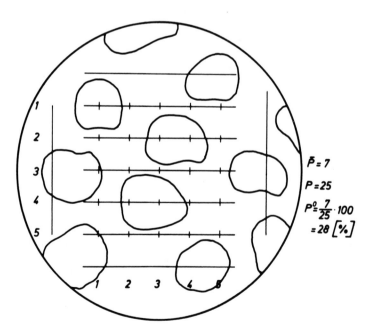

Fig. 4.4. The principle of point counting using an eyepiece graticule. If the islands are considered to be bone trabeculae, then there are 7 out of 25 points falling on bone, that is 28% of total tissue is bone

counted until a sufficient number of measurements has been made to give an accurate estimate of the true area of a feature as a percentage of the total tissue. If n_1, n_2, n_3 etc. are the numbers of points falling on bone trabeculae and N_1, N_2, N_3 etc. are the total possible numbers of points in each field, the area A, expressed as a percentage, can be calculated as:

$$A = \frac{n_1 + n_2 + n_3 \ldots n_x}{N_1 + N_2 + N_3 \ldots N_x} \times 100$$

where x is the number of fields necessary to obtain an accurate result.

The optimal number of points to count in order to achieve a reproducible result can be calculated by the formula developed by Hally (1964) for the relative standard error:

$$\text{Relative standard error} = \frac{\sqrt{1 - \text{area}}}{\sqrt{\text{number of points}}}$$

Details of this method are available in Aherne and Dunnill (1982). It is not actually possible to do this calculation without first having an idea either of the area or the number of points, so that in practice the count is performed and a provisional value for area calculated. This has to be expressed as a decimal rather than a percentage in the above formula. Using this value it is then possible to calculate the number of points needed to obtain results with a given error. The relationship between the number of points which must be counted and the areas has been described by Anderson and Dunnill (1965). Small objects require larger total counts than do large objects.

A simple way to decide how much to count is to calculate the mean value after a given number of fields, count more fields and recalculate the mean value, continuing until the mean value settles to a constant level. This value is described as the 'nominal value' (Fig. 4.5). A further question arises as to

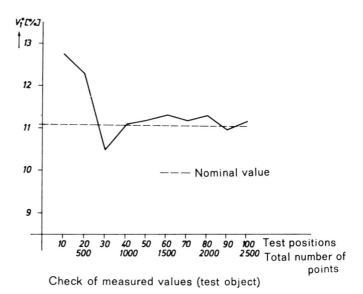

Check of measured values (test object)

Fig. 4.5. The effect of increasing the number of fields examined and points counted on the accuracy of the estimate obtained for a volume measurement. There is a considerable variation in the results when small numbers of points are counted, but the values gradually settle around a 'nominal' value (horizontal broken line)

whether it is better to sum the mean values obtained as quotients for each field
  i.e.

$$\frac{n_1}{N_1} + \frac{n_2}{N_2} + \frac{n_3}{N_3} \cdots \frac{n_x}{N_x}$$

or to use the means obtained from summing the individual values
  i.e.

$$\frac{n_1 + n_2 + n_3 \cdots n_x}{N_1 + N_2 + N_3 \cdots N_x}$$

These two values, the mean of the quotients and the quotient of the means, are not the same. The quotient of the means is preferable and is the method already quoted in this chapter.

Measurements are made on a two-dimensional object so that the value obtained is an area, better referred to as an area fraction (A_a) of the total area measured. Delesse, a French geologist in the middle of the last century (Delesse 1848) showed that area is an unbiased estimator of volume, that is, on average, the fractional volume (V_v) may be substituted for the fractional area, since $V_v = \bar{A}_a$. This concept is widely used in morphometry and is known as the Delesse principle.

Linear intercept method

Measurements of surface area or simple line length are performed by the linear intercept method. Superimposition on the microscope field of a series of lines using an eyepiece graticule is the basis of the procedure. The method should be readily understood by reference to Fig. 4.6. The number of intercepts (or more accurately intersections) that a feature makes with the reference lines are counted. Measurements are made on successive adjacent fields until an accurate estimate of the percentage of surface occupied by a particular feature is obtained. Repetition until a nominal value is achieved applies in the same way as for the point counting method for estimating areas already described. A different type of grid comprising a wave pattern of alternating semicircles has been developed by Merz (1968; Schenk et al. 1969; Fig. 4.7). This also incorporates a square array of points suitable for the point counting method. The grid overcomes problems associated with anisotropy of the material being examined.

Tetracycline labelling

The fluorescent line at the mineralisation front after tetracycline labelling of the biopsy is measured by the linear intercept method with UV light microscopy. Double-labelling of the biopsy with tetracycline enables the measurement of the distance between the two labels using a calibrated micrometer eyepiece to obtain an appositional rate. This measurement is performed at four equidistant points along each double-labelled surface, as illustrated in Fig. 4.8, and the measurement repeated a sufficient number of times at other sites (Frost 1976; Frost and Meunier 1976; Parfitt et al. 1976; Teitelbaum

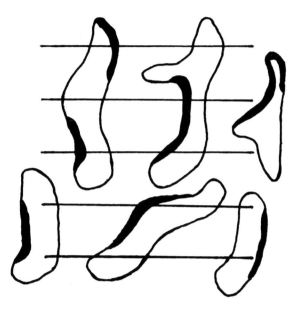

Fig. 4.6. Use of the linear intercept method for measuring surface lengths. The *broad black areas* represent osteoid. There are 5 places where lines intersect with osteoid-covered surface and 20 places where lines intersect trabecular surface, so that osteoid surface is 25% of trabecular surface.

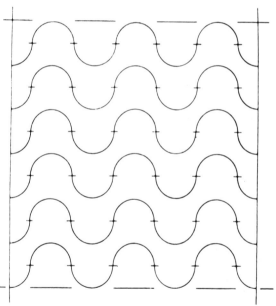

Fig. 4.7. Merz graticule comprising alternating semicircles to form a wave pattern

and Nichols 1976). The rate of apposition of bone is obtained by dividing the mean distance between the labels (d), by the time interval between administration of labels (t). The true appositional rate is calculated by the application of a correction factor since the two lines of tetracycline label will always be sectioned in random planes varying between right angles and nearly parallel (Fig. 4.8). The mathematical method for the derivation of this correction factor is available in papers by Frost (1976) and Teitelbaum and Nichols (1976). The true separation between the two markers, d, is related to the apparent (or measured) separation, x, in the equation, $d = x \, \text{cosine} \, \theta$ (Fig. 4.8). Frost has demonstrated that the distribution of values for θ is skewed, with smaller fractions of the total pairs of lines occurring as the angle θ increases, until

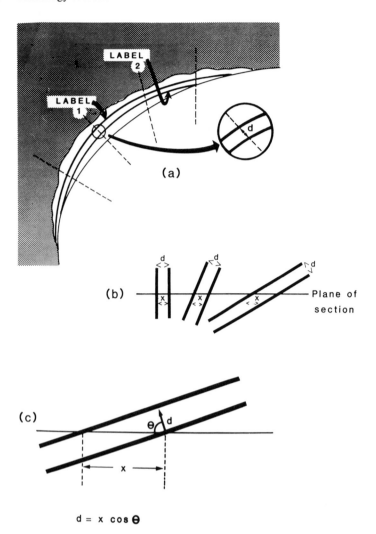

Fig. 4.8a–c. Diagrams illustrating the method of measuring appositional rate using a double tetracycline label. **a** The distance (d) between fluorescent tetracycline labels is measured at four equidistant points, with a calibrated eyepiece graticule. **b** Because the label will be orientated at a variety of angles to the plane of section, the distance actually measured is x. **c** The actual distance between labels may be calculated as $d = x \cos \theta$, where θ is the angle shown (see text)

few or no double lines are distinguishable when $\theta = 85°$ or $90°$ and the tetracycline label is parallel to the plane of section. Trabecular thickness, difference in time interval between labels and differences in the apposition rate will all accentuate the skewness away from high values of θ. Frost adopted a maximum θ value of $75°$ and recommended a correction factor of 0.74, assuming a range of θ from $0°$ to $75°$ (Frost 1976), so that the true appositional rate may be calculated as $\dfrac{0.74x}{t}$. If this correction factor is not applied, then the value obtained for the appositional rate will be approximately 35% too high.

Measurements made and terms used in bone morphometry

The main types of measurement made on bone are those of volume and surface. There is considerable variation in the literature with respect to the terms used for the various values obtained. The volume of trabecular bone as a proportion of total tissue (bone and bone marrow) is variously termed the trabecular bone volume, absolute volume of trabecular bone, fractional bone volume, fractional trabecular bone volume, volume density of bone or relative trabecular volume. Table 4.1 is an attempt to list some of these terms. There are difficulties with respect to some of them. For example, surface density is

Table 4.1. Various terms used in bone morphometry

VOLUME:
  Trabecular
  Trabecular bone volume (TBV)
  Absolute volume of trabecular bone (AVTB)
  Fractional bone volume (tV fract; or tV fract (b))
  Fractional trabecular bone volume (tV fract)
  Volume density of bone (Vv)
  Relative trabecular bone volume (Vv)

  Osteoid
  (Relative) osteoid volume (OV or Vo)
  Volume density of osteoid (Vvo)
  Absolute volume of osteoid $(AOV) = \dfrac{OV \times AVTB}{100}$
  Relative trabecular osteoid volume (RTOV)

SURFACES:
  Osteoid
  (Relative) osteoid surface (OS)
  Surface density of osteoid seams (S vos)
  Relative trabecular osteoid surface (RTOS)
  % trabecular surface occupied by osteoid seams (OS%)

  Osteoblastic/formation
  Active osteoblastic surface (AOS)
  Fractional formation surface (S fract (f))
  Surface density of osteoblasts/bone surface (Svho)
  % trabecular surface covered by osteoblasts (OB%)

  Osteoclastic/resorption
  Resorption surface (RS)
  Osteoclastic resorption surface (ORS) (HO)
  Trabecular osteoclastic resorption surface (RS)
  Surface density of Howship's lacunae (Svht)
  Fractional resorption surface (S fract (r))
  Relative trabecular total resorption surface (RTRS)

OSTEOID THICKNESS
Mean osteoid seam thickness (s̄ or s)
Mean width of osteoid seams (WOS)
Thickness index, osteoid seams or osteoid index (TIOS or OI)

OSTEOCLASTS
Number of osteoclasts per mm² bone tissue (NO/mm²)
Index of osteoclasts (OI)

MINERALISATION FRONT (S fract (lab))
Mineralisation or calcification front (MF, CF)
Appositional rate (uM/t)
Mineralisation rate (MR)

Table 4.2. Measurements and ratios used by author

Trabecular bone volume	$= \dfrac{\text{Volume of trabeculae}}{\text{Volume of trabeculae and marrow}} \times 100$
Osteoid volume	$= \dfrac{\text{Volume of osteoid}}{\text{Volume of osteoid and mineralised bone}} \times 100$
Osteoid surface	$= \dfrac{\text{Length of surface occupied by osteoid}}{\text{Total length of trabecular surface}} \times 100$
(Active) osteoblastic surface	$= \dfrac{\text{Length of trabecula occupied by active osteoblasts}}{\text{Total length of trabecular surface}} \times 100$
Resorption surface	$= \dfrac{\text{Length of trabecular surface occupied by resorption lacunae}}{\text{Total length of trabecular surface}} \times 100$
Osteoclastic resorption surface	$= \dfrac{\text{Length of surface occupied by osteoclasts}}{\text{Length of resorption lacunae}} \times 100$
Mineralisation front	$= \dfrac{\text{Line length of mineralisation (tetracycline fluorescence)}}{\text{Total length of trabecular surface}} \times 100$
Osteoid index	$= \dfrac{\text{Osteoid volume}}{\text{Osteoid surface}} \times 100$
Appositional rate (see p. 95, correction factor)	$= \dfrac{\text{Distance between labels}}{\text{Time}} \mu\text{m/day}$
Osteoclastic index	$=$ Estimate of numbers of osteoclasts as either osteoclasts per high-power field, osteoclasts per mm^2 or cm^2 of tissue or osteoclasts per mm trabecular surface

strictly a measure of surface area as related to volume and it is expressed in mm^2/cm^3 (Bordier et al. 1964; Merz and Schenk 1970a, b; Olah 1976), but 'surface density' and the abbreviation S_v are used sometimes more loosely instead of surface area. Other difficulties arise because different authors relate individual surface measurements to different total surface measurements. Thus osteoblasts may be related to the osteoid surface (Svob) or total trabecular surface (OB%). It is important to have a clear idea of exactly what is being measured when examining a particular set of results. The author's preference is to use the measurements and ratios shown in Table 4.2.

The osteoid index is a guide to the thickness of osteoid seams obtained mathematically from the osteoid volume and osteoid surface. The osteoid index has been shown to correlate well with the actual measurement of osteoid seam width (Meunier et al. 1976). Rapid and fairly reliable assessment of osteoid seams is obtained by polarised light microscopy, and counting the number of birefringent lamellae (bright lines) in the osteoid. Up to four such lamellae are present in normal bone (Woods et al. 1968; Ellis and Peart 1972).

Normal values

Generalisations about normal values in bone morphometry are impossible to give. It is essential that each laboratory measures normal bone obtained at autopsy from the iliac crest of previously ambulant cases dying suddenly with cardiovascular disease and having no other known pathology. Quantitation of these specimens enables a normal range to be obtained for the laboratory using its own methods of observation and measurement. Examples of fairly typical normal values are presented in Table 4.3; in practice, those obtained

Table 4.3. Normal values for iliac crest bone

TRABECULAR BONE VOLUME

Age	Male	Female	Age	Male	Female
10–19	24.5 ± 1.7	31.8 ± 2.7	15–19	23.0 ± 4.1	22.9 ± 4.5
20–29	24.6 ± 2.3	26.8 ± 1.7	20–29	22.4 ± 4.8	23.6 ± 4.1
30–39	22.9 ± 1.1	26.5 ± 2.4	30–39	19.5 ± 4.9	23.3 ± 4.1
40–49	17.4 ± 1.9	22.5 ± 3.5	40–49	19.3 ± 3.1	21.9 ± 3.3
50–59	20.4 ± 1.2	20.1 ± 2.4	50–59	19.1 ± 4.7	20.0 ± 3.6
60–69	13.7 ± 1.2	15.5 ± 1.8	60–69	17.4 ± 5.6	15.3 ± 4.6
70–79	16.2 ± 2.4	17.0 ± 2.0	70–79 ⎫		14.8 ± 3.3
>80	15.4 ± 2.8	17.7 ± 3.2	80–89 ⎬ 17.8 ± 4.3		12.5 ± 2.1
			90–99 ⎭		14.0 ± 4.0

(Melsen et al. 1978b)   (Courpron et al. 1978)

OSTEOID VOLUME

Age	Male	Female	Age	Male	Female
10–19	2.6 ± 0.6	2.1 ± 0.7	10–29	3.9 ± 2.3	2.1 ± 1.4
20–29	2.5 ± 0.3	2.4 ± 0.4	30–49	2.7 ± 1.3	2.0 ± 1.2
30–39	1.8 ± 0.3	1.7 ± 0.4	50–69	2.8 ± 1.8	1.6 ± 0.7
40–49	2.2 ± 0.9	1.3 ± 0.5	>70	2.2 ± 1.7	2.2 ± 1.4
50–59	3.0 ± 0.5	1.9 ± 0.4		(Meunier et al. 1976)	
60–69	1.6 ± 0.3	2.0 ± 0.6			
70–79	1.8 ± 0.5	2.1 ± 0.5			
>80	0.9 ± 0.2	1.3 ± 0.2			

(Melsen et al. 1978b)

OSTEOID SURFACE

Age	Male	Female	Age	Male	Female
10–19	17.8 ± 2.8	14.7 ± 1.9	10–29	18.2 ± 9.3	11.0 ± 6.8
20–29	18.8 ± 2.5	16.7 ± 1.6	30–49	14.4 ± 5.9	11.3 ± 6.8
30–39	14.9 ± 2.2	14.1 ± 2.6	50–69	15.5 ± 6.1	8.6 ± 6.9
40–49	17.2 ± 5.5	14.1 ± 1.7	>70	15.3 ± 9.4	12.1 ± 7.5
50–59	20.3 ± 1.2	19.3 ± 3.1		(Meunier et al. 1976)	
60–69	16.0 ± 2.4	19.8 ± 3.4			
70–79	18.3 ± 2.5	18.2 ± 3.4			
>80	12.0 ± 3.2	12.7 ± 0.8			

(Melsen et al. 1978b)

RESORPTION SURFACE

Age	Male	Female
10–19	3.9 ± 0.4	3.2 ± 0.3
20–29	4.0 ± 0.5	3.9 ± 0.3
30–39	3.7 ± 0.3	4.0 ± 0.4
40–49	4.1 ± 0.8	3.4 ± 0.2
50–59	4.0 ± 0.3	5.1 ± 0.6
60–69	4.1 ± 0.6	3.6 ± 0.6
70–79	5.0 ± 0.6	4.3 ± 0.5
>80	6.0 ± 0.1	3.7 ± 0.6

(Melsen et al. 1978b)

by different centres fall within the same general range. For example, the mean values for trabecular bone volume in various series lie around the 15%–20% level and have similar standard deviations. Several workers have demonstrated a gradual decrease in the trabecular bone volume of normal bone with increasing age (Rasmussen and Bordier 1974; Courpron et al. 1976; Melsen et al. 1978b). Normal females have a slightly higher trabecular bone volume than normal males in the younger age groups but have values the same as (Melsen et al. 1978a, b) or lower than males (Courpron et al. 1976) over the age of 60 years (see Table 4.3). Sample normal values for osteoid volume, osteoid surface and resorption surface are shown in Table 4.3. The mineralisation front normally occupies more than 80% of the osteoid surface but decreases slightly in older subjects (Rasmussen and Bordier 1974). Although there may be wide variation in mineralisation front making it difficult to decide the significance of values in an individual case, it is safe to say that a mineralisation front of less than 20% represents a definite calcification defect. The mineralisation rate (appositional rate), measured by the double-labelling technique, is normally around 0.6 or 0.7 μm/day. Exact values will vary from centre to centre. Melson and Mosekilde (1978) and Vedi et al. (1982) showed that there was no significant variation in appositional rate with age or sex. Osteoid formation by active osteoblasts usually comprises about 5% of the total trabecular surface and active resorption less than 1% of total trabecular surface (Rasmussen and Bordier 1974). Resorptive activity can be evaluated by counting osteoclasts and expressing the results as cells per stated number of high-power fields, or per square millimetre of tissue. Alternatively, if measurements of actual trabecular surface are being obtained by semi-automated image analysis techniques (see p. 108), the osteoclast count can be expressed as a value related to trabecular surface length. We have found there to be a good correlation between osteoclast numbers expressed in this way and measurements of resorbing surface (Fig. 4.9).

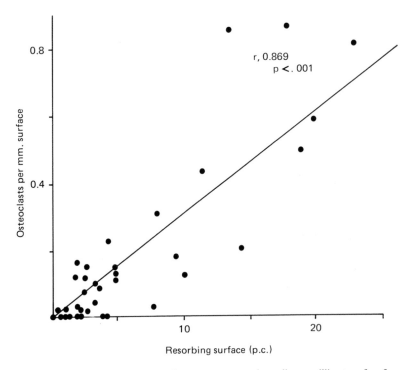

Fig. 4.9. Correlation between osteoclast count expressed as cells per millimetre of surface and resorbing surface in 37 cases of renal osteodystrophy

Variation and reproducibility

Variability in results and the reproducibility of the methods applied to bone quantitation need to be carefully considered. Important considerations are differences (1) between sites in the same bone; (2) between bones in the same patient; (3) between methods, such as staining techniques and magnification used; (4) between observers; and (5) between laboratories.

Numerous studies have compared different sites in the iliac crest. Insignificant or no differences have been demonstrated between adjacent sites in the same iliac crest (Beck and Nordin 1960; Rasmussen and Bordier 1964; Garner and Ball 1966; Melsen et al. 1978a), although differences occurred when the bone was more than 2 cm away from the standard site of biopsy (Melsen et al. 1978a), and differences with depth from the iliac crest surface were noted by Ellis and Peart (1972). No systematic differences have been demonstrated between the left and right iliac crests in comparisons performed by several workers (Ritz et al. 1973; Giroux et al. 1975; Courpron et al. 1976; Melsen et al. 1978a; Visser et al. 1976, 1980). No difference was demonstrable between vertical and transverse methods of iliac crest biopsy (Visser et al. 1976).

There is relatively little information about differences between bones. A comparison of Haversian bone in rib and iliac crest by Villanueva et al. (1976) showed no variations between these two sites. A good correlation between iliac trabecular bone volume and vertebral bone volume was shown by Giroux et al. (1975). The vertebral bone volume was much lower than that in the iliac crest. Lower values for trabecular bone volume in the vertebrae compared with the iliac crest were noted in the study of ankylosing hyperostosis of the spine made in the author's laboratory (Revell and Pirie 1981). The Quantimet method was used on random autopsy cases to make a comparison of trabecular bone volume measurements for the iliac crest and the eleventh thoracic vertebra. The results of this previously unpublished study are shown in Fig. 4.10. There is a good correlation between the two sites, and the results confirm the finding of Giroux and his colleagues that the vertebral body results are similar to those for the iliac crest. Knowledge of the comparability of morphometric values obtained at different sites in the skeleton is of considerable importance in the assessment of such conditions as osteoporosis. The applicability of quantitative studies of iliac crest bone to the assessment of the likelihood of vertebral crush fractures in osteopenic patients is discussed elsewhere (see p. 185). Giroux and his colleagues (1976) also showed that trabecular bone volume measurements on the iliac crest are comparable with those for the manubrium sterni.

Staining methods may influence results, as has already been mentioned (see this chapter, Staining methods). Comparability is good between solochrome and von Kossa for measurements of osteoid volume, and less reliable between solochrome and trichrome methods. Higher values for osteoid volume and osteoid surface were found using Masson trichrome compared with toluidine blue by Melsen et al. (1978a).

Some questions arise with respect to tetracycline labelling of bone. Any tetracycline administered at doses within the therapeutic range will label bone, but extremely high doses should be avoided since tetracyclines have an inhibitory effect on mineralisation, which is quantity dependent (Saxen 1966; Harris et al. 1968). The timing of administration of label and biopsy are

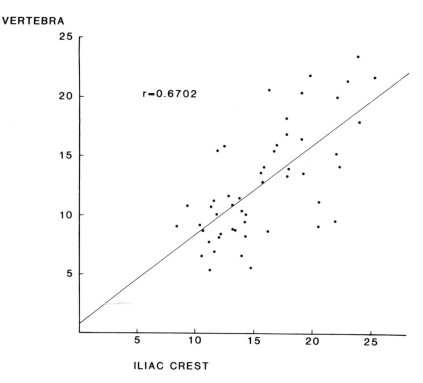

VERTEBRA

r−0.6702

ILIAC CREST

Fig. 4.10. Comparison of trabecular bone volume of iliac crest and 11th thoracic vertebra in 50 random autopsy cases.

important, and biopsy should normally follow the last label by 2 or 3 days (see p. 91). An interval between two labels much longer than 3 weeks results in a decrease in the percentage of osteoid bearing two labels. This is because the normal apposition rate is around 1 μm per day, so that an average osteoid seam of 8 μm thickness will take about 8 days for the process of mineralisation to be completed (Jaworski 1980). Biopsy performed within 24 h of the last label also gives rise to problems, especially if the specimen is placed in aqueous fixatives, when there may be significant loss of fluorescence. Differences in the tetracycline labelling pattern also occur in different pathological processes (see, for example, Baylink et al. 1970; Teitelbaum et al. 1976; Takahashi et al. 1980).

The effect of microscopic resolution in morphometry of bone has been described by Olah (1976). Magnification changes between 25 and 400 times did not influence estimations of volume (volume density), but over the same range of magnification there was a systematic increase in the estimate of surface density (Fig. 4.11). This effect of magnification on measurements of osteoid in bone biopsies had previously been reported by Woods et al. (1968).

That there is a greater variability in results obtained for surface measurements compared with volume measurements has been shown by Delling and his colleagues (1980). This occurred particularly where cellular details at trabecular surfaces were being measured, and many more fields had to be examined to obtain reproducibility under these circumstances. Contributory factors are the relatively small amount of cellular activity at trabecular surfaces and the irregular distribution of surfaces changes. Repeated measurement in exactly the same area showed maximum variation to occur in the evaluation of cellular

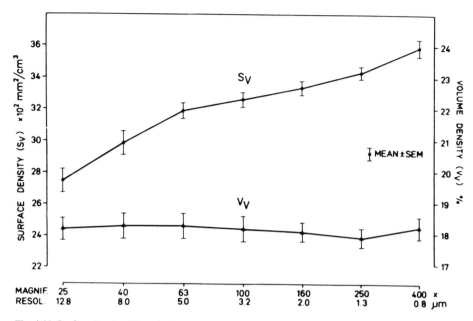

Fig. 4.11. Surface density (S_v) and volume density (V_v) of iliac crest cancellous bone at different magnifications, showing the systematic increase in the estimate of surface density as magnification changes, but no difference in volume density.

surfaces (surface density of osteoblasts/osteoid; surface density of osteoclasts/ bone). Greater variability also occurred with cellular parameters when sections were compared within the same biopsy. Such variation is somewhat disease dependent, since, for example, in advanced renal bone disease there may be much cellular activity requiring measurement of far fewer fields to achieve a reproducible result than, say, in osteoporosis, where there are practically no active osteoblastic or osteoclastic surfaces present.

Comparisons between observers and laboratories have been performed (Delling et al. 1980). The experience of the observer was found to be important, especially with respect to those surface measurements relating to osteoblastic and osteoclastic activity. The volume and surface densities of trabecular bone were not affected greatly by observer experience since comparison of a student with himself and the student with an experienced pathologist both showed good statistical correlation (Fig. 4.12). It is interesting to note that the line for the student/student comparison, made on the same 16 biopsies, but after an intervening examination of 150 biopsies, does not pass through zero but is shifted, indicating that on the second occasion the student was seeing features not originally recognised. The further shift in the line for the pathologist/ student comparison suggests that the pathologist was recognising features which were not recognised by the student.

There are differences between centres looking at the same biopsies. These were found to be considerable with respect to values obtained for osteoid surface measurements when four different morphometry groups were asked to assess ten biopsies, though volume density of trabecular bone showed a much smaller variation (Delling et al. 1980).

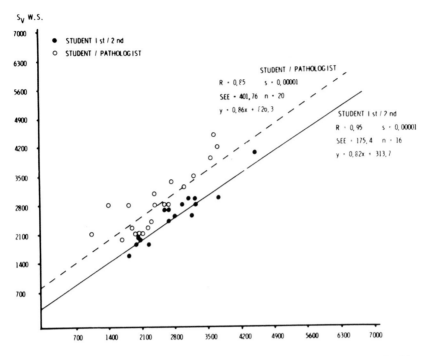

Fig. 4.12. Determination of surface density (S_v) of trabecular bone. ○, 16 values obtained by a student at the beginning and end of the study of 150 normal cases. ●, 20 values obtained by a student compared with an experienced pathologist on the same biopsies.

Semi-automatic and automatic methods in bone quantitation

The performance of morphometry on large numbers of specimens is laborious using the simple eyepiece graticule methods. An alternative approach to bone quantitation is offered by automated and semi-automated computer-linked systems. Both types of equipment enable a much greater throughput of information. Disadvantages include the amount of time which may be required in setting up the fully automatic equipment and the need to stain sections in a way which is suitable for automated image analysis (see below).

Automatic image analysers may be divided into different categories, analysis being achieved by:

1. Source-plane-scanning, in which scanning of the object is achieved with the movement of the light source, for example a flying spot system
2. Specimen-plane-scanning, in which light source and sensor are fixed in alignment in the optical axis of the equipment and the specimen is moved
3. Image-plane-scanning, in which the specimen is scanned by a sensor and both the light source and specimen remain stationary

All television-linked systems use image-plane-scanning. The best known is the Quantimet 720 (Fig. 4.13), and the following account is based on its use in the author's laboratory.

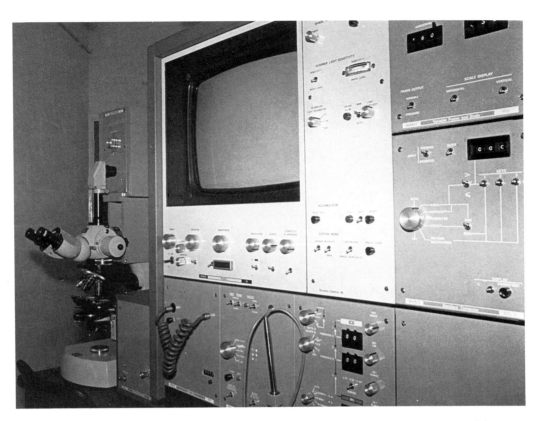

Fig. 4.13. Quantimet 720 image analysis system, showing light microscopy with television camera, screen, light pen and controls for selecting various functions, including densitometer

The function of the Quantimet may be considered in three stages. Input is by means of a closed-circuit television linked to a light microscope (Fig. 4.14). The signals from the scanning of the microscope image by the television camera are used to produce an image on a television screen and to provide information for computer analysis of the image. The results of the computer analysis are displayed numerically at the top of the television screen and it is also possible to superimpose the computer analysis display as an image on the television screen. Different modules are available to perform different functions and these vary from machine to machine, depending on the needs of the user.

The particular machine in the author's laboratory has television display, standard function computer, a control system to set light sensitivity and shade correction, variable frame and scale settings and densitometer function. It interfaces with a desk-top microcomputer. Area, intercept, perimeter and size can be measured, and a programmer module enables the machine to run automatically through a series of measurements on each field.

In the author's laboratory, osteoid volume and trabecular bone volume are measured using the densitometer function. Signals from the television camera pass to the detection module, in which grey level thresholds are set in 64 steps from black to white. The image being analysed has to be resolved into clearly distinguishable grey levels. The preference is to use von Kossa-stained sections counterstained with Van Gieson and treated in such a way that coloration of the bone marrow features is deliberately leached out to give a uniform pale-yellow background. It is then possible to resolve the image into black, grey and white areas corresponding to mineralised bone, osteoid and bone marrow, which are black, red and pale yellow respectively in the stained microscope slide. Careful selection of the grey level settings enables accurate detection at the precisely correct boundary point for the three features which are to be detected and measured. Analysis can then be made of all the features darker

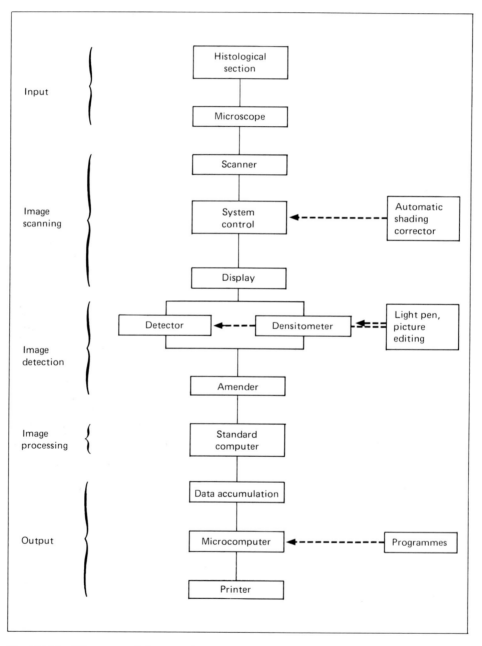

Fig. 4.14. The different stages in image analysis using a Quantimet 720

or lighter than a chosen grey level. A computer module enables selection of the measurement required.

There are 500 000 picture points in each frame (field) on the television screen. By selecting the area mode it is possible to determine the number of picture points at which there is a particular grey level and thus obtain measurements of areas of 'white, grey and black' present in the simplified image of bone. Data for the areas of osteoid, mineralised bone and total tissue are then routed to the desk-top computer (output terminal). The process is repeated for adjacent fields and all the data accumulated in the output computer. Osteoid volume and trabecular bone volume are then calculated automatically by a programme in this computer. A light pen 'screen-editing' facility enables the editing out of unwanted features such as small cracks in bone trabeculae or tissue fragments in the bone marrow. Appropriate care in processing and staining of sections for analysis minimises the need for such editing, and it is obvious that editing reduces the speed of analysis.

It is possible to obtain surface measurements using the same densitometric function with selection of perimeter mode, but the author has preferred to use the Quantimet as a semi-automatic image analyser when quantitating surface features of bone. This is partly because of problems in obtaining suitable definition of outlines and staining of sections, and partly because the use of a light pen enables the observer to measure cellular features at bone surfaces, which is not possible in a fully automated system. Toluidine blue- or thionin-stained sections give the clearest definition of features on the television screen. It is possible to outline trabecular surface, osteoid and resorption surfaces and lengths occupied by active osteoblasts and osteoclasts with the light pen (Fig. 4.15). The line lengths of each outlined feature are routed to the output

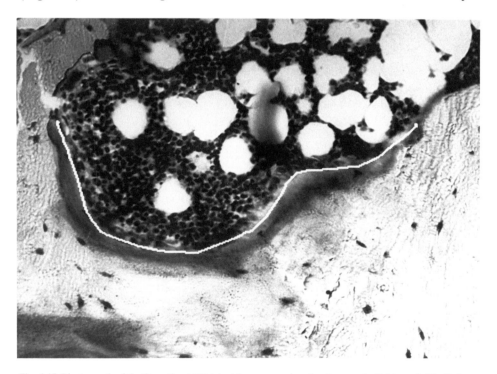

Fig. 4.15. Photograph of the Quantimet 720 television screen, showing the use of a light pen (*white line*) to outline that part of the trabecular surface occupied by osteoid

computer for each field examined, and the measurements calibrated, so that it is possible to obtain an absolute value for the lengths measured. The output computer programme accumulates data for each measurement made and, after a previously specified number of fields has been examined, calculates osteoid surface, active osteoblastic surface, resorption surface, osteoclastic resorption surface and total length of trabecular surface measured. The number of osteoclasts seen at each resorption surface is typed into the output computer as each field is examined and summated, so that it is possible to obtain an osteoclast index, expressed as osteoclasts per millimetre of trabecular surface.

Semi-automatic systems for quantitative analysis of histology consist of a 'digitising tablet', which is an electronic drawing board linked to a micro-computer. The microscopic field may be projected on to this drawing board, or a side-arm drawing tube used to reproduce the image. Commercially available equipment designed for this purpose includes the Leitz ASM, Reichert-Jung MOP and Videoplan, but it is also possible to combine an independent digitising tablet and desk-top microcomputer to produce equivalent equipment for less cost. The digitising tablet enables the outlining of features seen in the microscope field, and measurements of line length, perimeter, intercept or area are then rapidly obtained. Previous calibration enables measurements to be expressed in absolute terms. Area and surface measurements for each field may be summed and the various bone morphometry parameters calculated by use of a suitable programme in the microcomputer. Articles by Birkenhager-Frenkel et al. (1980), Malluche et al. (1980), and Manaka and Malluche (1981) describe the use of digitising tablets for bone quantitation.

Comparison of methods used in bone quantitation

Differences resulting from the use of different staining techniques with the same counting technique have already been discussed (see this chapter, Staining methods; Variation and reproducibility). Reproducible results are best obtained by uniform preparation and staining of samples and examination of sufficient fields in sufficient numbers of sections.

Ellis and Peart (1972) found a good correlation between the actual volume of bone measured by water displacement and that obtained by the point counting technique. Similarly good correlations were obtained by Schwartz and Recker (1980), using displacement methods and point counting with respect to volume density and surface density of bone.

A difference of 1.5% was found between the use of the Zeiss eyepiece graticule and the Quantimet method by Giroux et al. (1975). There was no difference in accuracy between point counting and a semi-automatic method with a digitiser tablet, according to Malluche et al. (1980). Fewer fields were needed in the semi-automatic method to achieve the same coefficients of variance with respect to both non-cellular and cellular (bone formation and resorption) parameters.

References

Aherne WA, Dunnill MS (1982) Morphometry. Edward Arnold, London

Anderson JA, Dunnill MS (1965) Observations on the estimation of the quantity of emphysema in the lungs by the point-sampling method. Thorax 20:462–466

Baud CA, Dupont DH (1962) Histologie intrastructurale sur la bifluorescence du tissu, osseux tonité par les tetracyclines. CR Seances Acad Sci 254:3129–3130

Baylink D, Stauffer M, Wergedal J, Rich C (1970) Formation, mineralisation and resorption of bone in vitamin D deficient rats. J Clin Invest 49:1122–1134

Beck JS, Nordin BEC (1960) Histological assessment of osteoporosis by iliac crest biopsy. J Pathol Bacteriol 80:391–397

Birkenhager-Frenkel DH, Clermonts ECGM, Richter H (1980) Histomorphometry by means of an x-y tabloid. Design of a computer programme; disposition of equipment. In: Jee WSS, Parfitt AM (eds) Bone histomorphometry. 3rd international workshop. Metab Bone Dis Relat Res 2 (Suppl):453–457

Bordier P, Matrajt H, Miravet B, Hioco D (1964) Mesure histologique de la masse et de la résorption des travées osseuses. Pathol Biol (Paris) 12:1238–1243

Bordier PJ, Marie P, Miravet L, Ryckewaert A, Rasmussen H (1976) Morphological and morphometrical characteristics of the mineralization front. A vitamin D regulated sequence of the bone remodelling. In: Meunier PJ (ed) Bone histomorphometry. 2nd international workshop. Armour Montagu, Paris, pp 335–354

Courpron P, Meunier P, Bressot C, Giroux JM (1976) Amount of bone in iliac crest biopsy. Significance of the trabecular bone volume. Its values in normal and in pathological conditions. In: Meunier PJ (ed) Bone histomorphometry. 2nd international workshop. Armour Montagu, Paris, pp 39–53

DeHoff RT, Rhines FN (1968) Quantitative microscopy. McGraw-Hill, New York

Delesse MA (1848) Procédé mechanique pour determiner la composition des roches. Ann Mines 13:379–388

Delling G, Luehmann H, Baron R, Mathews CHE, Olah A (1980) Investigation of intra and inter-reader reproducibility. In: Jee WSS, Parfitt AM (eds) Bone histomorphometry. 3rd international workshop. Metab Bone Dis Relat Res 2 (Suppl):419–427

Duncan J, Dao SD, Parfitt AM (1980) Complications of bone biopsy. In: Jee WSS, Parfitt AM (eds) Bone histomorphometry. 3rd international workshop. Metab Bone Dis Relat Res 2 (Suppl):483–486

Ellis HA, Peart KM (1972) Quantitative observations on mineralised and non-mineralised bone in the iliac crest. J Clin Pathol 25:277–286

Evans RA, Dunstan CR, Hills EE (1980) Extent of resorbing surfaces based on histochemical indentification of osteoclasts. In: Jee WSS, Parfitt AM (eds) Bone histomorphometry. 3rd international workshop. Metab Bone Dis Relat Res 2 (Suppl):29–34

Flora L (1976) Idiosyncrasies of the measurement of bone dynamics with fluorescent labels. In: Meunier PJ (ed) Bone histomorphometry. 2nd international workshop. Armour Montagu, Paris, pp 321–326

Frost HM (1962) Tetracycline labelling of bone and the zone of demarcation. Can J Biochem 40:485–489

Frost HM (1969) Tetracycline-based histological analysis of bone remodelling. Calcif Tissue Res 3:211–237

Frost HM (1976) Histomorphometry of trabecular bone. I. Theoretical correction of appositional rate measurements. In: Meunier PJ (ed) Bone histomorphometry. 2nd international workshop. Armour Montagu, Paris, pp 361–370

Frost HM, Meunier PJ (1976) Histomorphometry of trabecular bone. II. An empirical test of the theoretical correction for appositional rate measurements. In: Meunier PJ (ed) Bone histomorphometry. 2nd international workshop. Armour Montagu, Paris, pp 371–381

Garner A, Ball J (1966) Quantitative observations on mineralised and unmineralised bone in chronic renal azotaemia and intestinal malabsorption syndrome. J Pathol Bacteriol 91:545–561

Giroux JM, Courpron P, Meunier P (1975) Histomorphometrie de l'osteopenie physiologique senile. Monographie du Laboratoire de Researches sur l'Histodynamique Osseuse, Lyon

Goland P (1965) Permanent staining of tooth and bone by the in vivo use of reactive procion and remazol dyes. Int Assoc Dent Res 43:70 (abstr)

Hally AD (1964) A counting method for measuring the volumes of tissue components in microscopical sections. Q J Microsc Sci 105:503–517

Harris WH (1960) A microscopic method for determining rates of bone growth. Nature 188:1038–1039

Harris WH, Jackson RH, Jowsey J (1962) The in vivo distribution of tetracycline in canine bone. J Bone Joint Surg [Am] 44:1308–1320

Harris WH, Lavorgna J, Hamblen DL, Haywood EA (1968) The inhibition of ossification in vivo. Clin Orthop 61:52–60

Ibsen KH, Urist MR (1962) Complexes of calcium and magnesium with oxytetracycline. Proc Soc Exp Biol Med 109:797–801

Irving JT (1958) A histological stain for newly calcified tissues. Nature 181:704–705

Irving JT (1963) The sudanophil material at sites of calcification. Arch Oral Biol 8:735–745

Jaworski ZFG (1980) Three dimensional aspects of lamellar bone formation and interpretation of tetracycline labels in bone biopsy section. In: Jee WSS, Parfitt AM (eds) Bone histomorphometry. 3rd international workshop. Metab Bone Dis Relat Res 2 (Suppl):189–199

Jaworski ZFG, Lok E, Wellington JL (1975) Impaired osteoclastic function and linear bone erosion rate in secondary hyperparathyroidism associated with chronic renal failure. Clin Orthop 107:298–310

Johnson KA, Kelly PH, Jowsey J (1977) Percutaneous biopsy of the iliac crest. Clin Orthop 123:34–36

Klein L, Jackman KV (1976) Assay of bone resorption in vivo with ^{3}H-tetracycline. Calcif Tissue Res 20:275–290

Malluche HH, Sherman D, Manaka R, Massey SG (1980) Comparison between different histomorphometric methods. In: Jee WSS, Parfitt AM (eds) Bone histomorphometry. 3rd international workshop. Metab Bone Dis Relat Res 2 (Suppl):449–451

Manaka RC, Malluche HH (1981) A program package for quantitative analysis of histologic structure and remodelling dynamics of bone. Comput Programs Biomed 13:191–201

Matrajt J, Hioco D (1972) Solochrome cyanine R as an indicator dye of bone morphology. Stain Technol 41:97–100

Matrajt J, Bordier P, Martin J, Hioco D (1967) Technique pour l'inclusion des biopsies osseuses nondecalci-fies. J Microscopie 6:499–504

Melsen F, Mosekilde L (1978) Tetracycline double-labeling of iliac trabecular bone in 41 normal adults. Calcif Tissue Res 26:99–102

Melsen F, Mosekilde L (1980) Interpretation of single labels after in vivo labeling. In: Jee WSS, Parfitt AM (eds) Bone histomorphometry. 3rd international workshop. Metab Bone Dis Relat Res 2 (Suppl):171–178

Melsen F, Melsen B, Mosekilde L (1978a) An evaluation of the quantitative parameters applied in bone histology. Acta Pathol Microbiol Scand 86:63–69

Melsen F, Melsen B, Mosekilde L, Bergmann S (1978b) Histomorphometric analysis of normal bone from the iliac crest. Acta Pathol Microbiol Scand 86:70–81

Merz WA (1968) Strechenmessung an gerichteten Strukturen im Mikroskop und ihre Anwendung zur Bestimmung von Oberflächen—Volumen—Relationen im Knochengeweke. Mikroscopie 22:132 (Cited by Aherne and Dunnill 1982)

Merz WA, Schenk RK (1970a) Quantitative structural analysis of human cancellous bone. Acta Anat (Basel) 75:54–66

Merz WA, Schenk RK (1970b) A quantitative histological study on bone formation in human cancellous bone. Acta Anat 76:1–15

Meunier P, Edouard C (1976) Quantification of osteoid tissue in trabecular bone. Methodology and results in normal iliac bone. In: Jaworski ZFG (ed) Proceedings of the 1st workshop on bone histomorphometry, 1972. University of Ottawa Press, Ottawa, pp 191–196

Meunier P, Edouard C, Courpron P, Toussaint F (1975) Morphometric analysis of osteoid in iliac trabecular bone. Methodology. In: Norman AW et al. (eds) Dynamical significance of the osteoid parameters in vitamin D and problems related to uremic bone disease. Gruyter, Berlin, pp 149–155

Meunier PJ, Edouard C, Richard D, Laurent J (1976) Histomorphometry of osteoid tissue. The hyperosteoidoses. In: Meunier PJ (ed) Bone histomorphometry. 2nd international workshop. Armour Montagu, Paris, pp 249–262

Milch RA, Hall DP, Tobie JE (1958) Fluorescence of tetracycline antibiotics in bone. J Bone Joint Surg [Am] 40:897–910

Olah AJ (1976) Influence of microscopic resolution on the estimation of structural parameters in cancellous bone. In: Meunier PJ (ed) Bone histomorphometry. 2nd international workshop. Armour Montagu, Paris, pp 55–61

Parfitt AM, Villanueva AR, Crouch MM, Mathews CHE, Duncan H (1976) Classification of osteoid seams by combined use of cell morphology and tetracycline labelling. Evidence for intermittency of mineraliza-tion. In: Meunier PJ (ed) Bone histomorphometry. 2nd international workshop. Armour Montagu, Paris, pp 299–310

Rasmussen H, Bordier P (1974) The physiological and cellular basis of metabolic bone disease. Williams and Wilkins, Baltimore

Revell PA, Pirie CJ (1981) The histopathology of ankylosing hyperostosis of the spine. Rhumatologie 33:99–104

Ritz E, Krempien B, Mehls O, Malluche J (1973) Skeletal abnormalities in chronic renal insufficiency before and during maintenance hemodialysis. Kidney Int 4:116–127

Saxen L (1966) Drug induced teratogenesis in vitro: inhibition of calcification by different tetracyclines. Science 153:1384–1387

Schenk RK, Merz WA, Muller J (1969) A quantitative histological study on bone resorption in human cancellous bone. Acta Anat (Basel) 74:44–53

Schwartz MP, Recker RR (1980) Direct and histomorphometric determinations of surface density and volume. In: Jee WSS, Parfitt AM (eds) Bone histomorphometry. 3rd international workshop. Metab Bone Dis Relat Res 2 (Suppl):279–280

Takahashi H, Norimatsu H, Konno T, Inoue J, Yanagi K (1980) Different patterns of tetracycline uptake in varying forms of rickets and osteomalacia. In: Jee, WSS, Parfitt AM (eds) Bone histomorphometry. 3rd international workshop. Metab Bone Dis Relat Res 2 (Suppl):87–93

Teitelbaum SL, Nichols SH (1976) Tetracycline-based morphometric analysis of trabecular bone kinetics. In: Meunier PJ (ed) Bone histomorphometry. 2nd international workshop. Armour Montagu, Paris, pp 311–319

Teitelbaum SL, Rosenberg EM, Bates M, Avioli LV (1976) The effects of phosphate and vitamin D therapy on osteopenic, hypophosphatemic osteomalacia of childhood. Clin Orthop 116:38–47

Treharne RW, Brighton CT (1979) The use and possible misuse of tetracycline as a vital stain. Clin Orthop 140:240–246

Urist MR, Ibsen KH (1963) Chemical reactivity of mineralised tissue with oxytetracycline. Arch Pathol 76:484–496

Vedi S, Compston JE, Webb A, Tighe JR (1982) Histomorphometric analysis of bone biopsies from the iliac crest of normal British subjects. Metab Bone Dis Relat Res 4:231–236

Villanueva AR, Parfitt AM, Duncan H (1976) Comparison of Haversian bone dynamics between 11th rib and iliac trephine biopsies. In: Meunier PJ (ed) Bone histomorphometry. 2nd international workshop. Armour Montague, Paris, pp 75–77

Visser WJ, Niermans HJ, Roelofs JMM, Raymakers JA, Duursma SA (1976) Comparative morphometry of bone biopsies obtained by two different methods from the right and left iliac crest. In: Meunier PJ (ed) Bone histomorphometry. 2nd international workshop. Armour Montagu, Paris, pp 79–87

Visser WJ, Roelofs JMM, Peters JPJ, Lentferink MHF, Duursma SA (1980) Sampling variation in bone histomorphometry. In: Jee WSS, Parfitt AM (eds) Bone histomorphometry. 3rd international workshop. Metab Bone Dis Relat Res 2 (Suppl):429–434

Williams MA (1977) Quantitative methods in biology. North Holland, Amsterdam

Woods CG, Morgan DB, Paterson CR, Gossman HH (1968) Measurement of osteoid in bone biopsy. J Pathol Bacteriol 95:441–447

Chapter 5

Metabolic Bone Disease

Vitamin D metabolism

The vitamin D compounds all have the basic steroid ring structure. Splitting of one of the rings is brought about by ultraviolet light, a reaction which occurs in the skin (Holick et al. 1977; Esvelt et al. 1978), and previtamin D_3 so formed from 7-dehydrocholesterol is equilibrated to vitamin D_3 in the skin (Holick et al. 1977). Vitamin D_3 (cholecalciferol) and its metabolites are the main naturally occurring compounds in man and animals, but vitamin D_2 (ergocalciferol) and its metabolites are also present in man, because of fortification of the diet. Vitamin D_3 is converted to 25-hydroxycholecalciferol (25-OH-D_3) in the liver by means of a mitochondrial 25-hydroxylase (Bhattacharyya and DeLuca 1974; Olson et al. 1976; Madhok et al. 1978). Studies using tritiated 25-OH-D_3 have demonstrated its further hydroxylation to 1,25-dihydroxyvitamin D_3 (1,25(OH)$_2$$D_3$) (Cousins et al. 1970; Holick et al. 1971; Lawson et al. 1971), a process which occurs in the kidney, the necessary enzyme system being localised in the proximal tubules (Fraser and Kodicek 1970; Midgett et al. 1973; Brunette et al. 1978). Since 1,25(OH)$_2$$D_3$ is an inhibitor of the renal 1-hydroxylase, there is a short-loop negative feedback control of the hydroxylation process (Larkins et al. 1974; Omdahl 1978; Omdahl and Hunsaker 1978; Henry 1979). Vitamin D metabolites bind specifically to receptors with high affinity at end-organ sites and appear in the nuclei of cells of target tissues (intestine, bone) and other cells (Weber et al. 1971; Chen and DeLuca 1973; Brumbaugh and Haussler 1975; Zile et al. 1978; Lawson and Wilson 1979; Stumpf et al. 1979).

Vitamin D increases both mineralisation and resorption of bone. The effect on mineralisation is apparent in vitamin D deficiency, when wide osteoid seams result from defective calcification; excessive resorption of bone results when there is vitamin D excess. Radiolabelled vitamin D (25-OH-D or 1,25(OH)$_2$$D_3$) is localised to osteoblasts, chondrocytes and osteocytes, as demonstrated by autoradiography (Wezeman 1976; DeLuca 1979). However, vitamin D also has effects on collagen and proteoglycan synthesis (Stern 1980), so that it is difficult to be certain of its direct role in mineralisation processes. A recent source of further information about vitamin D and its effects in animals and cell culture experiments is the review by Raisz and Kream (1983a).

Studies of vitamin D-deficient animals suggest that it is decreased intestinal transport of calcium and phosphorus that is responsible for impaired bone mineralisation. Diets low in calcium or phosphorus can also result in defective mineralisation (Shipley et al. 1921; Shohl 1936; Howe et al. 1940; Weinman and Schour 1945). Vitamin D deficiency fails to cause changes in bone enzyme activity or mineralisation of osteoid in animals carefully prevented from becoming hypocalcaemic or hypophosphataemic (Wergedal and Baylink 1971; Taylor et al. 1976; Howard and Baylink 1980). Furthermore, it has been shown that rachitic bone calcifies when placed in a solution containing calcium and phosphorus (Cousins and DeLuca 1972).

The position is a little clearer with respect to the effect of vitamin D on bone resorption. Hypercalcaemia, hyperphosphataemia, hypercalciuria and hyperphosphaturia occur in vitamin D toxicity, and much of the excess of these two electrolytes is derived from bone. Using radioactive labelling techniques it has been shown that physiological doses of vitamin D cause mobilisation of calcium from bone. Animal experiments and clinical observations suggest that parathyroid hormone is required for the bone-resorbing effects of vitamin D, but there appears to be a reciprocal relationship, vitamin D being required for the resorbing effects of parathyroid hormone (Stern 1980).

The mechanism by which vitamin D affects bone is not yet clearly understood. $1,25(OH)_2D$ and 25-OH-D bind to homogenates of bone and isolated bone cells (Kream et al. 1977; Mellow et al. 1978; Chen et al. 1979). The exact nature of this binding and of the interactions between vitamin D and parathyroid hormone on bone have yet to be elucidated. Increases in osteoclast number and size, nuclear area, surface membrane ruffled border and clear zone after treatment with vitamin D and $1,25(OH)_2D_3$ have been reported by Thompson et al. (1975), Holtrop and Raisz (1979) and Stern (1980).

Parathyroid hormone

Parathyroid hormone is an 84 amino acid polypeptide, the amino acid sequence of which is now well established (Potts 1983). Biological activity is present in the first 34 residues (Tregear et al. 1973), since the intact hormone and 1-34 amino acid fragments have equivalent activity. The intact hormone is the predominant molecular species in the blood, together with a large, biologically inert, carboxyl fragment. Parathyroid hormone metabolism involves proteolysis of the polypeptide into two or more fragments, a cleavage which takes place both within the gland and in the liver. Amino terminal fragments may be present in the circulation or even produced locally within target tissues where they may be of considerable significance even if only present in small amounts. References to the metabolism of parathyroid hormone in the liver and kidney are available in the recent review by Potts (1983). The kidney appears responsible for the removal of carboxyl fragments formed by cleavage of the intact hormone in the liver.

Parathyroid hormone secretion is controlled by the level of circulating calcium ions (Sherwood et al. 1968), a fall in calcium causing increased hormone secretion. Hypomagnesaemia also stimulates parathyroid hormone secretion (Sherwood et al. 1970). The function of parathyroid hormone is the maintenance of physiological levels of calcium in the extracellular fluid and the prevention of hypocalcaemia. The effects of the hormone are brought about by its direct action on bone and the kidneys. The main action on bone is to increase resorptive activity (Forland et al. 1968; Dalen and Hjern 1974; Tougaard et al. 1977; Knop et al. 1980), although the actual numbers of osteoblasts and osteoclasts are also increased (King et al. 1978; Melsen and Mosekilde 1980). Parathyroid hormone stimulates activity by the recruited osteoclasts (Melsen and Mosekilde 1980), and increases reabsorption of calcium by the renal tubules (Haas et al. 1971), thereby raising the calcium level in the blood. It also has effects on inorganic phosphate metabolism by increasing renal phosphate excretion, which results in elevation of serum calcium. This action on phosphate clearance, it should be pointed out, is not homeostatic, since there is no feedback mechanism for phosphate on the parathyroid gland. In target tissues and organs, parathyroid hormone reacts with hormone-specific receptors on the plasma membrane of cells. A series of intracellular events is brought about by this interaction at the cell surface, commencing with the generation of cyclic AMP. Details of the role of adenylate cyclase activation in relation to hormone receptors on cells are available elsewhere (Rodbell 1980; Ross and Gilman 1980; Raisz and Kream 1983a).

Primary hyperparathyroidism

Parathyroid adenoma is the commonest cause of hyperparathyroidism and is responsible for around 80% of cases of primary hyperparathyroidism. In a small number of cases, probably less than 5%, more than one adenoma is present. Adenomas of the parathyroid show a preponderance in females, in whom the peak age of incidence is 45 years. Adenomas may, however, present at any age. Primary hyperplasia of the parathyroid gland is an unusual cause of primary hyperparathyroidism, while parathyroid carcinoma is rare, although when present nearly always shows evidence of functional activity, the hyperparathyroidism being more severe than with an adenoma.

The onset of hyperparathyroidism was often insidious in the past, presentation being with either renal or bone disease. Most cases nowadays are asymptomatic and detected during the biochemical screening procedures of modern medicine (Purnell et al. 1974). The biochemical changes of hyperparathyroidism comprise a raised serum or plasma calcium level and low phosphorus level, with elevation of the alkaline phosphatase level depending on how extensive is the bone involvement. Due attention should be paid to the correction of calcium levels in relation to the plasma albumin. Patients with symptomatic bone involvement may have pain and fractures (Byers and Smith 1971).

Cystic lesions are apparent on radiological examination in advanced disease but are in fact solid tumour-like lesions simulating osteoclastomas rather than true cysts. Radiographic evidence of primary hyperparathyroidism is often most readily demonstrated as resorptive changes in the fingers, particularly the tufts of the terminal phalanges and periosteal erosion of the sides of the other phalanges.

Histological examination of bone in hyperparathyroidism shows increased numbers of osteoblasts and osteoclasts, increased resorption lacunae and fibrosis in the intertrabecular spaces (Fig. 5.1). Quantitative examination of bone showed trabecular bone volume to be normal, according to Mosekilde and Melsen (1978), and normal in males, according to Courpron et al. (1976), who found the trabecular bone volume significantly decreased in females with primary hyperparathyroidism up to the age of 50 years. There may occasionally be osteosclerosis (Genant et al. 1975). Examination of the trabecular surfaces shows increased numbers of osteoclasts and increase in resorption lacunae, but it may not be generally recognised that an increase in osteoblasts also occurs, together with an increase in the percentage of trabecular surface covered by osteoid, so that the unwary may be tempted into considering the possibility of osteomalacia. The cellular rate of mineralisation, determined by double-labelling with tetracycline is decreased (Mosekilde and Melsen 1978), that is the activity of each osteoblast is diminished compared with normal, but the overall rate of bone formation is increased because more osteoblasts are taking part in the process (Mosekilde and Melsen 1978). Increased osteoblastic activity over large areas of the skeleton is reflected in the raised plasma alkaline phosphatase level found in patients with extensive bone lesions in hyperparathyroidism. No problem should arise if due attention is paid to the increased osteoclastic activity and resorption lacunae. While there may

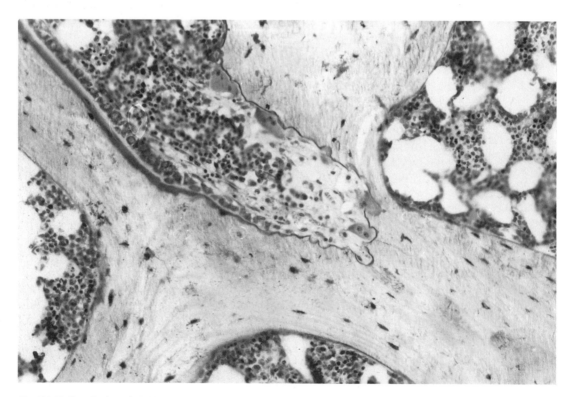

Fig. 5.1. Trabecular bone in hyperparathyroidism to show active osteoblastic and resorption surfaces with resorption lacunae occupied by osteoclasts. (Methylmethacrylate, thionin × 250)

be quite extensive marrow fibrosis, the presence of paratrabecular fibrosis, especially adjacent to resorption surfaces, is pathognomonic and helps to differentiate fibrosis of hyperparathyroidism from that occurring in relation to myelofibrosis, in which there may be secondary bone changes of osteosclerosis. Detection of fibrosis is particularly aided by the use of a reticulin stain (Figs. 5.2, 5.3), for example in early cases in which there may be no radiographic abnormalities, minimal biochemical changes and where the bone biopsy pro-

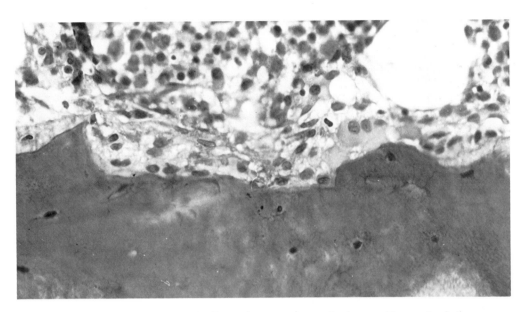

Fig. 5.2. High-power view of paratrabecular fibrous tissue near a resorption lacuna with one osteoclast. (H&E × 400)

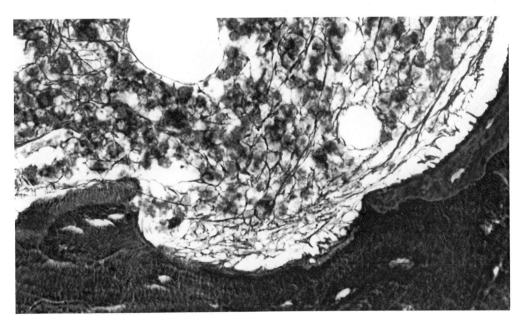

Fig. 5.3. High-power view of resorption lacuna showing paratrabecular fibroisis, which is more readily detected than in a haematoxylin/eosin-stained section. (Reticulin × 400)

vides the most sensitive method of detecting hyperparathyroidism. In just such a case seen by the author subsequent exploration of the neck revealed a parathyroid adenoma, which, but for the bone biopsy, might have gone undetected for a considerable time before obvious biochemical or radiological changes were present.

The so-called cystic lesion of hyperparathyroid bone disease closely resembles a giant cell tumour (osteoclastoma) of bone. This focal lesion, the brown tumour of hyperparathyroidism, is expansive, osteolytic and forms a mass with a variegated yellow, brown and haemorrhagic cut surface which may bulge beyond the thinned overlying cortex (Fig. 5.4). Histologically, the two lesions are virtually impossible to separate. Both comprise a spindle-celled stroma, in which there are numerous osteoclast-like multinucleate giant cells (Fig. 5.5), and both may contain areas of haemorrhage and haemosiderin and lipid-laden macrophages. The possibility of hyperparathyroidism must always be borne in mind when a diagnosis of osteoclastoma is being contemplated, and skeletal radiology, blood calcium and parathyroid hormone levels should be performed to exclude this. The site of the lesion may be helpful, since a solitary giant cell lesion at the end of a bone around the knee joint in a 20- to 30-year-old is most likely to be an osteoclastoma, while a brown tumour

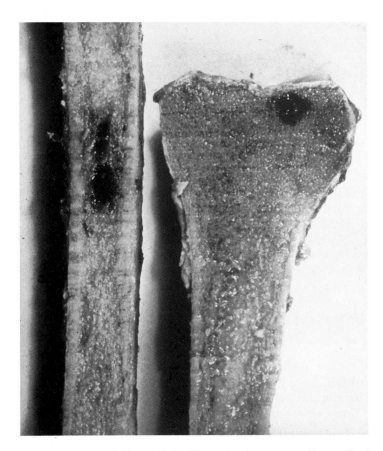

Fig. 5.4. Upper end of tibia and shaft of femur, showing presence of haemorrhagic cystic lesions which are brown tumours of hyperparathyroidism

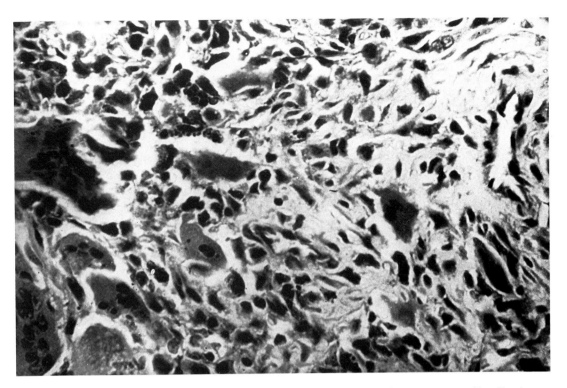

Fig. 5.5. Brown tumour of hyperparathyroidism, showing spindle-celled tissue containing numerous osteoclast-like giant cells. (H&E × 400)

of hyperparathyroidism generally develops in the diaphysis of a long bone, the ribs, the jaw or skull (Clark and Taylor 1972). Giant cell lesions in the jaw may introduce the further diagnostic possibility of reparative granuloma. Resolution of the bone lesions after parathyroidectomy has been observed many times, both radiologically and by subsequent biopsy or autopsy studies (Collins 1966).

The effects of hyperparathyroidism on other organs and tissues include nephrocalcinosis and renal calculus formation as a result of excessive calcium excretion, as well as metastatic calcification in such sites as the walls of arteries and the lung alveoli.

Secondary and tertiary hyperparathyroidism

Hyperplasia of the parathyroid glands occurs secondarily to chronic renal failure, hyperphosphataemia, hypocalcaemia, vitamin D deficiency and malabsorption syndromes. The bone changes related to chronic renal failure and vitamin D deficiency are considered later in this chapter (see Osteomalacia and rickets; Renal osteodystrophy). Parathyroid gland autonomy, that is the development of an adenoma, supervening on responsive hyperplasia is referred to as tertiary hyperparathyroidism.

Hypoparathyroidism

Hypoparathyroidism is characterised by low serum calcium, high serum inorganic phosphorus, absence of rickets or osteomalacia on radiological or histological examination, and chronic tetany, together with absence of renal insufficiency, steatorrhoea, chronic diarrhoea and alkalosis (Parfitt 1972a). Differences exist with respect to the development of bone disease in long-standing cases (see below). The above changes are seen in hypoparathyroidism following thyroid or parathyroid surgery, but phosphate excretion in response to exogenous parathyroid hormone and low serum parathyroid hormone levels in the presence of hypocalcaemia are features of idiopathic hypoparathyroidism (Strom and Winberg 1954). Some features of pseudo-hypoparathyroidism may also be present in patients with idiopathic hypoparathyroidism, including calcification and ossification of the soft tissues (Bronsky et al. 1958; Jimenea et al. 1971; Moses et al. 1974). Hypoparathyroidism sometimes leads to osteomalacia in man (Drezner et al. 1977), and parathyroidectomised rats show poor skeletal development with inhibition of osteoid formation, mineralisation and resorption (Wergedal et al. 1973). Thus, while it is true that clinical bone disease is uncommon in hypoparathyroidism, it is also likely that most patients with this disorder will present with the effects of hypocalcaemia before there has been time for the development of bone disease. The possible mechanism would comprise lack of parathyroid hormone leading to hypocalcaemia, hyperphosphataemia and insufficient conversion of 25-OH-D_3 to $1,25(OH)_2D_3$, with the development of clinically significant bone disease in long-standing cases. Decreased levels of $1,25(OH)_2D_3$ have been demonstrated in idiopathic and surgical hypoparathyroidism (Haussler et al. 1976; Lund et al. 1980). Radioimmuno-assay has shown there is failure of secretion of endogenous parathyroid hormone in idiopathic hypoparathyroidism (Reiss and Canterbury 1971).

Animal experiments have shown that parathyroid hormone stimulates the synthesis of $1,25(OH)_2D_3$ in the kidney and that parathyroidectomy eliminates the stimulatory effects of hypocalcaemia on renal 25-OH-D_3-1-hydroxylase, providing evidence that parathyroid hormone has an influence on the production of $1,25(OH)_2D_3$ (Garabedian et al. 1972; Fraser and Kodicek 1973; Henry et al. 1974; Booth et al. 1977).

Pseudohypoparathyroidism

Albright et al. (1942) introduced the term 'pseudohypoparathyroidism' to describe patients with a characteristic facies and physical appearance and hypo-calcaemia without evidence of hypoparathyroidism. Subsequently various other terms, such as 'pseudopseudohypoparathyroidism', 'pseudohypo-parathyroidism type 2', 'hypohyperparathyroidism' and 'pseudohypohyper-parathyroidism' have been used to describe various clinical conditions which show combinations of hypocalcaemia or normocalcaemia with or without bone changes of osteitis fibrosa cystica. The resulting confusion is apparent from the number of terms alone. Pseudopseudohypoparathyroidism, for example, was suggested for patients who were like those with pseudo-hypoparathyroidism except that they had normal serum calcium concentrations; however, both of these conditions have been recognised as manifestations of the same genetic abnormality (Beighton 1978).

In pseudohypoparathyroidism there is obesity, a 'moon face' appearance and some loss of stature associated with shortening of the tubular bones of the extremities. There may be cataracts, mental deficiency, tetany and heterotopic calcification, for example in the soft tissues and basal ganglia. Radiologically, cone-shaped epiphyses may be identified in the phalanges (Steinbach and Young 1966; Lewin et al. 1978; Beighton 1978). The condition usually becomes apparent in the first decade of life and most probably has an X-linked dominant inheritance (Mann et al. 1962; Lee et al. 1968), although there are descriptions of affected fathers producing affected sons (Weinberg and Stone 1972) and of kindreds in which the inheritance appears to be autosomally recessive (Reinhart et al. 1973; Kinard et al. 1979).

Pseudohypoparathyroidism is associated with defective generation of cyclic AMP by the kidney in response to exogenous parathyroid hormone (Chase et al. 1969) and absence of renal phosphorus excretion. A different group of patients, with type 2 pseudohypoparathyroidism, are able to synthesise cyclic AMP in the kidney in response to parathyroid hormone but do not excrete phosphorus in the urine (Drezner et al. 1973b). Skeletal resistance to parathyroid hormone may also be present in pseudohypoparathyroidism (Drezner et al. 1977; Lewin et al. 1978). Patients with pseudohypoparathyroidism are hyperphosphataemic and may have secondary hyperparathyroidism. This may help to explain the large number of different syndromes mentioned at the beginning of this section. For example, Frame et al. (1972) described phenotypically normal individuals with hypocalcaemia, hyperphosphataemia and osteitis fibrosa cystica as 'pseudohypohyperparathyroidism' and postulated a renal resistance to parathyroid hormone.

Histopathological examination of bone may show little abnormality, but many patients have evidence of secondary hyperparathyroidism. The epiphyses of affected children close prematurely.

It is probable that pseudohypoparathyroid patients also have abnormal vitamin D metabolism, since they have low blood levels of 1,25 dihydroxy-vitamin D (Drezner et al. 1977; Metz et al. 1977; Sinha et al. 1977). The position is complicated further by such cases as those described by Nusynowitz and Klein (1973), in which there were clinical features of idiopathic hypoparathyroidism and pseudohypoparathyroidism, in that parathyroid hormone was detectable in the serum by radioimmunoassay, without the physical stigmata of pseudohypoparathyroidism.

Osteomalacia and rickets

Osteomalacia (from Gk. *osteon*, bone + *malakia*, softness) is the skeletal manifestation of various metabolic abnormalities which result in defective mineralisation. Routine histological examination of undecalcified bone sections shows an increase in the amount of osteoid. This is manifest as an increase in the number of osteoid seams present, elevation in the percentage of trabecular bone surface covered by osteoid (osteoid surface) and usually an increase in the width of osteoid seams, so that the overall effect is to increase the osteoid volume (Woods 1966).

Caution is needed in interpreting increased osteoid content of bone as osteomalacia, since this occurs in other conditions such as Paget's disease and hyperparathyroidism. An increase in osteoid may result from either increased matrix formation or defective calcification, and it is necessary to demonstrate a mineralisation defect by use of tetracycline labelling methods before osteomalacia can be diagnosed with absolute certainty (see Chap. 4, Staining methods; Tetracycline labelling). Impaired mineralisation in children affects

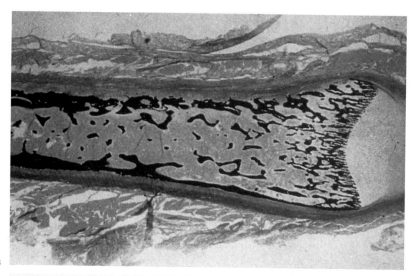

a

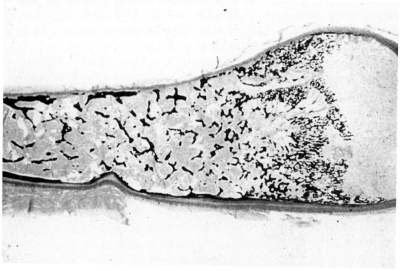

b

Fig. 5.6. a Normal costochondral junction of a child showing regular growth plate and orderly arrangement of the adjacent newly formed trabeculae. (Methylmethacrylate, von Kossa × 3.5) **b** Costochondral junction of a child with rickets showing irregularly shaped outline to the growth plate with large defects and disorderly arrangement of adjacent trabeculae. The costochondral region is expanded, and mineralised bone trabeculae extend along the outer surfaces to give a cup-like appearance. (Methylmethacrylate, von Kossa × 3.5)

endochondral ossification at the growth plate and results in the clinical picture of rickets (Fig. 5.6). The changes are otherwise the same as those in osteomalacia.

'Osteomalacia' and 'rickets' were originally used as terms to describe the skeletal effects of vitamin D deficiency. Both terms are now applied much more widely to include a large number of other disorders, all of which produce the same clinical, radiological and histological appearance.

The clinical features of osteomalacia include bone pain, which is worse on weight bearing or pressure, bone tenderness, and the development of such deformities as bowing of the limbs (Figs. 5.7, 5.8), pigeon chest, gibbus, scolio-

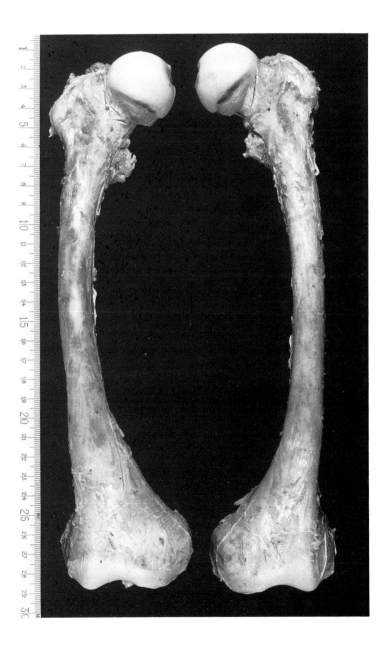

Fig. 5.7. Femur of a child with rickets due to Fanconi syndrome, showing bowing and widening of the metaphysis at the lower end of the bone

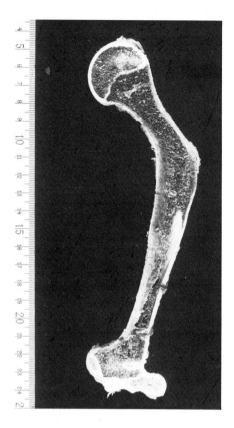

Fig. 5.8. Marked bowing deformity of the humerous in a child with Fanconi syndrome

sis or kyphosis because of bone softening and proximal muscle weakness. The biochemical abnormalities depend on the underlying cause of the osteomalacia and are summarised by Frame and Parfitt (1978). Serum calcium and phosphate may be low, normal or raised, and a further complication of the situation arises with the development of secondary hyperparathyroidism. Alkaline phosphatase is usually increased but may sometimes be normal (Chalmers 1968), whereas there is increased urinary excretion of hydroxyproline, which is greatest in those cases with the highest alkaline phosphatase levels (Anderson et al. 1967).

Radiological examination of the skeleton shows a non-specific decrease in radiodensity, sometimes wrongly described as 'demineralisation'. Osteosclerosis, as revealed in radiographs, may be real or apparent, the latter because the increased osteoid present has a greater density than bone marrow so that the bone may appear to be of increased density. The most distinctive radiological feature of osteomalacia is the presence of 'Looser's zones' or 'pseudofractures', which are radiolucent bands adjacent and perpendicular to the surface of the ribs, pubic rami, scapulae and ends of long bones. Such pseudofractures may show increased uptake of bone-seeking isotopes in bone scans (McFarlane et al. 1977).

The causes of osteomalacia and rickets form a long list and are clearly summarised in the article by Frame and Parfitt (1978). A simplified classification is given in Table 5.1, from which it will be seen that the causes may be divided into several broad categories. The following brief accounts give background information to these groups.

Table 5.1. Causes of osteomalacia and rickets

A. Vitamin deficiency
    1. Dietary lack (Dent and Smith 1969; Dent 1970)
    2. Low sunlight exposure (Hodkinson et al. 1973; Preece et al. 1975)
    3. Neonatal rickets (Felton and Stone 1966)
B. Vitamin D malabsorption
    1. Coeliac disease (Moss et al. 1965; Melvin et al. 1970)
    2. Postgastrectomy (Eddy 1971)
    3. Small bowel operations (Teitelbaum et al. 1977; Parfitt et al. 1978)
    4. Pancreatic disease (Prost et al. 1975)
C. Impaired vitamin D metabolism
    1. Impaired 25-hydroxylation in the liver
        a) Immaturity (Hillman and Haddad 1975)
        b) Neonatal hepatitis (Yu et al. 1971)
        c) Cirrhosis and chronic hepatitis (Long et al. 1976; Compston and Thompson 1977)
    2. Impaired 1-hydroxylation in the kidney
        a) Enzyme defect (vitamin D dependency) (Fraser et al. 1973)
        b) Chronic renal failure (Coburn et al. 1976; Haussler et al. 1976)
        c) Parathyroid hormone deficiency/resistance (Drezner et al. 1973a, b, 1977)
D. Increased catabolism
    Induction of microsomal enzymes by drugs (e.g. barbiturates; Pierides et al. 1976)
E. Phosphate depletion and hypophosphataemia, including renal tubular disorders
    1. As a complication of all the above because of excess parathyroid hormone or lack of vitamin D
    2. Negative phosphorous balance. Malabsorption, haemodialysis, antacids (Lotz et al.1968)
    3. Hypophosphataemia
        a) Primary—X-linked (familial, sporadic; Dent and Stamp 1971; Parfitt 1972; Fraser et al. 1973; Glorieux et al. 1980)
        b) Secondary—tumour related (Salassa et al. 1970; Dent and Stamp 1971; Evans and Azzopardi 1972)
    4. Metabolic acidosis (Cunningham et al. 1982)
    5. Fanconi's syndrome (Frame and Parfitt 1978)
    6. Cystinosis (Frame and Parfitt 1978)
F. Inhibition of mineralisation
    1. Diphosphonates (Jowsey et al. 1971)
    2. Sodium fluoride (Jowsey et al. 1972; Faccini and Teotia 1974)
    3. Aluminium (Ellis et al. 1979)
G. Others (see Frame and Parfitt 1978)
    1. Fibrogenesis imperfecta ossium
    2. Axial osteomalacia
    3. Hypophosphatasia

Vitamin D deficiency

The diet of modern man in the developed countries of the world is heavily fortified with vitamins, including vitamin D. The dietary requirement to prevent the development of disease is accepted as 10 μg/day (4000 IU) for children from infancy to adolescence and in pregnancy, while for the adult it is 2–5 μg/day (Dent and Smith 1969). Pure dietary deficiency of vitamin D does occur, though such factors as strict vegetarianism, as practised by some Asians resident in the UK, are the usual background to disease. The histological appearances of the bone from such a case are illustrated in Fig. 5.9. The ingestion by immigrants of whole grain cereals with high phytate content may interfere with calcium absorption (Wills et al. 1972). Decreased sunlight exposure may aggravate the effects of dietary deficiency, especially in housebound elderly people who have a generally low vitamin D intake (Hodkinson et al. 1973).

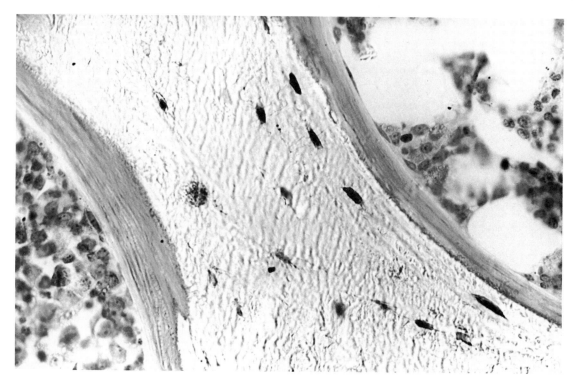

Fig. 5.9. Osteomalacia caused by dietary vitamin D deficiency in an Asian practising strict vegetarianism. Wide osteoid seams. (Thionin × 400)

Malabsorption of vitamin D

Absorption of vitamin D, which is fat soluble, takes place in the upper intestine, where there is rapid uptake by the mucosa followed by slower transfer to the lymphatics after combination with fatty acids and monoglycerides. Initial uptake requires the presence of bile salts. In addition, $25(OH)D_3$ produced in the liver is excreted in the bile and reabsorbed (Arnaud et al. 1975). Osteomalacia may complicate malabsorption states resulting from a variety of causes when there is interference with these mechanisms.

Vitamin D deficiency, bone disease and gastrointestinal disorders

Several different mechanisms may contribute to the development of metabolic bone disease in gastrointestinal disorders so that it may be misleading to simplify matters in the way described above. A brief but helpful review is provided by Sitrin et al. (1978).

Gastrectomy is sometimes followed by the development of osteomalacia (Eddy 1971; Garrick et al. 1971), in which the contributory factors include bypass of the duodenum through a gastrojejunal anastamosis with malabsorption of vitamin D, phosphate depletion induced by antacid use and poor dietary intake of vitamin D and calcium.

Metabolic bone disease complicates primary biliary cirrhosis, biliary atresia and other chronic cholestatic syndromes. Malabsorption of vitamin D caused by lack of bile salts is a major factor, but failure of 25-hydroxylation may also contribute (Wagonfeld et al. 1976; Compston and Thompson, 1977; Skinner et al. 1977). Bone disease occurs in chronic parenchymatous liver disease and especially in cirrhosis (Lancet 1977). Low circulating levels of $25(OH)D_3$ and decreased conversion of vitamin D to $25(OH)D_3$ (Long et al. 1976; Hepner et al. 1976) suggest failure of 25-hydroxylation under these circumstances, but there may also be malabsorption of vitamin D.

Osteomalacia occurs in a large number of different intestinal diseases where there is malabsorption, including coeliac and Crohn's diseases. Excessive faecal loss of $25(OH)D$ and refractoriness of the diseased bowel to the influence of $1,25(OH)D_3$ are further possible factors in both conditions. A combination of deficient intake and malabsorption of vitamin D has been suggested in cases of bowel resection (Compston and Creamer 1977). Malabsorption of vitamin D is the most likely reason for the development of bone disease following jejunoileal bypass surgery for obesity, but there is hepatic dysfunction after such an operation and this might also contribute, by impairing vitamin D metabolism.

Impaired vitamin D metabolism in the liver and kidney

The association between liver disease and osteomalacia is still poorly understood. Occasionally, hypocalcaemia and rickets in premature infants may be related to impaired production of $25(OH)D_3$ resulting from delayed production of the 25-hydroxylase for vitamin D. The occurrence of rickets in neonatal hepatitis has been described (Yu et al. 1971), while low levels of $25(OH)D_3$ in untreated cirrhosis and chronic liver disease in the adult have also been recorded (Long et al. 1976). Clearly there are good reasons why patients with liver disease may develop osteomalacia, though further study is required in this area.

The position is better understood with respect to the role of impaired renal 1-hydroxylation of $25(OH)D_3$ in the development of osteomalacia. Reduction in the synthesis of $1,25(OH)_2D_3$ as a result of destruction of the renal cortex is considered to play a major part in the development of the osteomalacic component of renal osteodystrophy. It also contributes to the hypocalcaemia, which in turn results in secondary hyperparathyroidism in renal disease. The changes of renal osteodystrophy are described later in this chapter (see p. 132). The fact that small doses of $1,25(OH)_2D_3$ are able to correct the defect in vitamin D-dependent rickets, while large amounts of other vitamin metabolites are required, has led to the postulation that this form of bone disease is due to a congenital deficiency in 1-hydroxylase in the kidney, especially since the low plasma levels of $1,25(OH)_2D_3$ do not increase after treatment with $25(OH)D_3$ (DeLuca 1978). Renal 1-hydroxylation is stimulated by parathyroid hormone and hypophosphataemia. Although clinical and radiological osteomalacia have not been reported in parathyroid hormone deficiency, mild osteomalacia has been found by bone biopsy in hypoparathyroidism (Drezner et al. 1977).

Vitamin D-dependent rickets

Vitamin D-dependent rickets (pseudovitamin D-deficiency rickets) is a disorder resulting from defective metabolism of 1,25-dihydroxyvitamin D $(1,25(OH)_2D)$. Rickets is present in affected individuals and there is hypocalcaemia, hypophosphataemia and decreased calcium absorption in the intestine with the development of secondary hyperparathyroidism. There are low blood levels of $1,25(OH)_2D$, and treatment with small amounts of $1,25(OH)_2D$ results in complete cure, although massive doses of vitamin D or 25-hydroxyvitamin D are also effective. This particular type of vitamin D-dependent rickets is considered to be due to defective conversion of 25(OH)D to $1,25(OH)_2D$. It is inherited as an autosomal recessive condition (Fraser et al. 1973; Scriver 1974) and may be referred to as type I vitamin D-dependent rickets, since a second type of disease has been described.

Patients with type II vitamin D-dependent rickets may be siblings of those with the type I disease, and sometimes the two disorders may coexist in an affected individual (Brooks et al. 1978; Marx et al. 1978, Zerwekh et al. 1979). These individuals (type II) have extremely high circulating levels of $1,25(OH)_2D$, and the metabolic problem consists of defective tissue sensitivity to this metabolite (Marx et al. 1978). Large doses of vitamin D, 25(OH)D or $1,25(OH)_2D$ are required for effective treatment.

The degree of mineralisation defect which manifests as osteomalacia or rickets and the biochemical abnormalities in type I and type II vitamin D-dependent disorders are similar (Bell 1980; Liberman et al. 1980; Tsuchiya et al. 1980).

Phosphate depletion and hypophosphataemia

In man, a low serum phosphate is more frequently associated with osteomalacia than a low serum calcium (Frame and Parfitt 1978). Poor dietary intake of phosphate and phosphate binding by antacids may lead to osteomalacia (Lotz et al. 1968), and such factors may therefore combine with others in an individual patient. Hypophosphataemia occurs in a variety of different conditions where there are renal tubular defects, including Fanconi's syndrome, in which there is dwarfism with rickets, albuminuria, aminoaciduria, renal glycosuria, hypophosphataemia and hyperphosphaturia (see Figs. 5.7, 5.8).

Familial hypophosphataemia

Familial hypophosphataemia (vitamin D-resistant rickets) has an X-linked dominant inheritance, although about one-third of cases are sporadic (Winters et al. 1958). There is decreased renal tubular phosphate reabsorption, even though blood phosphate levels are low, that is the kidney fails to conserve phosphate (Glorieux and Scriver 1972). The disorder becomes clinically evident during the second year of life, when rickets develops with growth retardation and bowing of the legs (Dent and Harris 1956). Histological examination of bone shows increased osteoid volume and a mineralisation defect using tetracycline labelling (Glorieux et al. 1980; Marie and Glorieux

1981), changes which are seen in any form of osteomalacia or rickets. Microradiographic studies and examination of thick ground bone sections show the presence of a 'halo effect' around osteocyte lacunae (Engfeldt et al. 1956; Frost 1963), regarded by Frost as a unique feature of the disorder. These perilacunar zones of hypomineralisation may reflect delayed osteocyte-mediated mineralisation (Frost 1963; Choufoer and Steendijk 1979). The 'hyp' mouse provides an X-linked hypophosphataemic animal model which is apparently identical with human vitamin-D resistant rickets (Cowgill et al. 1979; Meyer et al. 1980; Marie et al. 1981).

Other forms of hypophosphataemic bone disease

There are several forms of non-X-linked congenital hypophosphataemia which do not become manifest until adolescence and therefore present with osteomalacia rather than rickets (Dent and Harris 1956; Frymoyer and Hodgkin, 1977; Perry and Stamp 1978). Renal wasting of phosphate may be associated with a variety of neoplasms. Patients with carcinoma of the prostate were found to be hypophosphataemic and to have osteomalacia in a study by Lyles and colleagues (1980).

Inhibitors of mineralisation

Long-term administration of sodium fluoride leads to osteomalacia, the increase in unmineralised osteoid probably developing through the blocking of nucleation of calcium. Recently a form of calcification defect has been described in patients receiving haemodialysis for renal failure in areas where there is a high aluminium content in the water supply. There is deposition of aluminium in the bone, as demonstrated by histochemical staining methods, X-ray microanalysis, flameless atomic absorption spectroscopy and electron probe microanalysis (Ellis et al. 1979; Cournot-Witmer et al. 1980; Boyce et al. 1981, 1982; Ott et al. 1982; Smith and McClure 1982). Staining for aluminium in undecalcified sections reveals deposition at the junction between mineralised bone and osteoid, namely at the site of the mineralisation front. An example of aluminium-induced osteodystrophy is shown in Fig. 5.10.

Osteomalacia in metabolic acidosis

Osteomalacia has been recognised as a complication of chronic hyperchloraemic acidosis as a result of renal tubular disorders or surgery involving creation of continuity between the urinary tract and bowel (Albright et al. 1946; Pines and Mudge 1951). Healing of the osteomalacia has been reported following treatment with alkali alone or administration of vitamin D (Richards et al. 1972; Mautalen et al. 1976; Perry et al. 1977; McSherry and Morris 1978). The author has recently had the opportunity to study serial bone biopsies from two cases in which bowel and urinary tract were placed in continuity; there was osteomalacia and this healed with alkali treatment alone (Cunningham et al. 1982). One such case is illustrated in Fig. 5.11. Suggested mechanisms whereby chronic acidosis may cause bone disease include

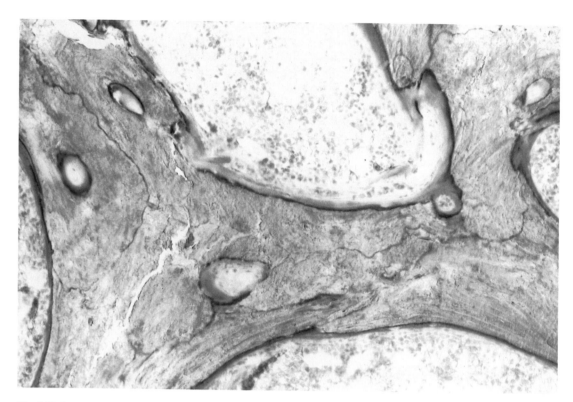

Fig. 5.10. Renal osteodystrophy with aluminium deposition, shown as black lines at the border between mineralised bone and osteoid. Some aluminium deposition is also present along cement lines within the bone trabecula. (Methylmethacrylate, method for aluminium × 400)

a direct effect of acidosis on bone (Lemann et al. 1966; Barzel and Jowsey 1969), augmentation of the effects of parathyroid hormone on bone resorption (Beck and Webster 1976), altered effect of parathyroid hormone on the kidney and changes in the renal handling of phosphate leading to hypophosphataemia (Cunningham et al. 1982). The osteomalacia of chronic renal failure does not respond to correction of acidosis (Stanbury and Lumb 1962).

Hypophosphatasia

Hypophosphatasia is a disorder in which there are low serum alkaline phosphatase levels with rickets or osteomalacia and increased excretion of phosphoethanolamine and pyrophosphate in the urine (Goldfischer et al. 1976; Whyte et al. 1979). It has been classified into 'congenita', 'juvenile', 'tarda' and 'adult' subtypes depending on age of onset. There is, however, considerable overlap, and there is controversy as to whether the various types represent variations in clinical expression of the same basic defect or whether they are separate genetic entities. On one hand, mild and severe cases have been reported in the same kindred, whereas, on the other hand, affected children in an inbred Hungarian community showed consistent clinical features (Beighton 1978).

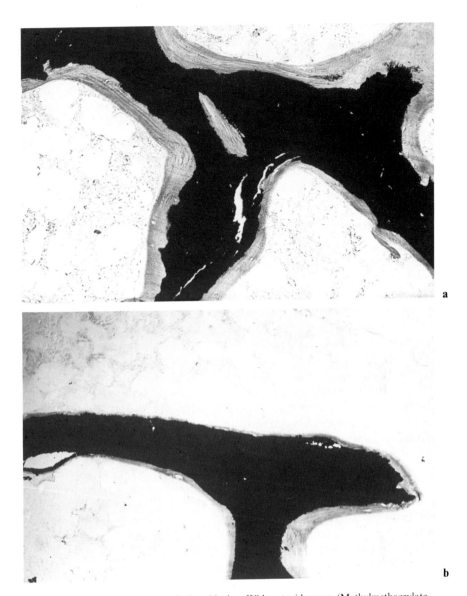

Fig. 5.11a,b. Osteomalacia in metabolic acidosis. **a** Wide osteoid seams. (Methylmethacrylate, von Kossa × 300)
b After treatment with alkali, same case as **a**, showing reduction in width of osteoid seams. (Methylmethacrylate, von Kossa × 300)

Congenital hypophosphatasia is inherited as an autosomal recessive disorder. Defective ossification of the calvaria gives rise to a caput membranaceum, and early death occurs with respiratory distress or intracranial bleeding. Differentiation from other lethal osseous dysplasias may be difficult since the limbs are shortened and deformed and the metaphyses are seen as irregular in a poorly ossified skeleton on radiological examination. Hypophosphatasia is one condition in which recognition of the heterozygote is simple and certain on the basis of the demonstration of a low serum alkaline phosphatase level and increased urinary phosphoethanolamine excretion (Rathbun et al. 1961). Hypophosphatasic patients often lose their permanent teeth at an early age, and in children there is early loss of the anterior deciduous teeth (Pimstone

et al. 1966). Infants presenting after the age of 6 months are less severely affected, and a possibly separate juvenile form of the disease may exist. Presentation
in adulthood is recognised (Whyte et al. 1979; Weinstein and Whyte 1981),
and cases described by Silverman (1962) and Danovitch et al. (1968) raise the
possibility of dominant inheritance in some forms of hypophosphatasia.
Patients with hypophosphatasia developing in childhood through to adult life
often have a history of multiple fractures and develop bowing of the long
bones. Examination of the bones shows changes indistinguishable from rickets
in childhood, including altered endochondral ossification, while in adults the
features are those of osteomalacia. (For further details see Chap. 3,
Hypophosphatasia.)

Renal osteodystrophy

The occurrence of bone disease in patients with renal failure has been
recognised for many years, and the basic descriptions of the histological
appearances still hold true. Our understanding of the endocrine changes and
more detailed analysis of histological features using quantitative methods (see
Chap. 4) have advanced the subject over recent years. Although, in the past,
bone disease in renal failure was well recognised, it was uraemia which was
the most important clinical feature of chronic renal disease. The advent of
dialysis and transplantation procedures has meant that skeletal changes have
now assumed greater clinical importance.

It is convenient to refer to the bone disease of chronic renal failure by the
broad term 'renal osteodystrophy', especially since a mixture of different features may be present in any individual case. Thus changes of osteomalacia
and/or osteitis fibrosa cystica occur in bone which may have decreased, normal
or increased trabecular bone volume (see Fig. 7.1, p. 170). Occasionally, pure
osteoporosis occurs. The exact incidence of the different features seen in renal
osteodystrophy seems to vary from place to place. The commonest feature
in the USA is osteitis fibrosa, while in parts of the UK osteomalacia predominates (Pierides et al. 1979), as is also borne out by the author's own study
of a large series of cases in London. In the series reported by Palma et al.
(1983), just over half of the undialysed and non-transplanted cases of chronic
renal failure had osteitis fibrosa, while a further one-third had both osteitis
fibrosa and osteomalacia. Eastwood (1982) reported histological evidence of
hyperparathyroidism in twice as many cases as that of osteomalacia in a series
of patients with advanced renal failure. The situation is complicated by such
factors as the aluminium content of the water supply used for dialysis (see
this chapter, Inhibitors of mineralisation). The bone biopsy may show wide
osteoid seams with little osteoblastic activity, few resorption lacunae and no
marrow fibrosis. This is the appearance of osteomalacic renal osteodystrophy,
and there is a calcification defect demonstrable in the tetracycline-labelled
biopsy. If a biopsy shows osteoid seams with plentiful active osteoblastic surfaces, many resorption lacunae with osteoclasts actively removing bone and
paratrabecular fibrosis in the region of the resorption lacunae, there is little
difficulty in recognising the effects of hyperparathyroidism, especially if tetracycline labelling is available to show that there is no calcification defect. In

practice, many biopsies from patients with renal failure show a mixed picture with features suggesting both osteomalacia and hyperparathyroidism (Fig. 5.12). Certainly caution is required in interpreting wide osteoid seams as representing osteomalacia, since this change may be due to accelerated synthesis of bone in many cases (Teitelbaum et al. 1980; Frost et al. 1981) and a reflection of secondary hyperparathyroidism (Ellis and Peart 1973). The availability of a tetracycline-labelled specimen enables the pathologist to make a clearer statement about any calcification defect and helps in unscrambling what may be a complicated histological picture. Other simple methods of assessing the significance of osteoid seams are the counting of the maximum number of lamellae using polarisation microscopy and calculation of the osteoid index from knowledge of the osteoid volume and osteoid surface (see Chap. 4, Measurements made and terms used in bone morphometry; Meunier et al. 1976). Cases of pure osteomalacia have more than five lamellae and high values for osteoid index, whereas the 'hyperosteoidosis' of hyperparathyroidism shows an increase in osteoid surfaces and more osteoblastic and osteoclastic activity.

The pathogenesis of the different elements in renal osteodystrophy is undoubtedly complex. Altered mineral metabolism in uraemia is manifest as hypocalcaemia, hyperphosphataemia, hypermagnesaemia, parathyroid gland hyperplasia with raised serum immunoreactive parathyroid hormone levels, skeletal resistance to parathyroid hormone, decreased renal metabolism of parathyroid hormone and vitamin D, and defective intestinal absorption of calcium. The possible reasons for the development of secondary

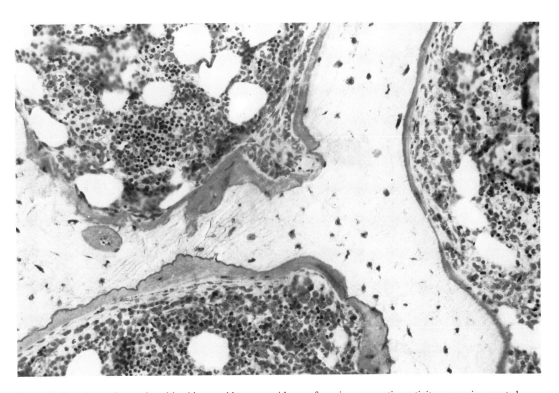

Fig. 5.12. Renal osteodystrophy with wide osteoid seams, evidence of previous resorptive activity as seen in crenated outline to lower margin of mineralised bone, and active osteoblasts (*centre top*). Adjacent bone shows active resorption by osteoclasts. (Methylmethacrylate, thionin × 400)

hyperparathyroidism are reviewed by Massry and Ritz (1978). Phosphate retention with hyperphosphataemia plays an important role even in the early stages of renal failure, according to Slatopolsky et al. (1978). If each small decrease in renal function were accompanied by a small increase in serum phosphorus, then the corresponding decrease in serum calcium level would bring about a homeostatic increase in parathyroid gland activity. A new steady state would then be reached for the calcium and phosphorus levels at the expense of the setting of a higher parathyroid hormone level. Skeletal resistance to the action of parathyroid hormone is also considered to play a role in the development of hyperparathyroidism. Deficiency of $1,25(OH)_2D_3$ and uraemia itself are thought to be factors responsible for skeletal resistance to parathyroid hormone (Massry and Ritz 1978), the former because vitamin D plays some role in the action of parathyroid hormone on bone (Arnaud et al. 1966).

Phosphate retention with hypocalcaemia is, however, considered to be the main reason for the initial increase in parathyroid gland activity in chronic renal failure (see above; Slatopolsky et al. 1971, 1979; Rutherford et al. 1977). Impairment of $1,25(OH)_2D_3$ production by the kidney occurs in advancing renal failure (Fraser and Kodicek 1973) and in turn leads to decreased absorption of calcium by the intestine (Rutherford et al. 1975; Colodro et al. 1978). In addition, impaired degradation of parathyroid hormone by the damaged kidney also contributes to the elevation of circulating parathyroid hormone levels (Freitag et al. 1978). Figure 5.13 is an attempt at a simplified scheme of the likely mechanisms in the development of renal osteodystrophy.

Patients receiving chronic dialysis may accumulate large amounts of aluminium in their bones, with deposition mainly at the mineralisation front (see this chapter, Inhibitors of mineralisation), although aluminium may some-

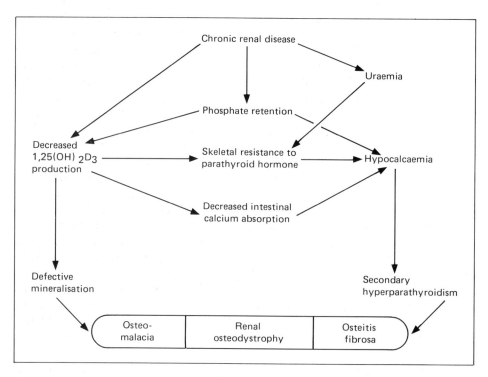

Fig. 5.13. Diagram to show possible mechanisms in the development of renal osteodystrophy

times also be seen at reversal lines within trabeculae. The role of aluminium in the development of osteomalacia has been well demonstrated by Ellis and his colleagues (1979), who were also able to produce severe osteomalacia in rats by the administration of aluminium.

Osteosclerosis may be a significant component of renal osteodystrophy and was present in 30% of the cases studied by Ellis and Peart (1973). The thickened trabeculae in osteosclerosis have wide osteoid seams and there is also evidence of osteitis fibrosa. Significantly higher levels of circulating parathyroid hormone have been found in uraemic patients with vertebral osteosclerosis compared with similar patients without overt osteosclerosis (Campos et al. 1976), and it seems likely that increased parathyroid hormone production is the most significant factor in the development of this change (Teitelbaum et al. 1980). Anaemia in renal failure may result from several different causes, but it is pertinent to mention that there may be sufficient fibrosis of the bone marrow and osteosclerosis of the bone for this to make a significant contribution in severe renal osteodystrophy (Weinberg et al. 1977).

Calcitonin

Calcitonin is a polypeptide hormone which has calcium-lowering effects on the plasma and which is produced by the parafollicular or 'C' cells of the thyroid gland, as first suggested by Foster et al. (1963) and later demonstrated in the human (McMillan et al. 1974; Wolfe et al. 1974). Calcitonin in pharmacological doses almost completely inhibits osteoclastic resorption of bone in organ culture. Loss of ruffled borders of osteoclasts is detectable within 15 min of the introduction of calcitonin and this becomes significant in extent by 1 h (Kallio et al. 1972; Holtrop et al. 1974). More recently the effect of calcitonin on isolated osteoclasts in vitro has been demonstrated by Chambers and Magnus (1982), while Warshawsky and his colleagues (1980) have presented evidence that osteoclasts have receptors for calcitonin. The question of whether calcitonin stimulates osteoblastic bone formation is at present unresolved (see review by Austin and Heath 1981 for references). Apart from its action on bone, the decrease in serum calcium and phosphate occurring after calcitonin may also be due to increased renal clearance of calcium and phosphate. There are specific renal receptors for calcitonin, and activation of adenylate cyclase occurs (Heersche et al. 1974; Ardaillon 1975). Calcitonin also alters gastrointestinal function (Austin and Heath 1981) but at higher than physiological levels of the hormone (Gray et al. 1976). Indeed, one of the problems with our present knowledge of the hormone is that there is little information available with respect to its effects at physiological concentrations on bone, kidney or the gut. Soon after it was described, calcitonin was said to be a 'hormone in search of a function'. Naturally occurring experiments, namely disease states where there are abnormal levels of calcitonin, do not apparently clarify the position. Thyroidectomy is associated with a reduction in calcitonin levels (Silva et al. 1978), but although thyroidectomised patients dispose of large calcium loads more slowly than normal, they are not hypercalcaemic and have apparently adapted to the absence of calcitonin (Austin and Heath 1981). Plasma levels of the hormone are lower in women than men, and the calcitonin response to calcium may decrease with age in women (Heath and Sizemore 1977; Deftos et al. 1980), so that the possibility of a role for calcitonin deficiency in the development of senile osteoporosis has been raised. There is at present, however, no agreement as to whether such hormone deficiency actually occurs in osteoporosis (Austin and Heath 1981).

The position is no clearer with respect to the effects of calcitonin excess. Patients with medullary carcinoma of the thyroid may have greatly raised calcitonin levels and indeed assays of the circulating hormone levels provide a sensitive method of detecting this tumour. There is, however, no evidence that such patients suffer any deleterious effects, and calcitonin levels 20 000 times the physiological concentration are tolerated with hypocalcaemia (Austin and Heath 1981). The possible reasons for this are briefly discussed by these authors. There is no evidence of osteosclerosis in bone biopsies of individuals with sustained elevation of plasma calcitonin, and in fact some show osteopenia. This finding is made all the more difficult to interpret when some authors believe that calcitonin promotes mineralisation (Boris et al. 1979), while others suggest that it suppresses bone formation (Baylink et al. 1969; Krane et al. 1973).

Supposedly vestigial organs have, in the light of further investigation, been proved to have vital functions (for example, the thymus). Mammalian physiology appears to be so finely tuned in the better understood areas that experience should caution against dismissing calcitonin as being of little importance.

The bones and other hormones

Relatively little detailed information is available about the effects of other hormones and vitamins on bone. The following is a brief description of some of them.

Growth hormone and acromegaly

Overproduction of growth hormone by a pituitary adenoma is responsible for acromegaly, a name meaning enlargement of the extremities, so called because the condition is characterised from the skeletal point of view by enlargement of the hands, feet and face. The appearances are described by Collins (1966). The orbital ridges and cheek bones become more prominent and exophthalmos may develop. Changes in the jaw result from increase in length and height of the mandible. The bones of the hands and feet become heavier and thicker, but in fact all bones are affected to some degree. The ribs become longer because of reactivation of endochondral ossification at the costochondral junction, and the joints are affected by proliferation of articular cartilage, which is abnormally thickened and undergoes secondary changes with the development of osteoarthritis. The vertebral bodies show cortical thickening, mainly anteriorly and laterally (Erdheim 1931).

The microscopic changes in bone are not yet clearly defined, since Jowsey and her colleagues considered that osteopenia develops in acromegaly (Riggs et al. 1972), a point of view also mentioned by Collins (1966) for long-standing cases; however, a morphometric study of iliac crest biopsies from 24 cases by Delling and Schultz (1977) showed thickened trabeculae with the trabecular bone volume in the normal range. These authors showed increased amounts of active osteoblastic and osteoclastic surfaces in some of their cases. Ramser and his colleagues (1966) considered that increased bone turnover in the presence of excess growth hormone was related to the formation of more sites of bone remodelling, a finding consistent with the results of Delling and Schultz. The differences between results may not be real, since it is possible that long-standing stimulation of both bone formation and resorption might ultimately lead to osteopenia if the two functions were slightly out of balance and there was gradual removal of bone.

Animal studies have shown the influence of growth hormone on cartilage and bone formation, both of which are stimulated. Hypophysectomy of young animals results in cessation of growth with diminution in the width of the epiphyseal plate and increase in the number of chondrocyte columns. Vascularisation of the growth plate disappears and transverse bridging between trabeculae occurs, resulting in an appearance similar to that thought to occur with the development of Harris' lines of growth arrest (Harris 1926). Administration of growth hormone to hypophysectomised growing animals results in chondrocyte proliferation, synthesis of cartilage matrix and widening of the growth plate. The metaphysis becomes revascularised and the transverse bone plate is resorbed as endochondral ossification is resumed (Urist 1972).

Thyroid hormone, hyperthyroidism and hypothyroidism

Thyroid hormone is important in skeletal growth and maturation, as is evident from both animal experiments and knowledge of the effects of thyroid deficiency and cretinism. The best and largest accumulation of skeletons from cretins is in the collection which was brought together early this century by Uehlinger in Zurich. These skeletons of adult cretins are of short stature, being around 1 m in height, and have disproportionate shortening of the limbs in relation to the trunk.

The effects of hypothyroidism on the growing child are delayed appearance and retarded growth of postnatal centres of ossification, retarded development and persistence of growth plates beyond the age at which they would normally disappear (Jaffe 1972). Dwarfism results mainly from effects on endochondral ossification. Radiologically the postnatal centres of ossification show irregular calcification giving the appearance of 'stippled epiphyses', which is not a diagnosis but a radiographic appearance also seen in various other conditions (see Chap. 2, Stippled epiphyses and chondrodysplasia punctata). This 'epiphyseal dysgenesis' was described in 23 out of 25 hypothyroid children by Wilkins (1941). Replacement treatment with thyroid hormone may bring about the virtual disappearance of the fragmented appearance within 2 years (Jaffe 1972), and epiphyses with ossification dates later than the time of treatment ossify normally (Collins 1966). Adults with hypothyroidism show evidence of depressed cellular activity in bone with inactive trabecular surfaces having few osteoblasts and osteoclasts and showing little uptake of tetracycline (Bordier et al. 1967; Jowsey and Detenbeck 1969).

Osteoporosis (osteopenia) has been regarded as the most regular feature of the bones in hyperthyroidism (Askanazy and Rutishauser 1933; Follis 1953; Adams and Jowsey 1967; Mosekilde et al. 1977) and this may be so pronounced as to lead to vertebral collapse or kyphosis. It was demonstrated many years ago that there is negative mineral balance in hyperthyroidism, and the loss of calcium is a reflection of both increased bone resorption (Mundy et al. 1976) and decreased intestinal absorption (Lekkerkerker and Doorenbos 1973; Haldimann et al. 1980).

Hyperthyroid patients have low $1,25(OH)_2D$ levels, may have hypercalcaemia and also decreased serum levels of parathyroid hormone (Parfitt and Dent 1970; Bouillon and DeMoor 1974; Castro et al. 1975; Maxon et al. 1978; Bouillon et al. 1980). There are occasional cases recorded in which hyperthyroidism and hypercalcaemia are accompanied by hyperparathyroidism (Frame and Durham 1959; Parfitt and Dent 1970). The precise mechanisms involved in the development of bone changes in hyperthyroidism are not easy to understand, since thyroxine itself enhances bone remodelling and promotes the effects of $1,25(OH)_2D$ and parathyroid hormone on bone (Castro et al. 1975; Pavlovitch et al. 1977; Melsen and Mosekilde 1978; High et al. 1981). Bone biopsies by Cook et al. (1959) showed osteopenia without excessive resorptive activity or osteomalacia, while older autopsy studies showed evidence of osteoblastic and osteoclastic activity at endosteal surfaces (Askanazy and Rutishauser 1933; Follis 1953), and more recent work has confirmed increased numbers of resorption lacunae and osteoclastic resorption (Melsen and Mosekilde 1978; Mosekilde and Melsen 1978; High et al. 1981). It is resorptive activity in compact bone which gives rise to 'cancellisation' of the cortex (Collins 1966). Although there may be some wide osteoid seams, they always represent new bone formation as judged by tetracycline labelling and are not due to true osteomalacia (Adams et al. 1967). The osteopenia of hyperthyroidism is therefore characterised by increased bone resorption with normal or increased bone formation.

Adrenal cortical steroids and Cushing's syndrome

The presence of osteoporosis as one of the features of Cushing's syndrome is familiar to the most junior medical student. Similarly it is well established that osteoporosis is an important complication of the long-term corticosteroid treatment of various diseases. The development of osteoporosis in association with glucocorticoids is described in more detail in Chapter 8, pp. 195–196, while references to tissue culture and basic research are available in Raisz and Kream (1983b).

Diabetes mellitus

Radiological studies in children with diabetes mellitus of recent onset have shown that the postnatal ossification centres develop slightly in advance of chronological age and that stature is likely to be somewhat above average. However, in children with long-standing diabetes, the ossification centres are not as fully developed as in normal children of comparable age, the long bones are gracile with thinned cortices, and there are frequently Harris's growth arrest lines in the metaphyses (Jaffe 1972). Both insulin-dependent and maturity onset diabetics show evidence of osteopenia and this may be detectable within 5 years of the onset of the disease (Levin et al. 1976; McNair et al. 1978). Studies of experimentally induced diabetes in the rat have shown decreased tetracycline uptake and minimal cellular activity (Hough et al. 1981; Shires et al. 1981). Further information about the effects of insulin on bone in animals and tissue culture is available in Raisz and Kream (1983b).

References

Adams P, Jowsey J (1967) Bone and mineral metabolism in hyperthyroidism: an experimental study. Endocrinology 81:735–740

Adams PH, Jowsey J, Kelly PJ, Riggs BL, Kinney VR, Jones JD (1967) Effects of hyperthyroidism on bone and mineral metabolism in man. Q J Med 36:1–15

Albright F, Burnett CH, Smith PH, Parson W (1942) Pseudo-hypoparathyroidism: example of 'Seabright-bantam syndrome': a report of three cases. Endocrinology 30:922–932

Albright F, Burnett CH, Parson W, Reifenstein FC, Roos A (1946) Osteomalacia and late rickets. Medicine (Baltimore) 25:399–479

Anderson J, Bannister DW, Parsons V, Tomlinson RWS (1967) Total urinary hydroxyproline in osteomalacia. Calcif Tissue Res 1:183–191

Ardaillon R (1975) Kidney and calcitonin. Nephron 15:250–260

Arnaud C, Rasmussen J, Anast C (1966) Further studies on the inter-relationship between parathyroid hormone and vitamin D. J Clin Invest 45:1955–1964

Arnaud SR, Goldsmith RS, Lambert RW, Go VLW (1975) 25 hydroxyvitamin D_3: evidence of an entero-hepatic circulation in man. Proc Soc Exp Biol Med 149:570–572

Askanazy M, Rutishauser E (1933) Die Knochen der Basedow Kranken. Beitrag zur latenten Osteodystrophia fibrosa. Virchows Arch [A] 291:653–681

Austin LA, Heath H (1981) Calcitonin. Physiology and patho-physiology. N Engl J Med 304:269–278

Barzel US, Jowsey J (1969) The effect of chronic acid and alkali administration on bone turnover in adult rats. Clin Sci 36:517–524

Baylink D, Morey E, Rich C (1969) Effect of calcitonin on the rates of bone formation and resorption in the rat. Endocrinology 84:261–269

Beck N, Webster SK (1976) Effect of acute metabolic acidosis on parathyroid hormone action and calcium mobilization. Am J Physiol 230:127–131

Beighton P (1978) Inherited disorders of the skeleton. Churchill Livingstone, Edinburgh

Bell NH (1980) Vitamin D-dependent rickets type II. Calcif Tissue Int 31:89–91

Bhattacharyya M, DeLuca HF (1979) Subcellular localisation of rat liver calciferol-25-hydroxylase. Arch Biochem Biophys 160:58–62

Booth BE, Tsai HC, Morris ERC (1977) Parathyroidectomy reduces 25-hydroxyvitamin D_3-1-hydroxylase activity in the hypocalcaemic vitamin D-deficient chick. J Clin Invest 60:1314–1320

Bordier P, Miravet L, Matrajt H, Hioco D, Ryckewaert A (1967) Bone changes in adult patients with abnormal thyroid function (with special reference to ^{45}Ca kinetics and quantitative histology). Proc R Soc Med 60:1132–1134

Boris A, Hurkey JF, Trinal T, Mallon JP, Matuszewski DS (1979) Inhibition of diphosphonate-blocked bone mineralization. Evidence that calcitonin promotes mineralization. Acta Endocrinol (Copenh) 91:351–361

Bouillon R, De Moor P (1974) Parathyroid function in patients with hyper- and hypothyroidism. J Clin Endocrinol Metab 38:999–1004

Bouillon R, Muls E, De Moor P (1980) Influence of thyroid function on the serum concentration of 1,25-dihydroxyvitamin D_3. J Clin Endocrinol Metab 51:793–797

Boyce BF, Elder HY, Fell GS, Nicholson WAP, Smith GD, Dempster DW, Gray CC, Boyle IT (1981) Quantitation and localisation of aluminium in human cancellous bone in renal osteodystrophy. Scan Electron Microsc III:329–337

Boyce BF, Fell GS, Elder HY, Junar BJ, Elliot HL, Beastall G, Fogelman I, Boyle IT (1982) Hypercalcaemic osteomalacia due to aluminium toxicity. Lancet II:1009–1012

Bronsky D, Kushner DS, Dubin A, Snapper I (1958) Idiopathic hypoparathyroidism: case reports and review of the literature. Medicine (Baltimore) 37:317–352

Brooks MH, Bell NH, Love L, Stern PH, Orfei E, Queener SF, Hamstra AJ, DeLuca HF (1978) Vitamin D-dependent rickets type II. Resistance of target organs to 1,25-dihyroxy-vitamin D. N Engl J Med 298:996–999

Brumbaugh PF, Haussler MR (1975) Specific binding of 1 alpha, 25 dihydroxycholecalciferol to nuclear components to chick intestine. J Biol Chem 250:1588–1595

Brunette MG, Chan M, Ferriere C, Roberts KO (1978) Site of 1,25-dihydroxyvitamin D_3 synthesis in the kidney. Nature 276:287–289

Byers PD, Smith R (1971) Quantitative histology of bone in hyperparathyroidism. Its relation to clinical features, X-ray and biochemistry. Q J Med 40:471–486

Campos C, Arata RO, Mautalen CA (1976) Parathyroid hormone and vertebral osteosclerosis in uraemic patients. Metabolism 25:495–501

Castro JH, Genuth SM, Klein L (1975) Comparative response to parathyroid hormone in hyperthyroidism and hypothyroidism. Metabolism 24:840–848

Chalmers J (1968) Osteomalacia. J R Coll Surg Edinb 13:255–275

Chambers TJ, Magnus CJ (1982) Calcitonin alters behaviour of isolated osteoclasts. J Pathol 136:27–39

Chase LR, Melsen GL, Aurbach GD (1969) Pseudohypoparathyroidism: defective excretion of 3'5'-AMP in response to parathyroid hormone. J Clin Invest 48:1832–1844

Chen TC, DeLuca HF (1973) Receptors of 1,25 dihydroxycholecalciferol in rat intestine. J Biol Chem 248:4890–4895

Chen TC, Hirst MA, Feldman D (1979) A receptor-like binding macromolecule of 1α21 dihydroxy-cholecalciferol in cultured mouse bone cells. J Biol Chem 254:7491–7494

Choufoer JH, Steendijk R (1979) Distribution of the perilacunar hypomineralized areas in cortical bone from patients with familial hypophosphatemic (vitamin D-resistant) rickets. Calcif Tissue Int 27:101–104

Clark OH, Taylor S (1972) Osteoclastoma of the jaw and multiple parathyroid tumors. Surg Gynecol Obstet 135:188–192

Coburn JW, Hartenbower DL, Birchman AS (1976) Advances in vitamin D metabolism as they pertain to chronic renal disease. Am J Clin Nutr 29:1283–1299

Collins DH (1966) Pathology of bone. London, Butterworths

Colodro IH, Brickman AS, Coburn JW, Osborn TW, Norman AW (1978) Effect of 25-hydroxyvitamin D_3 on intestinal absorption in normal man and patients with renal failure. Metabolism 27:745–753

Compston JE, Creamer B (1977) Plasma levels and intestinal absorption of 25-hydroxyvitamin D in patients with small bowel resection. Gut 18:171–175

Compston JE, Thompson RPH (1977) Intestinal absorption of 25-hydroxyvitamin D and osteomalacia in primary biliary cirrhosis. Lancet II:721–724

Cook PB, Nassim JR, Collins J (1959) The effects of thyrotoxicosis upon the metabolism of calcium, phosphorus and nitrogen. Q J Med 28:505–529

Cournot-Witmer G, Plachot JJ, Lefevre R, Bourdon R, Galle P, Drueke T, Balsan S (1980) Aluminium in bone from haemodialysed patients: relationship to bone histology and localization by electron microprobe and secondary ion microscopy. Metab Bone Dis Relat Res 25:491

Courpron P, Meunier P, Bressot C, Giroux JM (1976) Amount of bone in iliac crest biopsy. Significance of the trabecular bone volume. Its values in normal and in pathological conditions. In: Meunier PJ (ed) Bone histomorphometry. 2nd international workshop. Armour Montagu, Paris, pp 39–53

Cousins RJ, DeLuca HF (1972) Vitamin D and bone. In: Bourne GH (ed) The biochemistry and physiology of bone, 2nd edn, Vol 2 Physiology and pathology. Academic, New York, pp 282–335

Cousins RJ, DeLuca HF, Gray RW (1970) Metabolism of 25-hydroxycholecalciferol in target and nontarget tissues. Biochemistry 9:3649–3652

Cowgill LD, Goldfarb S, Lau K, Slatopolsky E, Agus ZS (1979) Evidence for an intrinsic renal tubular defect in mice with genetic hypophosphatemic rickets. J Clin Invest 63:1203–1210

Cunningham J, Fraher LJ, Clemens TL, Revell PA, Papapoulos SE (1982) Chronic acidosis with metabolic bone disease. Effect of alkali on bone morphology and vitamin D metabolism. Am J Med 73:199–204

Dalen M, Hjern B (1974) Bone mineral content in patients with primary hyperparathyroidism without radiological evidence of skeletal changes. Acta Endocrinol (Copenh) 75:297–304

Danovitch SH, Baer PN, Laster L (1968) Intestinal alkaline phosphatase activity in familial hypophosphatasia. N Engl J Med 278:1253–1260

Deftos LJ, Weisman MH, Williams GW, Karpf DB, Frumar AM, Davidson BJ, Pothenmore JG, Judd HL (1980) Influence of age and sex on plasma calcitonin in human beings. N Engl J Med 302:1351–1353

Delling GR, Schultz A (1977) Bone cells and remodelling surfaces in acromegaly. Calcif Tissue Res (Suppl) 22:255–259

DeLuca HF (1978) Vitamin D metabolism and function. Arch Intern Med 138:836–847

DeLuca HF (1979) The vitamin D system in the regulation of calcium and phosphorous metabolism. Nutr Rev 37:161–193

Dent CE (1970) Rickets (and osteomalacia), nutritional and metabolic. Proc R Soc Med 63:401–408

Dent CE, Harris H (1956) Hereditary forms of rickets and osteomalacia. J Bone Joint Surg [Br] 38:204–226

Dent CE, Smith R (1969) Nutritional osteomalacia. Q J Med 38:195–209

Dent CE, Stamp JCB (1971) Hypophosphataemic osteomalacia presenting in adults. Q J Med 40:303–329

Drezner MK, Neelon FA, Haussler M, McPherson HT, Lebovitz HE (1973a) 1,25-dihydroxycholecalciferol deficiency: the probable cause of hypercalcaemia and metabolic bone disease in pseudohypoparathyroidism. J Clin Endocrinol Metab 42:621–628

Drezner MK, Neelon FA, Lebovitz HE (1973b) Pseudohypoparathyroidism type II. A possible defect in the reception of the cyclic AMP signal. N Engl J Med 289:1056–1060

Drezner MK, Neelon FA, Jowsey J, Lebovitz HE (1977) Hypoparathyroidism: a possible cause of osteomalacia. J Clin Endocrinol Metab 45:114–122

Eastwood JB (1982) Quantitative bone histology in 38 patients with advanced renal failure. J Clin Pathol 35:125–134

Eddy RL (1971) Metabolic bone disease after gastrectomy. Am J Med 50:442–449

Ellis HA, Peart KM (1973) Azotaemic renal osteodystrophy: a quantitative study on iliac bone. J Clin Pathol 26:83–101

Ellis HA, McCarthy JH, Herrington J (1979) Bone aluminium in haemodialysed patients and in rats injected with aluminium chloride: relationship to impaired bone mineralisation. J Clin Pathol 32:832–844

Engfeldt B, Zetterstrom R, Winberg T (1956) Primary vitamin D resistant rickets. III Biophysical studies of skeletal tissue. J Bone Joint Surg [Am] 38:1323–1334

Erdheim J (1931) Über Wirbelsäutenwenänderungen bei Akromegalie. Virchows Arch [A] 281:197–296

Esvelt RP, Schnoes HK, DeLuca HF (1978) Vitamin D_3 from rat skins irradiated in vitro with ultraviolet light. Arch Biochem Biophys 188:282–286

Evans DJ, Azzopardi JG (1972) Distinctive tumours of bone and soft tissue causing acquired vitamin D resistant osteomalacia. Lancet I:353

Faccini JM, Teotia SP (1974) Histopathological assessment of endemic skeletal fluorosis. Calcif Tissue Res 16:45–57

Felton DJC, Stone WD (1966) Osteomalacia in Asian immigrants during pregnancy. Br Med J I:1521–1522

Follis RH (1953) Skeletal changes associated with hyperthyroidism. Bull John Hopkins Hosp 92:405–421

Forland M, Strandjord NM, Paloyan E, Cox A (1968) Bone density studies in primary hyperparathyroidism. Arch Intern Med 122:236–240

Foster GV, MacIntyre I, Pease AGE (1963) Calcitonin production and the mitochondrion-rich cells of the dog thyroid. Nature 203:1029–1030

Frame B, Durham RH (1959) Simultaneous hyperthyroidism and hyperparathyroidism. Am J Med 27:824–828

Frame B, Parfitt AM (1978) Osteomalacia: current concepts. Ann Intern Med 89:966–982

Frame B, Hanson CA, Frost HM, Block M, Arnstein AR (1972) Renal resistance to parathyroid hormone with osteitis fibrosa: "pseudohypoparathyroidism". Am J Med 52:311–321

Fraser D (1957) Hypophosphatasia. Am J Med 22:730–746

Fraser DR, Kodicek E (1970) Unique biosynthesis by kidney of a biologically active vitamin D metabolite. Nature 228:764–766

Fraser DR, Kodicek E (1973) Regulation of 25-hydroxycholecalciferol-1-hydroxylase activity in the kidney by parathyroid hormone. Nature 241:163–166

Fraser D, Koch SW, Kind HP, Holick MF, Tanaka Y, DeLuca HF (1973) Pathogenesis of hereditary vitamin-D-dependent rickets. An inborn error of vitamin D metabolism involving defective conversion of 25-hydroxyvitamin D to 1,25-dihydroxyvitamin D. N Engl J Med 289:817–824

Freitag J, Martin KJ, Hruska KA, Anderson C, Conrades M, Ladenson J, Klahr S, Slatopolsky E (1978) Impaired parathyroid hormone metabolism in patients with chronic renal failure. N Engl J Med 298:29–32

Frost HM (1963) A unique histological feature of vitamin D resistant rickets observed in four cases. Acta Orthop Scand 33:220–226

Frost HM, Griffith DL, Jee WSS, Kimmel DB, McCandlis RP, Teitelbaum SL (1981) Histomorphometric changes in trabecular bone of renal failure patients treated with calcifediol. Metab Bone Dis Relat Res 2:285–293

Frymoyer JW, Hodgkin W (1977) Adult-onset vitamin D-resistant hypophosphatemic rickets. J Bone Joint Surg [Am] 59:101

Garabedian M, Holick MF, DeLuca HF, Boyle IT (1972) Control of 25-hydrocholecalciferol metabolism by parathyroid glands. Proc Natl Acad Sci USA 69:1673–1676

Garrick R, Ireland AW, Posen S (1971) Bone abnormalities after gastric surgery. Ann Intern Med 75:221–225

Genant HK, Baron JM, Straus FH, Paloyan E, Jowsey J (1975) Osteosclerosis in primary hyperparathyroidism. Am J Med 59:104–113

Glorieux F, Scriver CR (1972) Loss of a parathyroid hormone-sensitive component of phosphate transport in X-linked hypophosphatemia. Science 175:997–1000

Glorieux FH, Marie PJ, Pettifor JM, Delvin EE (1980) Bone response to phosphate salts, ergocalciferol and calcitrol in hypophosphatemic vitamin D-resistant rickets. N Engl J Med 303:1023–1031

Goldfischer S, Johnson A, Morecki R (1976) Hypophosphatasia. A cytochemical study of phosphate activities. Lab Invest 35:55–62

Gray TK, Brannan P, Juan D, Morawski SG, Fordtran JS (1976) Ion transport changes during calcitonin-induced intestinal secretion in man. Gastroenterology 71:392–398

Haas HG, Dambacher MA, Guncaga J, Lauffenburger T (1971) Renal effects of calcitonin and parathyroid hormone extract in man. J Clin Invest 50:2689–2702

Haldimann B, Kaptein EM, Singer FR, Nicoloff JT, Massry SG (1980) Intestinal absorption in patients with hyperthyroidism. J Clin Endocrinol Metab 51:995–997

Harris HA (1926) The growth of the long bones in childhood, with special reference to certain bony striations of the metaphysis and to the role of vitamins. Arch Intern Med 38:785–806

Haussler MR, Baylink DJ, Hughes MR (1976) The assay of $1a$, 25-dihydroxyvitamin D_3: physiologic and pathologic modulation of circulating hormone levels. Clin Endocrinol 5:151S–165S

Heath H III, Sizemore GW (1977) Plasma calcitonin in normal man: differences between men and women. J Clin Invest 60:1135–1140

Heersche JNM, Marcus R, Aurbach GD (1974) Calcitonin and the formation of 3'5'-AMP in bone and kidney. Endocrinology 94:241–247

Henry HL (1979) Regulation of hydroxylation of 25-hydroxyvitamin D_3 in vivo and in primary cultures of chick kidney cells. J Biol Chem 254:2722–2729

Henry HL, Midgett RJ, Norman AW (1974) Regulation of 25-hydroxyvitamin D_3-1-hydroxylase in vivo. J Biol Chem 249:7584–7592

Hepner GW, Roginsky M, Moo HF (1976) Abnormal vitamin D metabolism in patients with cirrhosis. Am J Dig Dis 21:527–532

High WB, Capen CC, Black HE (1981) Effects of thyroxine on cortical bone remodeling in adult dogs. A histomorphometric study. Am J Pathol 102:438–446

Hillman LS, Haddad JG (1975) Perinatal vitamin D metabolism. II serial 25-hydroxyvitamin D concentrations in the sera of term and premature infants. J Pediatr 86:928–935

Hodkinson HM, Stanton BR, Round P, Morgan C (1973) Sunlight, vitamin D and osteomalacia in the elderly. Lancet I:910–912

Holick MF, Schnoes HK, DeLuca HF (1971) Identification of 1,25-dihydroxycholecalciferol, a form of vitamin D_3 metabolically active in the intestine. Proc Natl Acad Sci USA 68:803–804

Holick MF, Frommer J, McNeill S, Richt N, Henley J, Potts JT (1977) Photometabolism of 7-dehydrocholesterol to previtamin D_3 in skin. Biochem Biophys Res Commun 76:107–114

Holtrop ME, Raisz LG (1979) Comparison of the effects of 1,25-dihydroxycholecalciferol, prostaglandin E_2 and osteoclast-activity factor with parathyroid hormone on the ultrastructure of osteoclasts in cultured long bones of fetal rats. Calcified Tissue Int 29:201–205

Holtrop ME, Raisz LG, Simmons HA (1974) The effects of parathyroid hormone, colchicine and calcitonin on the ultrastructure and the activity of osteoclasts in organ culture. J Cell Biol 60:346–355

Hough S, Avioli LV, Bergfeld MA, Fallon MD, Slatopolsky E, Teitelbaum SL (1981) Correction of abnormal bone and mineral metabolism in chronic streptozotocin-induced diabetes mellitus in the rat by insulin therapy. Endocrinology 108:2228–2234

Howard G, Baylink D (1980) Matrix formation and osteoid maturation in vitamin D-deficient rats made normocalcaemic by dietary means. Miner Electrolyte Metab 3:44–50

Howe PR, Wesson LG, Boyle PE, Wolbach SD (1940) Low calcium rickets in the guinea pig. Proc Soc Exp Biol Med 45:298–301

Jaffe HL (1972) Metabolic, degenerative and inflammatory diseases of bones and joints. Lea and Febiger, Philadelphia

Jimenea CV, Frame B, Chaykin LB, Sigler JW (1971) Spondylitis of hypoparathyroidism. Clin Orthop 74:84–89

Jowsey J, Detenbeck LC (1969) Importance of thyroid hormones in bone metabolism and calcium homeostasis. Endocrinology 85:87–95

Jowsey J, Riggs BL, Kelly PJ, Hoffman DL, Bordier PH (1971) The treatment of osteoporosis with disodium ethane-1-hydroxyl-1, 1-diphosphonate. J Lab Clin Med 78:574–584

Jowsey J, Riggs BL, Kelly PJ, Hoffman DL (1972) Effects of combined therapy with sodium fluoride, calcium, vitamin D on the lumbar spine in osteoporosis. Am J Med 53:43–49

Kallio DM, Garant PR, Minkin C (1972) Ultrastructural effects of calcitonin on osteoclasts in tissue culture. J Ultrastruct Res 39:205–216

Kinard RE, Walton JE, Buckwalter JA (1979) Pseudohypoparathyroidism. Report on a family with four affected sisters. Arch Intern Med 139:204–207

King GJ, Holtrop ME, Raisz LG (1978) The relation of ultrastructural changes in osteoclasts to resorption in bone cultures stimulated with parathyroid hormone. Metab Bone Dis Relat Res 1:67–72

Knop J, Mantz R, Schneider C, Striktzke P, Dorn-Quint G, Nordmeyer JP, Kruse HP, Kohlencordt F (1980) Bone calcium exchange in primary hyperparathyroidism as measured by [47]calcium kinetics. Metabolism 29:819–825

Krane SM, Harrie ED, Singer FR, Potts JT (1973) Acute effects of calcitonin on bone formation in man. Metabolism 22:51–58

Kream BE, Jose M, Yamada S, DeLuca HF (1977) A specific high affinity binding macromolecule for 1,25-dihydroxyvitamin D_3 in fetal bone. Science 197:1086–1088

Lancet (1977) Hepatic osteodystrophy. Lancet I:988 (editorial)

Larkins RG, MacAuley SJ, MacIntyre I (1974) Feedback control of vitamin D metabolism by a nuclear action of 1,25-dihydroxycholecalciferol on the kidney. Nature 252:412–413

Lawson DEM, Fraser DR, Kodicek E, Morris HR, Williams DH (1971) Identification of 1,25-dihydroxycholecalciferol, a new kidney hormone controlling calcium metabolism. Nature 230:228–230

Lawson DEM, Wilson PW (1979) Intranuclear localization and receptor proteins for 1,25-dihydroxycholecalciferol in chick intestine. Biochem J 144:573–592

Lee JB, Tashjian AH, Streeto JM, Fratz AG (1968) Familial pseudohypoparathyroidism. Role of parathyroid hormone and thyrocalcitonin. N Engl J Med 279:1179–1184

Lekkerkerker JFF, Doorenbos H (1973) The influence of thyroid hormone on calcium absorption from the gut in relation to urinary calcium excretion. Acta Endocrinol (Copenh) 73:672–680

Lemann J, Litzow JR, Lennon EJ (1966) The effects of chronic acid loads in normal man: further evidence for the participation of bone mineral in the defense against chronic metabolic acidosis. J Clin Invest 45:1608–1614

Levin ME, Boisseau VC, Avioli LV (1976) Effects of diabetes mellitus on bone mass in juvenile and adult-onset diabetes. N Engl J Med 294:241–245

Lewin IG, Papapoulos SE, Tomlinson S, Hendy GN, O'Riordan JLH (1978) Studies of hypoparathyroidism and pseudohypoparathyroidism. Q J Med 47:533–548

Liberman UA, Halabe A, Samuel R, Kauli R, Edelstein S, Weisman Y, Papapoulos SE, Fraher LJ, Clemens TL, O'Riordon JLH (1980) End-organ resistance to 1,25-dihydroxycholecalciferol. Lancet I:504–506

Long RG, Shiver RD, Wills MR, Sherlock S (1976) Serum 25-dihydroxyvitamin D in untreated parenchymal and cholestatic liver disease. Lancet II:650–652

Lotz M, Zisman E, Bartter FC (1968) Evidence for a phosphorus depletion syndrome in man. N Engl J Med 278:409–414

Lund Bj, Sorenson OH, Lund Bi, Bishop JE, Norman AW (1980) Vitamin D metabolism in hypoparathyroidism. J Clin Endocrinol Metab 51:606–610

Lyles KW, Berry WR, Haussler M, Harrelson JM, Drezner MK (1980) Hypophosphatemic osteomalacia: association with prostatic carcinoma. Ann Intern Med 93:275–278

Mann JB, Alterman S, Hills SG (1962) Albright's hereditary osteodystrophy, comprising pseudo-hypoparathyroidism and pseudo-pseudohypoparathyroidism, with a report of two cases representing the complete syndrome occurring in successive generations. Ann Intern Med 56:315–342

Marie PJ, Glorieux FH (1981) Histomorphometric study of bone remodeling in hypophosphatemic vitamin D-resistant rickets. Metab Bone Dis Relat Res 3:31–38

Marie PJ, Travers R, Glorieux FH (1981) Healing of rickets with phosphate supplementation in the hypophosphatemic male mouse. J Clin Invest 67:911–914

Marx SJ, Spiegel AM, Brown EM, Gardner DG, Downs RW Jr, Attie M, Hamstra AJ, DeLuca HF (1978) A familial syndrome of decrease in sensitivity to 1,25-dihydroxyvitamin D. J Clin Endocrinol Metab 47:1303–1310

Massry SG, Ritz E (1978) The pathogenesis of secondary hyperparathyroidism of renal failure. Is there a controversy? Arch Intern Med 138:853–856

Mautalen C, Montoreano R, Labarrere C (1976) Early skeletal effect of alkali therapy upon the osteomalacia of renal tubular acidosis. J Clin Endocrinol Metab 42:875–881

Maxon HR, Apple DJ, Goldsmith RE (1978) Hypercalcaemia in thyrotoxicosis. Surg Gynecol Obstet 147:694–696

McFarlane JD, Lutkin JE, Burwood MA (1977) The demonstration by scintography of fractures in osteomalacia. Br J Radiol 50:369–371

McMillan PJ, Hooker WM, Deftos LJ (1974) Distribution of calcitonin-containing cells in the human thyroid gland. Am J Anat 140:73–79

McNair P, Madsbad S, Christiansen C, Faber OK, Transbol I, Binder C (1978) Osteopenia in insulin treated diabetes mellitus. Its relation to age at onset, sex and duration of disease. Diabetologia 15:87–90

McSherry E, Morris RC (1978) Attainment and maintenance of normal stature with alkali therapy in infants and children with classical renal tubular acidosis. J Clin Invest 61:509–527

Mellow AM, Stosich GV, Stern PH (1978) Dissociation of specific binding of 25-OH-D$_3$ and resorption in fetal rat bones. Mol Cell Endocrinol 10:149–158

Melsen F, Mosekilde L (1978) Dynamic studies of trabecular bone formation and osteoid maturation in normal and certain pathological conditions. Metab Bone Dis Relat Res 1:45–48

Melsen F, Mosekilde L (1980) Trabecular bone mineralisation lag time determined by tetracycline double-labelling in normal and certain pathological conditions. Acta Pathol Microbiol Immunol Scand [A] 88:83–88

Melvin KEW, Hepner GW, Bordier P, Neale G, Joplin GF (1970) Calcium metabolism and bone pathology in adult coeliac disease. Q J Med 39:83–113

Metz SA, Baylink DJ, Hughes MR, Haussler MR, Robertson RP (1977) Selective deficiency of 1,25-dihydroxycholecalciferol. A cause of isolated skeletal resistance to parathyroid hormone. N Engl J Med 297:1084–1090

Meunier P, Edouard C, Richard D, Laurent J (1976) Histomorphometry of osteoid tissue. The hyperosteoidoses. In: Meunier PJ (ed) Bone histomorphometry. 2nd international workshop. Armour Montagu, Paris. pp 249–262

Meyer RA, Gray RW, Meyer MH (1980) Abnormal vitamin D metabolism in the X-linked hypophosphatemic mouse. Endocrinology 107:1577–1581

Midgett RJ, Spielvogel AM, Coburn JW, Norman AW (1973) Studies on calciferol metabolism. VII The renal production of the biologically active form of vitamin D, 1,25-dihydroxycholecalciferol; species, tissue and subcellular distribution. J Clin Endocrinol Metab 36:1153–1161

Mosekilde L, Melsen F (1978) A tetracycline-based histomorphometric evaluation of bone resorption and bone turnover in hyperthyroidism and hyperparathyroidism. Acta Med Scand 204:97–102

Mosekilde L, Melsen F, Bagger JP, Myrhe-Jensen O, Sorenson NS (1977) Bone changes in hyperthyroidism: inter-relationships between bone morphometry, thyroid function and calcium-phosphorus metabolism. Acta Endocrinol (Copenh) 85:515–525

Moses AM, Rao KJ, Coulson R, Miller M (1974) Parathyroid hormone deficiency with Albright's hereditary osteodystrophy. J Clin Endocrinol Metab 39:496–500

Moss AJ, Waterhouse, C, Terry R (1965) Gluten-sensitive enteropathy with osteomalacia but without steatorrhoea. N Engl J Med 272:825–830

Mundy GR, Shapiro JL, Bandelin JG, Canalis EM, Raisz LG (1976) Direct stimulation of bone resorption by thyroid hormones. J Clin Invest 58:529–534

Nusynowitz ML, Klein MH (1973) Pseudoidiopathic hypoparathyroidism. Hypoparathyroidism with ineffective parathyroid hormone. Am J Med 55:677–686

Olson EB, Knutson JC, Bhattacharyya MH, DeLuca HF (1976) Effect of hepatectomy on synthesis of 25 hydroxyvitamin-D_3. J Clin Invest 57:1213–1220

Omdahl JL (1978) Interaction of the parathyroid and 1,25-dihydroxyvitamin D_3 in the control of renal 25-hydroxyvitamin D_3 metabolism. J Biol Chem 253:8474–8478

Omdahl JL, Hunsaker LA (1978) Direct modulation of 25-hydroxyvitamin D_3 hydroxylation in kidney tubules by 1,25-dihydroxyvitamin D_3. Biochem Biophys Res Commun 81:1073–1079

Ott SM, Maloney NA, Coburn JW, Alfrey AC, Sherrard DJ (1982) The prevalence of bone aluminium deposition in renal osteodystrophy and its relation to the response to calcitriol therapy. N Engl J Med 307:709–713

Palma FJM, Ellis HA, Cook DB, Dewar JH, Ward MK, Wilkinson R, Kerr DNS (1983) Osteomalacia in patients with chronic renal failure before dialysis or transplantation. Q J Med 52:332–348

Parfitt AM (1972a) The spectrum of hypoparathyroidism. J Clin Endocrinol Metab 34:152–158

Parfitt AM (1972b) Hypophosphatemic rickets and osteomalacia. Orthop Clin North Am 3:653–680

Parfitt AM, Dent CE (1970) Hyperthyroidism and hypercalcaemia. Q J Med 39:171–187

Parfitt AM, Miller MJ, Frame B, Villanueva AR, Rao DS, Oliver I, Thomson DL (1978) Metabolic bone disease after intestinal by-pass for treatment of obesity. Ann Intern Med 89:193–199

Pavlovitch H, Presle V, Balsani S (1977) Decreased bone sensitivity of thyroidectomized rats to the calcaemia effects of 1,25-dihydroxycholecalciferol. Acta Endocrinol (Copenh) 84:774–779

Perry W, Stamp TCB (1978) Hereditary hypophosphataemic rickets with autosomal recessive inheritance and severe osteosclerosis. J Bone Joint Surg [Br] 60:430–434

Perry W, Allen LN, Stamp TCB, Walker PG (1977) Vitamin D resistance in osteomalacia after ureterosigmoidostomy. N Engl J Med 297:1110–1112

Pierides AM, Ellis HA, Ward M, Simpson W, Peart KM, Alvares-Ude F, Uldall PR, Kerr DNS (1976) Barbiturate and anticonvulsant treatment in relation to osteomalacia with haemodialysis and renal transplantation. Br Med J I:190–193

Pierides AM, Skillen AW, Ellis HA (1979) Serum alkaline phosphatase in azotemic and hemodialysis osteodystrophy: a study of isoenzyme patterns, their correlation with bone histology and their changes in response to treatment with $1OHD_3$ and $1,25(OH)_2D_3$. J Lab Clin Med 93:899–909

Pimstone B, Eisenberg E, Silverman S (1966) Hypophosphatasia: genetic and dental studies. Ann Intern Med 65:722–729

Pines KL, Mudge GH (1951) Renal tubular acidosis with osteomalacia. Am J Med 11:302–322

Potts JT (1983) Calcium metabolism. In: Osteoporosis. A multidisciplinary problem. Royal Society of Medicine International Congress and Symposium Series No 55. Academic Press and Royal Society of Medicine, London, pp 3–18

Preece MA, Tomlinson S, Ribot CA, Pietrek J, Korn HT, Davies DM, Ford JA, Dunnigan MG, O'Riordan JLH (1975) Studies of vitamin D deficiency in man. Q J Med 44:575–580

Prost A, Hanniche M, Bordier P, Miravet L, DeSeze S, Rambaud JC (1975) Osteomalacia in chronic pancreatitis. Nouv Presse Med 4:1561–1566

Purnell DC, Smith LH, Scholz DA, Elveback LR, Arnaud CD (1971) Primary hyperparathyroidism. A prospective clinical study. Am J Med 50:670–678

Purnell DC, Scholz DA, Smith LH, Sizemore GH, Black BM, Goldsmith RS, Arnaud CD (1974) Treatment of primary hyperparathyroidism. Am J Med 56:800–809

Raisz LG, Kream BE (1983a) Regulation of bone formation. N Engl J Med 309:29–35

Raisz LG, Kream BE (1983b) Regulation of bone formation. N Engl J Med 309:83–89

Ramser JR, Frost H, Smith R (1966) Tetracycline-based measurement of the tissue and cell dynamics in rib of a 25 year old man with active acromegaly. Clin Orthop 49:151–162

Rathbun JC, MacDonald JW, Robinson HMC, Wanklin JM (1961) Hypophosphatasia: a genetic study. Arch Dis Child 36:540–542

Reinhart R, Brickman AS, Kurokawa K, Coburn JW, Massry SG (1973) Studies in three generations of a kindred with pseudohypoparathyroidism. Clin Res 21:255–261

Reiss E, Canterbury JM (1971) Genesis of hyperparathyroidism. Am J Med 50:679–685

Richards P, Chamberlain MJ, Wrong OM (1972) Treatment of osteomalacia of renal tubular acidosis by sodium bicarbonate. Lancet II:994–997

Riggs BL, Randall RV, Wahner HW, Jowsey J, Kelly PJ, Singh M (1972) The nature of the metabolic bone disorder in acromegaly. J Clin Endocrinol Metab 34:911–918

Rodbell M (1980) The role of hormone receptors and GTP regulatory proteins in membrane transduction. Nature 284:17–22

Ross EM, Gilman AG (1980) Biochemical properties of hormone sensitive adenylate cyclase. Annu Rev Biochem 49:533–564

Rutherford WE, Blendin J, Hruska K (1975) Effect of 25 hydroxycholecalciferol on calcium absorption in chronic renal disease. Kidney Int 8:320–324

Rutherford WE, Bordier P, Marie P, Hruska K, Harter H, Greenwalt A, Blondin J, Haddad J, Bricker N, Slatopolsky E (1977) Phosphate control and 25 hydroxycholecalciferol administration in preventing experimental renal osteodystrophy in the dog. J Clin Invest 60:332–341

Salassa RM, Jowsey J, Arnaud CD (1970) Hypophosphatemic osteomalacia associated with non-endocrine tumours. N Engl J Med 283:65–70

Scriver CR (1974) Rickets and the pathogenesis of impaired tubular transport of phosphate and other solutes. Am J Med 57:43–49

Sherwood LH, Mayer GP, Ramberg CF, Kronfeld DS, Aurbach GD, Potts JT (1968) Regulation of parathyroid hormone secretion: proportional control by calcium, lack of effect of phosphate. Endocrinology 83:1043–1051

Sherwood LM, Herrman I, Bassett CA (1970) Parathyroid hormone secretion in vitro: regulation by calcium and magnesium ions. Nature 225:1056–1058

Shipley PG, Park EA, McCollum EV, Simmons N (1921) Studies on experimental rickets. III A pathological condition bearing fundamental resemblances to rickets of the human being resulting from diets low in phosphorus and fat soluble A. The phosphate ion in its prevention. Bull Johns Hopkins Hosp 32:160–166

Shires R, Teitelbaum SL, Bergfeld MA, Fallon MD, Slatopolsky E, Avioli LB (1981) The effect of streptozotocin-induced chronic diabetes mellitus on bone and mineral homeostasis in the rat. J Lab Clin Med 97:231–240

Shohl AT (1936) Rickets in rats. XV. The effect of low calcium—high phosphorus diets at various levels and ratios upon the production of rickets and tetany. J Nutr 11:275–291

Silva OL, Wisneski LA, Cyrus J, Snider RH, Moore CF, Becker KL (1978) Calcitonin in thyroidectomised patients. Am J Med Sci 275:159–164

Silverman JL (1962) Apparent dominant inheritance of hypophosphatasia. Arch Intern Med 110:191–198

Sinha TK, DeLuca HF, Bell NH (1977) Evidence for a defect in the formation of 1,25 dihydroxyvitamin D in pseudohypoparathyroidism. Metabolism 26:731–738

Sitrin M, Meredith S, Rosenberg IH (1978) Vitamin D deficiency and bone disease in gastrointestinal disorders. Arch Intern Med 138:886–888

Skinner RK, Long RG, Sherlock S (1977) 25-hydroxylation of vitamin D in primary biliary cirrhosis. Lancet I:720–721

Slatopolsky E, Calgar S, Pennell JP, Taggart DD, Canterbury JM, Reiss E, Bricker NS (1971) On the pathogenesis of hyperparathyroidism in chronic experimental renal insufficiency in the dog. J Clin Invest 50:492–499

Slatopolsky E, Rutherford E, Hruska K, Martin K, Klahr S (1978) How important is phosphate in the pathogenesis of renal osteodystrophy? Arch Intern Med 138:848–851

Smith PS, McClure J (1982) Localisation of aluminium by histochemical and electron probe microanalytical techniques in bone tissues of cases of renal osteodystrophy. J Clin Pathol 35:1283–1293

Stanbury SW, Lumb GA (1962) Metabolic studies of renal osteodystrophy. I. Calcium, phosphorus and nitrogen metabolism in rickets, osteomalacia and hyperparathyroidism complicating chronic uremia and in the osteomalacia of the adult Fanconi syndrome. Medicine (Baltimore) 41:1–34

Steinbach HL, Young DA (1966) The roentgen appearance of pseudohyperparathyroidism (PH) and pseudohypoparathyroidism (PPH). Differentiation from other syndromes associated with short metacarpals, metatarsals and phalanges. Am J Roentgenol Radium Ther Nucl Med 97:49–66

Stern PH (1980) The D vitamins and bone. Pharmacol Rev 32:47–80

Strom L, Winberg J (1954) Idiopathic hypoparathyroidism. Acta Paediatr Scand 43:574–581

Stumpf WE, Sar M, Reid FA, Tanaka Y, DeLuca HF (1979) Target cells for 1,25 dihydroxyvitamin D_3 in intestinal tract, stomach, kidney, skin, pituitary and parathyroid. Science 206:1188–1190

Taylor CM, Hughes SE, de Silva P (1976) Competitive protein binding assay for 24,25 dihydroxycholecalciferol. Biochem Biophys Res Commun 70:1243–1249

Teitelbaum SL, Halverson JD, Bates BS (1977) Abnormalities of circulatory 25-OH vitamin D after jejunal-ileal bypass for obesity. Ann Intern Med 86:289–293

Teitelbaum SL, Bergfeld MA, Freitag J, Hruska KA, Slatopolsky E (1980) Do parathyroid hormone and 1,25-dihydroxyvitamin D modulate bone formation in uremia? J Clin Endocrinol Metab 51:247–251

Thompson ER, Baylink DJ, Wergedahl JE (1975) Increases in number and size of osteoclasts in response to calcium or phosphorus deficiency in the rat. Endocrinology 97:283–289

Tougaard L, Hau C, Rodbro P, Kitzel J (1977) Bone mineralization and bone mineral content in primary hyperparathyroidism. Acta Endocrinol (Copenh) 84:314–319

Tregear GW, Van Rietschoten J, Greene E, Kentmann HT, Niall HD, Reit B, Parsons JA, Potts JT (1973) Bovine parathyroid hormone: minimum chain length of synthetic peptide required for biological activity. Endocrinology 93:1349–1353

Tsuchiya Y, Matsuo N, Cho H, Kumagai M, Yasaka A, Suda T, Orimo H, Shiraki M (1980) An unusual form of vitamin D-dependent rickets in a child: alopecia and marked end-organ hyposensitivity to biologically active vitamin D. J Clin Endocrinol Metab 51:685–690

Urist MR (1972) Growth hormone and skeletal tissue metabolism. In: Bourne GH (ed) The biochemistry and physiology of bone, 2nd edn. Vol 2 Physiology and pathology. Academic, New York, pp 155–195

Wagonfeld JB, Nemchausky BA, Bolt M (1976) Comparison of vitamin D and 25-hydroxy-vitamin-D in the therapy of primary biliary cirrhosis. Lancet II:391–394

Warshawsky H, Goltzman D, Rouleau MF, Bergeron JJM (1980) Direct in vivo demonstration by autoradiography of specific binding sites for calcitonin in skeletal and renal tissues of the rat. J Cell Biol 85:682–694

Weber JC, Pons U, Kodicek E (1971) The localization of 1,25 dihydroxycholecalciferol in bone cell nuclei of rachitic chicks. Biochem J 125:147–153

Weinberg AG, Stone RT (1972) Autosomal dominant inheritance in Albright's hereditary osteodystrophy. J Pediatr Scand 79:996–999

Weinberg SG, Lubin A, Wiener SN, Deoras MP, Ghose MK, Kopelman RC (1977) Myelofibrosis and renal osteodystrophy. Am J Med 63:755–764

Weinman JP, Schour I (1945) Experimental studies in calcification III. The effect of parathyroid hormone on the alveolar bone and teeth of the normal and rachitic rat. Am J Pathol 21:857–875

Weinstein RS, Whyte MP (1981) Heterogeneity of adult hypophosphatasia. Report of severe and mild cases. Arch Intern Med 141:727–731

Wergedal JE, Baylink DJ (1971) Factors affecting bone enzymatic activity in vitamin D-deficient rats. Am J Physiol 220:406–409

Wezeman F (1976) 25 hydroxyvitamin D_3. Autoradiographic evidence of sites of action in epiphyseal cartilage and bone. Science 194:1069–1071

Whyte MP, Teitelbaum SL, Murphy WA, Bergfeld MA, Avioli LV (1979) Adult hypophosphatasia, clinical, laboratory and genetic investigation of a large kindred with review of the literature. Medicine (Baltimore) 58:329–347

Wilkins L (1941) Epiphyseal dysgenesis associated with hypothyroidism. Am J Dis Child 61:13–20

Wills MR, Phillips JB, Day RC, Bateman EC (1972) Phytic acid and nutritional rickets in immigrants. Lancet I:771–773

Winters RW, Graham JB, Williams TF, McFalls VW, Burnett CH (1958) A genetic study of familial hyperphosphatemic and vitamin D-resistant rickets with a review of the literature. Medicine (Baltimore) 37:97–142

Wolfe HJ, Voelkel EF, Tashjian AH Jr (1974) Distribution of calcitonin-containing cells in the normal adult human thyroid gland: a correlation of morphology with peptide content. J Clin Endocrinol Metab 38:688–705

Woods CG (1966) Histological studies in osteomalacia. J Bone Joint Surg [Br] 48:188 (abstr)

Yu JS, Walker-Smith JA, Burnard ED (1971) Rickets, a common complication of neonatal hepatitis. Med J Aust 1:790–792

Zerwekh JE, Glass K, Jowsey J, Pak CYC (1979) A unique form of osteomalacia associated with end organ refractoriness to 1,25 dihydroxyvitamin D and apparent defective synthesis of 25-hydroxyvitamin D. J Clin Endocrinol Metab 49:171–175

Zile M, Bunge EC, Barsness L, Yamada S, Schnoes HK, DeLuca HF (1978) Localization of 1,25 dihydroxyvitamin D_3 in intestinal nuclei in vivo. Arch Biochem Biophys 186:15–24

Chapter 6

Paget's Disease of Bone

Introduction

In 1877, Sir James Paget described a generalised bone disease resulting in marked deformities and gave it the name 'osteitis deformans'. Since this disease is not now considered to be an inflammatory condition and there may be little deformity, especially in individuals with monostotic disease, preference is given here to the name 'Paget's disease of bone'. There was some early confusion over similarities with osteitis fibrosa cystica before the two conditions were clearly defined. Important descriptions of Paget's disease made earlier this century are those by Schmorl (1932) and Jaffe (1977).

Examining the skeleton in a large number of autopsies, Schmorl found the post-mortem incidence of Paget's disease to be around 3% in those aged over 40 years (Schmorl 1932). Subsequent population surveys have shown an incidence varying between 0.1% and 3%, with the disease in many of these cases being asymptomatic (Krane 1977). There are occasional reports of so-called juvenile Paget's disease, but these are almost certainly examples of other bone diseases such as hypophosphatasia.

Clustering of cases of Paget's disease in families has been noted, as well as the occurrence of the condition in successive generations of the same family (McKusick 1972; Simon et al. 1975), but no association with a particular histocompatibility (HLA) antigen has been noted (Simon et al. 1975). Considerable interest centres on the regional variations in the incidence of Paget's disease, as noted in the USA, Europe and Australia (Rosenbaum and Hanson 1969; Barker et al. 1977, 1980; Detheridge et al. 1982). There is a higher incidence of Paget's disease in certain states in the USA, while in western Europe the disease occurs more frequently in the UK than in neighbouring countries on the mainland and in Scandinavia. Detheridge et al. (1982), using a postal questionnaire to radiologists and a subsequent radiological survey of 13 towns in 9 different countries, showed lowest rates in Sweden and Norway and highest in the UK with respect to the age- and sex-standardised prevalence of Paget's disease in the population aged 55 years and over. Only in three

French towns (Nancy 2%, Rennes 2.4%, Bordeaux 2.7%) did the prevalence approach the levels in the lowest prevalence towns in the UK (Aberdeen 2.3%, Carlisle 2.7%), and the overall figure for the UK was much higher at 4.6%. Particularly large numbers of cases of Paget's disease occur in certain Lancashire towns (Barker et al. 1977, 1980). The possible significance of this tendency for cases to occur in families and cluster geographically will be discussed later in this chapter (see Aetiology).

Clinical features

Abnormality of the skeleton passes unnoticed in most cases of Paget's disease, partly because there are no symptoms, signs or metabolic consequences related to the bone changes themselves when they occur in a site such as the pelvis. The principal serious clinical complications of Paget's disease are bone tumours and pathological fractures. There may, however, be neurological and cardiovascular changes, the development of deformities and joint disease and, occasionally, changes related to altered calcium metabolism. These manifestations of Paget's disease may be subdivided into focal, local and systemic changes, as outlined in Table 6.1.

The external appearance of a patient having widespread involvement with Paget's disease is fairly typical. The head is large, mainly over the calvaria, and usually shows little change in the facial bones. Prominent temporal vessels may be present. The spine is curved forward, predominantly in the thoracic region, and the femora and tibiae are bowed anteriorly and laterally, giving rise to a waddling gait and bow-legged appearance. The anterior convexity of the tibia results in the 'sabre-blade' appearance, while the neck of the femur is bent horizontally and may form a right angle with the shaft of the bone so that coxa vara results. The pelvis sometimes becomes markedly deformed.

Table 6.1 Clinical manifestations of Paget's disease

1. No clinical symptoms or signs
2. Focal manifestations:
   a) Skull—osteoporosis circumscripta
   b) Cranial enlargement, sometimes painful
   c) Hearing loss—temporal bone and ear ossicles involved
   d) Cranial nerve compression, e.g. trigeminal neuralgia
   e) Spinal disease—nerve root and spinal cord compression
   f) Pain, e.g. spinal, pelvic, limb bones
   g) Joint involvement—hip and knee
   h) Long bone involvement—femoral and tibial bowing
3. Local complications:
   a) Fractures—transverse and perpendicular to cortex, tibia and femur
   b) Neoplasia in Pagetic bone:
      i) Osteosarcoma, giant cell tumour
      ii) Others (chondrosarcoma, fibrosarcoma, malignant lymphoma, multiple myeloma etc.)
4. Systemic complications:
   a) Hypercalcaemia—in immobilised patients with fractures and extensive Paget's disease (rare)
   b) Hypercalciuria—development of renal stones
   c) Hyperuricaemia and gout
   d) Cardiovascular problems—high-output state and heart failure

An excellent description of the clinical appearances is presented in the early article by Jaffe, which is reproduced as Jaffe (1977).

'Osteoporosis circumscripta' is the term used for the initial resorptive phase of Paget's disease, occurring in the skull. There is localised well-demarcated rarefaction of the calvaria, often in the frontal or occipital region (Fig. 6.1), and the condition is usually painless. At a more advanced stage of involvement, the skull may become greatly thickened and there may sometimes be associated pain. Deafness of neurogenic origin may result from involvement of the petrous temporal bone, and hearing loss can also be caused by Paget's disease affecting the ear ossicles. Further details of the deafness in Paget's disease are available in Lindsay (1976).

Changes happen in the configuration of Pagetic bone because it is soft. In the skull, this may lead to invagination of the base of the skull from below by the vertebral column (so-called basilar invagination) and this in turn results in neurological difficulties with encroachment onto the brain stem, related cranial nerves and cerebellum and even vertebrobasilar insufficiency. Hydrocephalus and dementia have also been related to Paget's disease of the skull, caused most probably by impaired drainage of the cerebrospinal fluid through

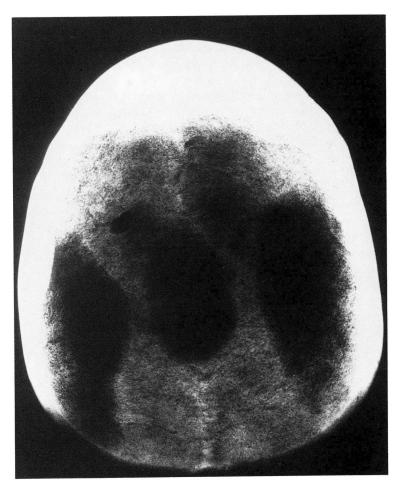

Fig. 6.1. Radiograph of a Pagetic calvaria showing large areas of rarefaction, caused by osteoporosis circumscripta

the aqueduct of Sylvius and the foramina at the base of the brain (Culebras et al. 1974).

Nerve compression resulting from bony encroachment may occur at various sites, most notably in the skull and spine. Cranial nerve involvement gives rise to anosmia, trigeminal neuralgia, vertigo, facial spasm and defects of the lower cranial nerves. Paget's disease of the cervical spine is relatively uncommon and cord compression at this level is rare. The upper thoracic spine is the site at which spinal cord compression most frequently occurs, the neural canal being narrowest here. There is gradual onset of sensory and motor loss in the lower limbs, which subsequently become spastic, and this may be accompanied by problems of sphincter control. Several adjacent thoracic vertebrae are usually involved by Paget's disease when cord compression occurs at this level. Involvement of the cauda equina at the level of the upper lumbar vertebrae sometimes gives rise to neurological deficits. The neurological effects of Paget's disease are described in more detail by Schmidek (1977) and Feldman and his colleagues (1979).

Paget's disease may be painless or give rise to considerable disability, either directly related to bone or arising from secondary changes in joints. A recent study of nearly 300 cases showed over 90% of patients with Paget's disease had signs suggestive of osteoarthritis in one or more joints, including a decreased range of movement, most commonly in the cervical spine, shoulder, hip and knee (Altman 1980). Long bone deformity was present in 45% of the patients, many of whom had lower backache or joint pain in the lower limb. Anterior and lateral bowing of the femur and tibia frequently caused a functional flexion deformity at the knee. Back pain was considered mostly to be related to accompanying degenerative spinal disease, and in only 2% of cases was Paget's disease the sole source of backache. Degenerative joint disease related to Paget's disease was present in 30% of cases at the hip and 11% at the knee (Altman 1980).

Fractures

The first manifestation of Paget's disease, and the commonest reason for a patient with this condition to be admitted to hospital, is the fracture of an involved long bone. Such fractures are typically transverse across long bones, perpendicular to the cortex and most frequently affect the femur or tibia. The upper femur (subtrochanteric and femoral neck) accounts for over one-third of fractures of that bone in Paget's disease, according to Barry (1980), who states that tibial fractures usually occur in the upper third of the shaft. Bone affected by either the osteolytic resorptive or the sclerotic phase of the disease may become fractured. Fracture healing occurs at the same rate as in normal bone, though there may be abundant callus formation, and non-union happens in around 10% of cases (Barry 1980).

Tumours

The other significant local complication of Paget's disease is the development of a malignant tumour, an occurrence recognised by Paget himself and well documented in the literature over many years. Nearly 70 references to bone neoplasia in Paget's disease are given in the introduction to the paper by Wick and his colleagues (1981). Early estimates put the incidence of sarcoma in Paget's disease at around 10%, but more recent studies show malignant change to be a much rarer event, occurring in 1% or less of Pagetic patients (Collins 1966; Barry 1969; Wick et al. 1981). An alternative way of presenting the frequency of sarcoma in Paget's disease is to say that in all patients with bone sarcoma over the age of 40 years about 20% have Paget's disease, according to McKenna et al. (1964), while Huvos and his colleagues (1983) found that 27% of osteogenic sarcomas occurring in patients over the same age arose in bones affected by Paget's disease. Almost any bone may be involved, but the vertebrae are often spared, even though there is otherwise a predilection for the axial skeleton. Commoner sites of involvement are the pelvis, skull, femur and humerus. All patients had polyostotic Paget's disease in the large series reported by Wick and his colleagues (1981), although occasional cases have been described with monostotic disease (see, for example Huvos et al. 1983). Recent onset, or sudden increase in severity, of pain at the site of the sarcoma are among the presenting features, together with development of a palpable mass or neurological impairment, the latter being particularly confusing since Paget's disease may cause this in the absence of sarcoma (Schmideck 1977; Shannon and Hopkins 1977; Feldman et al. 1979). The discovery of a bone sarcoma in a middle-aged or older person should initiate radiological examination of the skeleton in search of Paget's disease (Coley and Sharp 1931). Tumours arising in Pagetic bone have a poorer prognosis than those in bone without Paget's disease (Spjut et al. 1971; Dorfman 1973; Schwinn and McKenna 1973; Dahlin and Unni 1977; Wick et al. 1981; Huvos et al. 1983).

The vast majority of malignant bone tumours occurring in Paget's disease are osteosarcomas (Dahlin 1978; Wick et al. 1981), and these have sometimes been subdivided into osteoblastic, telangiectatic, chondrosarcomatous, fibrosarcomatous, fibrous histiocytomatous types. Fibrosarcoma, chondrosarcoma, malignant fibrous histiocytoma, giant cell tumour and multiple myeloma also occur in relation to Paget's disease (Reich and Brodsky 1948; Goldenberg 1951; Jaffe 1972; Dahlin 1978; Mirra et al. 1981; Schajowicz et al. 1983). There are reports of multicentric sarcomas in Paget's disease (Thompson et al. 1970; Taurel et al. 1973), though there is debate about whether these truly represent multifocal synchronous development of malignant change or simply metastases from one bone to another (Jaffe 1972; McKenna et al. 1964). This problem is virtually impossible to resolve, as the author also has found in the case of ordinary osteosarcomas presenting simultaneously at three separate sites in a young man not having Paget's disease.

Jaffe (1972) makes the point that there may be considerable variation in the histological appearances of biopsies from different areas of the same tumour, some showing osteosarcoma, others fibrosarcoma and yet others showing giant cell tumour. For this reason he prefers to designate the tumour as a sarcoma complicating Paget's disease. The significant prognostic point would seem to be the importance of defining those bone tumours arising in Pagetic rather than normal bone in those over the age of 40 years (as already mentioned above).

Cardiovascular effects

Marked changes in the dynamics of the cardiovascular system with increased blood flow to involved extremities were noted by Edholm et al. (1945). It has been suggested that increased blood flow is due to the presence of arterio-venous fistulae in Pagetic bone (Nagent de Deuxchaisnes and Krane 1964). Increased vascularity of the bone has been confirmed by biopsy, post-mortem dissection and angiography, but none of these methods have demonstrated evidence for arteriovenous fistulae, and neither has the injection of isotope-labelled microspheres (Edholm and Howarth 1953; Storsteen and Jones 1954; Rhodes et al. 1972). Much of the increased warmth and blood flow in Pagetic limbs may be accounted for by cutaneous vasodilation and blood flow, according to Heistad et al. (1975). The development of high-output heart failure occurs in patients with around one-third of the skeleton involved (i.e. polyostotic disease), though there may be increased cardiac output in those with a lesser degree of involvement (Krane 1977).

Biochemical changes

The biochemical changes of Paget's disease relate to the increased osteoclastic and osteoblastic activity in involved bone, demonstrated by raised hydroxyproline and alkaline phosphatase levels in urine and blood respectively. The main organic component of bone is type I collagen (see Chap. 1, p. 15). No definite abnormality of bone collagen in Paget's disease has been demonstrated. When bone collagen is resorbed, peptides are released which are excreted in the urine. Measurement of urinary levels of the amino acid hydroxyproline give some indication about collagen breakdown (Kivirikko 1970), and high rates of urinary hydroxyproline excretion have been shown in Paget's disease (Woodhouse 1972; Franck et al. 1974). Serum alkaline phosphatase levels are elevated in patients with Paget's disease. The increase correlates with disease activity, the extent of skeletal involvement, and the level of urinary hydroxyproline excretion (Nagent de Deuxchaisnes and Krane 1964; Woodhouse 1972). Patients developing osteosarcoma in Paget's disease may show a sudden large rise in alkaline phosphatase level (Woodward 1959), although in others no significant increase may be seen (Poretta et al. 1957).

The correlation between urinary hydroxyproline and serum alkaline phosphatase levels is indicative of the maintenance of coupling between resorption and bone formation, even though bone turnover is markedly increased. The equilibrium between the inflow and outflow of minerals for bone is maintained and blood calcium levels remain normal. However, some patients with Paget's disease are in negative balance, and factors which result in altered calcium balance in the normal skeleton are also responsible for changes in Paget's disease. Thus, for example, immobilisation of a Pagetic patient with a fracture may lead to hypercalcaemia and hypercalciuria. Increased urinary calcium excretion may lead to kidney stone formation. Another noteworthy metabolic disturbance in a significant proportion of patients with Paget's disease is the presence of hyperuricaemia, sometimes with clinical gout (Franck et al. 1974; Altman 1980).

Radiological appearances

Paget's disease may be divided into different radiological and pathological stages, namely an initial osteolytic, an active osteoblastic and a final inactive phase. Such division is obviously somewhat artificial, but nevertheless it is possible to see this spectrum of changes within an affected bone. The relationship of the radiology with the different pathological phases is described by Milgram (1977). The initial phase is seen at the junction between normal and Pagetic bone, which is clearly defined and obliquely rather than transversely orientated to give a 'V'-shaped interface. Resorbed pre-existing bone is replaced by a delicate mesh of fine trabeculae, and there is some endosteal new bone formation in long bones.

The localised radiolucent areas in the Pagetic skull are known as 'osteoporosis circumscripta' and also represent the resorptive stage of the process, with loss of the inner and outer tables together with intervening cancellous bone, over a well-demarcated area, most frequently in the frontal or occipital regions. The process crosses the cranial suture lines (Goldenberg 1951; Jaffe 1972; Milgram 1977).

In the region of actively osteoblastic disease, the outline of the bone is increased in size with widening of the cortex on both endosteal and periosteal surfaces (Fig. 6.2). Sometimes abundant spongy Pagetic bone is formed at the periosteal surface, and this 'pumice bone' (so called because of its texture)

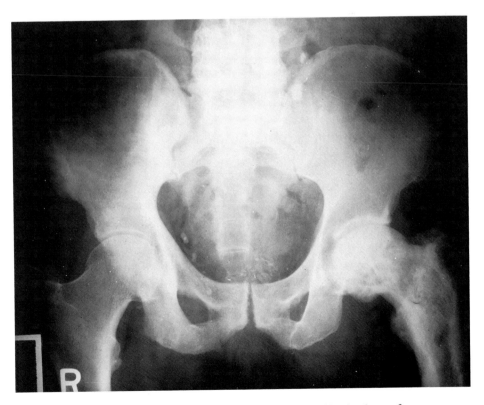

Fig. 6.2. Clinical radiograph showing Paget's disease of the left femoral head and upper femur

may very occasionally give rise to confusion in its differentiation from malignant change (Golding 1960). Such periosteal new bone is not usually more than a centimetre thick, covers an extensive surface area of the affected bone and should not normally give rise to a problem. A biopsy is indicated when there is any doubt about whether a periosteal outgrowth is Pagetic bone or osteosarcoma (Milgram 1977). Late in the involvement of a particular bone, Paget's disease reaches the inactive stage, in which radiological examination shows appearances little different from the more advanced part of the active osteoblastic phase.

There are particular terms used to describe the radiological appearances of Paget's disease in different bones. The vertebral bodies may show the osteolytic phase already mentioned, and there may be local mechanical failure with compression fractures; however, after years of remodelling within an affected bone, central areas become less dense, while the sides, upper and lower limits of the vertebral body become denser to form a sclerotic rectangle resembling a 'picture frame'. Sometimes, the vertebrae become decreased in height with convex upward and downward extensions of adjacent intervertebral discs to give 'fish vertebrae'. The variability in pathological stages present in different parts of the skull may mean that there are sclerotic radiopaque shadows intermingled with radiolucent streaks, or even large areas of porosity and the moderately diffuse radiopacity of pumice bone, so that the overall effect of the radiographic images is to create an appearance described as 'cotton wool'. This same appearance may be produced in radiographs of the involved iliac bones in the pelvis.

The usefulness of radioisotope scintillation scanning in the clinical assessment of Paget's disease has been examined by Wellman et al. (1977), who found that only 67% of lesions detected by scanning were visible on radiological examination, that those detected by scintillation methods alone were early lesions and that those seen on radiological examination alone were older sclerotic 'burned out' foci of disease.

Morbid anatomy and histopathology

The anatomical distribution of Paget's disease has already been outlined (see p. 148). Although almost any bone may be affected, the axial skeleton predominates where large series of cases have been studied, the sacrum and pelvis, spine, skull and femur accounting for around 75%–80% of the bone involved (Collins 1966; Jaffe 1977). The morbid anatomical appearances vary from bone to bone and depend on the stage the disease has reached. In the skull, an area of osteoporosis circumscripta is clearly defined and shows almost total absence of the compact bone of the inner and outer tables of the calvaria, the trabecular bone of the intervening diploic bone passing almost up to the surfaces. The osteolytic area has a purplish-red coloration, which is due to the continued presence of bone marrow and increased vascularity, either of which are visible through the overlying thinned bone, depending on the stage of the disease. The frontal and occipital bones are most frequently affected, and the process passes across cranial suture lines (Goldenberg 1951; Collins 1966; Jaffe 1977). The area of circumscribed osteoporosis may blend with more typical lesions of Paget's disease in which the skull is thickened and greyish-white in appearance. There may be alternating areas of bone showing lytic and osteoblastic phases of the disease. The changes are manifest mainly in the calvaria and most pronounced in the occipital region. There are graphic pictures in the literature of massive thickening of the skull causing considerable decrease in the space available for the brain (Fig. 6.3). Thickening of the bones of the face is unusual and when it does occur gives an appearance like that of leontiasis ossea, from which condition it should be differentiated (Jaffe 1972). Invagination of the softened bone of the skull with narrowing of the foramen magnum has already been mentioned, as has narrowing of nerve foramina (see p. 150).

Diffuse involvement of the innominate bones is seen most frequently in polyostotic disease. The pelvic outlet may be narrowed. The sacrum is often affected if there is pelvic involvement. According to Jaffe (1977), disease in the superior pubic ramus stops abruptly at the symphysis pubis. Involvement of vertebra, or the sacrum, is usually total in the segment(s) affected, but the change is more obvious in the bodies than in the neural arch and processes. The denser peripheral bone giving a framing appearance has already been mentioned (see p. 154), as have changes in shape of vertebrae.

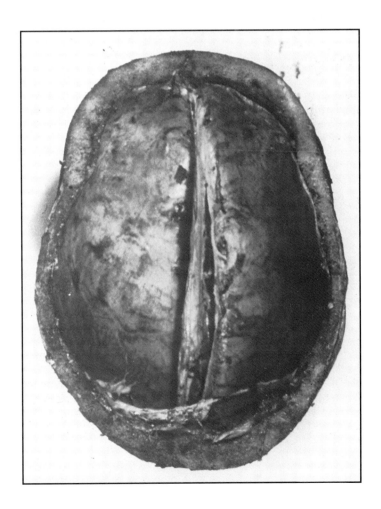

Fig. 6.3. Thickening of the skull involved by Paget's disease

Paget's disease in a long bone usually begins at one end and spreads towards the diaphysis (Fig. 6.4). The thickened cortex is grey-red in colour, in contrast to the normal cream colour, and the two appearances are easily demarcated. The 'V'-shaped interface between Pagetic and normal bone has already been described (see p. 153), as has thickening on the outside of the bone due to the periosteal woven bone formation, so-called pumice bone. There is some question about whether Paget's disease in bone immediately adjacent to a joint results in osteoarthritis (Jaffe 1977; Milgram 1977; Guyer and Dewbery 1978; Guyer 1979; Altman 1980), the radiological reviews of Guyer suggesting that the incidence of degenerative joint disease may not be high. An example of a femoral head with Paget's disease affecting the bone adjacent to the joint surface is shown in Figs. 6.5–6.7.

Histological examination of Pagetic bone reveals a variety of different appearances depending on the stage the disease has reached. The initial stage of osteoclastic resorption of existing bone is seen at the interface between the focus of involvement and adjacent normal bone. Existing bone trabeculae show increased numbers of resorption lacunae and there is accompanying inter-trabecular marrow fibrosis, although this is not always the case. Osteoclasts are larger than normal in Paget's disease and have considerable numbers of nuclei—up to 100. Cortical bone shows the same increase in osteoclastic activity as seen in the cancellum, and the Haversian systems also show the presence of some fibrosis. Increased vascularity occurs at both sites.

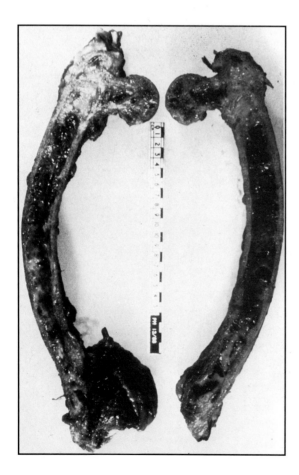

Fig. 6.4. Paget's disease involving the femur which shows bowing and loss of the normal angle between the neck and shaft of the femur

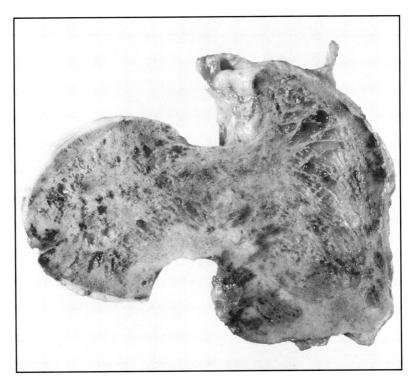

Fig. 6.5. Upper end of the femur, involved by Paget's disease. The femoral neck is approximately perpendicular to the axis of the femoral shaft

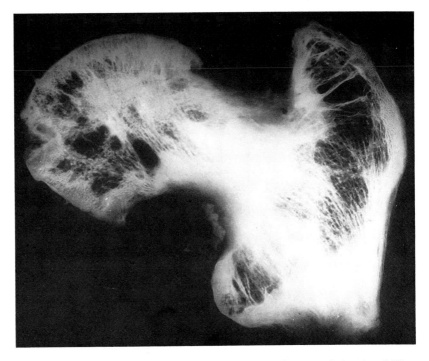

Fig. 6.6. Radiograph of the specimen shown in Fig. 6.5, showing areas of sclerosis and 90° angle between neck and shaft of femur. *Note:* there is little evidence of degenerative joint disease in this case

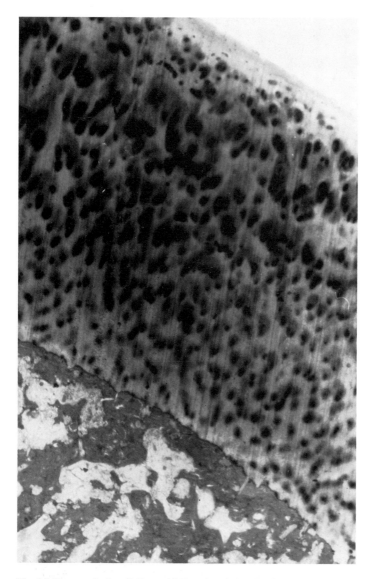

Fig. 6.7. Intact articular cartilage with Pagetic subchondral bone, from the case illustrated in Figs. 6.5 and 6.6. There is no evidence of degenerative joint disease. (H&E × 100)

Osteoclastic resorption always precedes osteoblastic activity (Fig. 6.8). Immediately adjacent to this zone of osteoclastic activity, there is osteoblastic activity with production of woven (Figs. 6.9, 6.10), followed later by lamellar, bone set down on the pre-existing trabecular framework. The inter-trabecular space contains vascular fibrous tissue in which new bone formation occurs. Small collections of haemopoietic cells may remain. This is the active or osteoblastic phase of the disease in which successive further periods of osteoclastic and osteoblastic activity take place so that the classic 'mosaic pattern' of Pagetic bone is developed (Fig. 6.11). This appearance, which is more or less specific to Paget's disease, results because bone is resorbed and replaced in a random fashion rather than in response to physiological needs. The mosaic appearance is usually apparent in haematoxylin/eosin-stained sections in

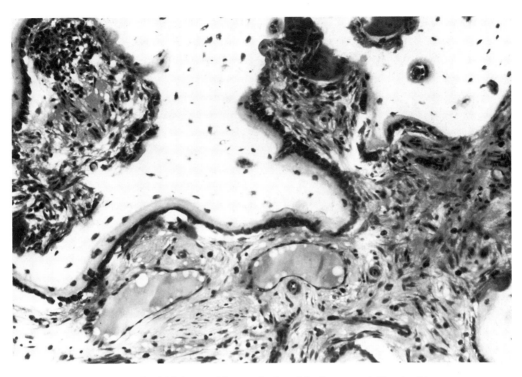

Fig. 6.8. Paget's disease showing initial stage with osteoclastic activity (*top, centre*), fibrosis of the marrow space and increased osteoblastic activity. (Methylmethacrylate, thionin × 760)

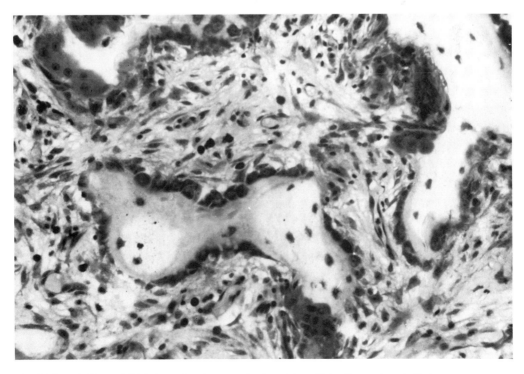

Fig. 6.9. Paget's disease, initial phase, showing osteoclastic activity, cellular fibrous tissue in the bone marrow space, and osteoblastic activity with the formation of new bone. (Methylmethacrylate, thionin × 950)

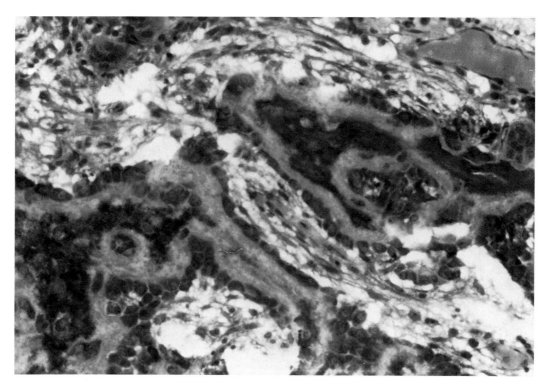

Fig. 6.10. Paget's disease. Vascular fibrous tissue containing trabeculae of newly formed bone with active osteoblasts. (Methylmethacrylate, H&E × 1000)

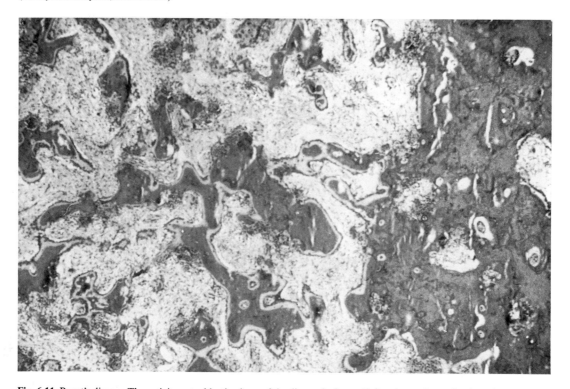

Fig. 6.11. Paget's disease. The activity osteoblastic phase of the disease is shown (*left and centre*), passing into the mosaic pattern (*right*). (H&E × 100)

which the cement lines within the disorganised bone are visible, but is also readily demonstrated by the use of polarisation microscopy when the orientation of lamellae within the bone is seen to be in different directions in adjacent areas of the same piece of bone (Figs. 6.12, 6.13). A little care is required in the interpretation of this appearance since fairly similar changes may result from repeated resorption and formation of bone in association with hyperparathyroidism, especially in renal osteodystrophy.

In the inactive phase of the disease, the coarse trabecular bone and thickened disorganised cortical bone are made up of randomly arranged blocks of bone giving the mosaic appearance (Fig. 6.14). Most of the bone surfaces lack osteoclasts or osteoblasts, though a small amount of residual cellular activity may be present (Milgram 1977). The intertrabecular spaces which had been filled in the active phase with fibrous tissue become repopulated with fat cells and haemopoietic tissue.

Although the appearance of Paget's disease is well known and obvious in the inactive final phase, it is important always to bear the condition in mind when examining bone biopsies from patients in the second half of life. The resorptive phase may not be readily recognised, especially since no mosaic pattern is then present in the bone. Possible confusion of periosteal new bone with osteosarcoma has already been mentioned, as also has that between the effects of hyperparathyroidism and Paget's disease. Confusion with fibrous dysplasia, callus and osteosclerotic metastatic carcinoma are also possible. Histomorphometric studies of Paget's disease have shown, with double tetra-

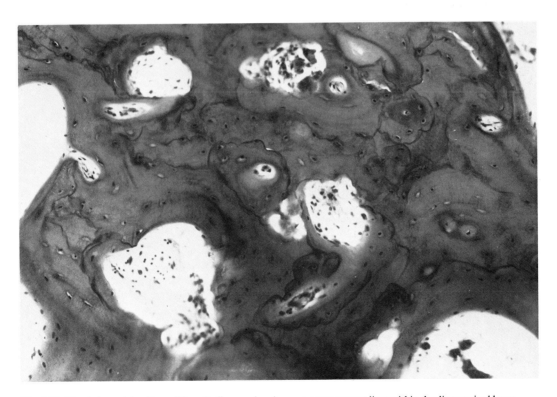

Fig. 6.12. Classic 'mosaic' pattern of Paget's disease, showing numerous cement lines within the disorganised bone. There is persistence of some cellular activity, shown by osteoclastic resorption (*top, centre*). (H&E × 640)

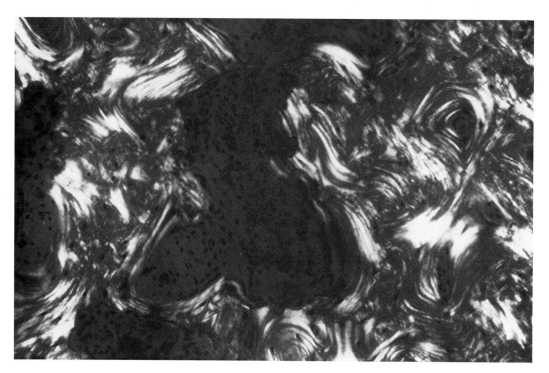

Fig. 6.13. Disorganised arrangement of collagen fibre lamellar pattern in Paget's disease, as viewed by polarisation microscopy. (Partially crossed polars, H&E × 640)

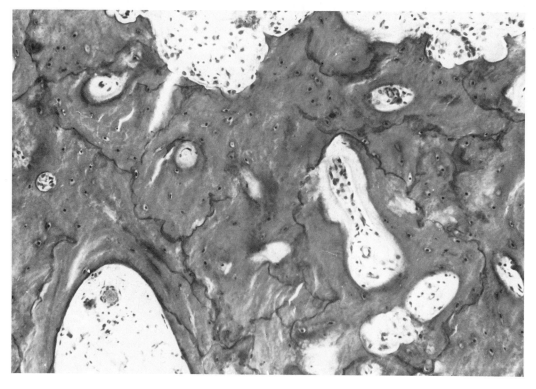

Fig. 6.14. Paget's disease in the inactive phase, showing dense bone with mosaic pattern and bone surfaces lacking cellular activity. (H&E × 640)

cycline labelling studies, that the increased density of bone results from over-production of bone by osteoblasts. Increased bone cell populations appear as a result of increased 'birth rate' of basic multicellular units (Lee 1967; Bordier et al. 1972; Meunier et al. 1980). Osteoblastic surfaces were found to be much increased by Bordier et al. (1972) and Guncaga et al. (1974) and give rise to increased osteoid volume and osteoid surface in Pagetic bone (Meunier et al. 1980). The calcification rate is nearly twice normal at a mean value of 1.36 μm/day, according to Meunier et al. (1980). There is a significant increase in trabecular resorption surfaces and periosteocytic enlargement (Belanger et al. 1968; Duriez et al. 1968), though this almost certainly reflects the difference between woven and lamellar bone rather than periosteocytic osteolysis (see Chap. 1, Osteocytes). A number of studies have appeared, and will continue to do so, in which the efficacy of particular forms of drug therapy for Paget's disease is assessed using histomorphometric methods. The potential hazards inherent in assessing a focal disease with variable appearances depending on the phase of activity as compared with evaluating a generalised bone disease should be self evident.

Aetiology

It is usual to discuss the aetiology of a disease near the beginning of a description, and even where the cause of a disease is unknown, as it is in Paget's disease, this is stated early in the account. It seems, however, more appropriate to mention aetiology at this point, since there is some evidence to suggest that Paget's disease may be related to viral infection and much of the evidence for this stems from the ultrastructural studies outlined below. Other aspects of relevance to this idea include the geographical distribution of the disease and the clustering of cases in families (see p. 147). In this connection, Sofaer et al. (1983) have examined the family histories of over 400 Pagetic patients and shown that the prevalence in parents and siblings is ten times higher than it is in the parents and siblings of spouses, thus indicating a possible genetic element. An alternative explanation is, of course, that exposure to a widespread environmental agent such as a virus early in life could be shared by families but not necessarily by other families (such as 'in-laws').

Onset of Paget's disease before the age of 40 years is exceptional and this is considered to be consistent with a long latent period following initial infection with the putative agent, a slow virus. Parallels are drawn with subacute sclerosing panencephalitis. Other possible causes for Paget's disease are outlined by Singer and Mills (1983). Included for consideration are an inborn error of connective tissue biosynthesis, hormonal dysfunction, autoimmune disease, vascular disorder and neoplastic disorder, should the viral theory of aetiology prove finally untenable.

Ultrastructural studies

Ultrastructural studies of bone cells in a large number of patients with Paget's disease have shown the presence of characteristic intranuclear and cytoplasmic inclusions in osteoclasts (Rebel et al. 1974; Mills and Singer 1976; Schulz et al. 1977; Gherardi et al. 1980; Rebel et al. 1980; Mills 1981; Harvey et al. 1982). The ultrastructural appearances of osteoblasts and osteoclasts in Paget's disease are described by Rebel et al. (1980), while a review of the evidence for a viral aetiology is provided by Singer and Mills (1983).

The inclusions found in osteoclasts are most often intranuclear and comprise randomly orientated bundles of microfilaments, about 15 nm in cross section, which on higher magnification are shown to be tubular structures and are hence also called microcylinders (Mills and Singer 1976; Rebel et al. 1974, 1980). The nuclear inclusions are sometimes arranged as a spherical or ovoid inclusion and sometimes have a paracrystalline organisation. Each microcylinder has an electron-lucent centre surrounded by 5-nm diameter dense peripheral globular structures and there is a longitudinal 5 nm periodicity (Rebel et al. 1980; Fig. 6.15). Intracytoplasmic inclusions have basically identical appearances. These inclusions are not like any known cell organelle in appearance and are not present in the osteoblasts of Pagetic bone, the ultrastructural appearances of which are described by Rebel et al. (1980). Such

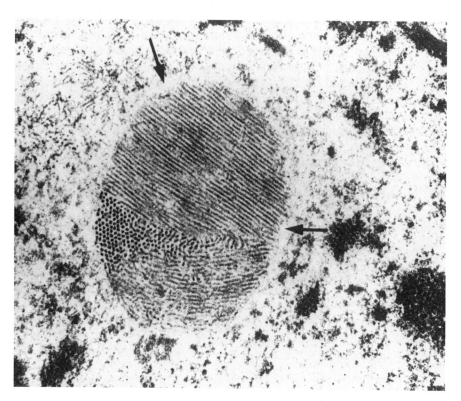

Fig. 6.15. Electron microscopic appearance of an osteoclast nucleus, showing an intranuclear inclusion with a paracrystalline organisation surrounded by a clear space (*arrows*) which separates it from the rest of the nucleoplasm. (× 35 000)

inclusions have been described in the osteoclasts of giant cell tumours of bone and in mononuclear cells of a Paget's sarcoma (Le Charpentier et al. 1977; Mills 1981; Mirra et al. 1981; Viola et al. 1982).

The similarity of the inclusions to nucleocapsids of paramyxoviruses has been noted, and parallels with subacute sclerosing panencephalitis (SSPE) and measles virus have been drawn (Mills and Singer 1976), although the resemblance of the inclusions to respiratory syncytial virus (RSV) has also been noted (Gherardi et al. 1980). Further careful analysis and measurement of the features of the possible nucleocapsids in Paget's osteoclasts showed these to be indistinguishable from RSV and different from measles virus (Howatson and Fornasier 1982).

However, RSV-infected cells did not contain intranuclear nucleocapsids, whereas measles virus inclusions are normally present in both nucleus and cytoplasm. Immunofluorescence and immunoperoxidase techniques have been applied and evidence given for the presence of measles virus antigens in osteoclasts of Paget's disease using rabbit antisera and sera from SSPE patients (Rebel et al. 1980). Mills and her colleagues (1980, 1981) showed the presence of intracytoplasmic RSV antigens and subsequently, using serial sections, showed that both measles and RSV antigens were demonstrable in the same osteoclasts (Mills et al. 1982). Raised antibody levels against measles in the peripheral blood have not been demonstrated (Morgan-Capner et al. 1981; Winfield and Sutherland 1981), and cell culture studies have so far been unsuccessful in demonstrating inclusions by electron microscopy in long-term cultures; however co-culture experiments with Hep-2 cells have shown the presence of RSV in the latter, which is evidence for passage of virus (Singer and Mills 1983). The question of whether Paget's disease is due to a slow virus infection must remain open for the time being. Present evidence suggests that if this is the case, paramyxoviruses are involved and that there may either be a mixed infection, as yet undetected, shared antigenic properties between measles virus and RSV, or a separate virus for Paget's disease which has yet to be discovered. The results available at present do not amount to a fully coherent picture, and it has been pointed out that any helical structure of dimensions similar to those under discussion will resemble the paramyxovirus nucleoprotein helix by electron microscopy (Editorial 1982).

References

Altman RD (1980) Musculoskeletal manifestations of Paget's disease of bone. Arthritis Rheum 23:1121–1127

Barker DJP, Clough PWL, Guyer PB, Gardner MJ (1977) Paget's disease of bone in 14 British towns. Br Med J I:1181–1183

Barker DJP, Chamberlain AT, Guyer PB, Gardner MJ (1980) Paget's disease of bone: the Lancashire focus. Br Med J I:1105–1107

Barry HC (1969) Paget's disease of bone. Williams and Wilkins, Baltimore

Barry HC (1980) Orthopedic aspects of Paget's disease of bone. Arthritis Rheum 23:1128–1130

Belanger LF, Jarry L, Uthoff HK (1968) Osteocytic osteolysis in Paget's disease. Rev Can Biol Exp 27:37–44

Bordier P, Woodhouse NHY, Joplin GF, Tunchot S (1972) Quantitative bone histology in Paget's disease. J Bone Joint Surg [Br] 54:553–554

Coley BL, Sharp GS (1931) Paget's disease: a predisposing factor to osteogenic sarcoma. Arch Surg 23:918–936

Collins DH (1966) Pathology of bone. Butterworths, London

Culebras A, Feldman RG, Fager C (1974) Hydrocephalus and dementia in Paget's disease of the skull.

J Neurol Sci 23:307–321

Dahlin DC (1978) Bone tumors, general aspects and data on 6221 cases, 3rd edn. Thomas, Springfield, Ill

Dahlin DC, Unni KK (1977) Osteosarcoma of bone and its important recognizable varieties. Am J Surg Pathol 1:61–72

Detheridge FM, Guyer PB, Baker DJP (1982) European distribution of Paget's disease of bone. Br Med J 285:1005–1008

Dorfman HD (1973) Malignant transformation of benign bone lesions. Proc Natl Cancer Conf 7:901–913

Duriez J, Flautre B, Ghosez JP (1968) Etude microscopique du tissu osseux pagetique. Presse Med 76:431–434

Edholm OG, Howarth S (1953) Studies on the peripheral circulation in osteitis deformans. Clin Sci 12:277–285

Edholm OG, Howarth S, McMichael J (1945) Heart failure and bone blood flow in osteitis deformans. Clin Sci 5:249–260

Editorial (1982) Viruses and Paget's disease of bone. Lancet II:1198–1199

Feldman RG, Culebras A, Schmideck HH (1979) Paget's disease and the nervous system. J Am Geriatr Soc 27:1–8

Franck WA, Bress NM, Singer FR, Krane SM (1974) Rheumatic manifestations of Paget's disease of bone. Am J Med 56:592–603

Gherardi G, Lo Cascio V, Bonucci E (1980) Fine structure of nuclei and cytoplasm of osteoclasts in Paget's disease of bone. Histopathology 4:63–74

Goldenberg RR (1951) The skull in Paget's disease. J Bone Joint Surg [Am] 33:911–922

Golding C (1960) Museum pages IV on the differential diagnosis of Paget's disease. J Bone Joint Surg [Br] 42:641–643

Guncaga J, Lauffenburger T, Lentner C, Dambacher MA, Haas HG, Fleisch H, Olah AJ (1974) Diphosphonate treatment of Paget's disease of bone. Horm Metab Res 6:62–69

Guyer PB (1979) The clinical relevance of radiologically revealed Paget's disease of bone (osteitis deformans). Br J Surg 66:438–443

Guyer PB, Dewbury KC (1978) The hip joint in Paget's disease (Paget's "Coxopathy"). Br J Radiol 51:574–578

Harvey L, Gray T, Beneton MNC, Douglas DL, Kanis JA, Russell RGG (1982) Ultrastructural features of the osteoclasts from Paget's disease of bone in relation to a viral aetiology. J Clin Pathol 35:771–779

Heistad DD, Abbond FM, Schmid PG, Mark AL, Wilson WR (1975) Regulation of blood flow in Paget's disease of bone. J Clin Invest 55:69–74

Howatson AF, Fornasier VL (1982) Microfilaments associated with Paget's disease of bone. Comparison with nucleocapsids of measles virus and respiratory syncytial virus. Intervirology 18:150–159

Huvos AG, Butler A, Bretsky SS (1983) Osteogenic sarcoma associated with Paget's disease of bone. A clinicopathologic study of 65 patients. Cancer 52:1489–1495

Jaffe HL (1972) Metabolic, degenerative and inflammatory diseases of bones and joints. Lea and Febiger, Philadelphia

Jaffe HL (1977) The classic Paget's disease of bone. Clin Orthop 127:4–23

Kivirikko KI (1970) Urinary excretion of hydroxyproline in health and disease. Int Rev Connect Tissue Res 5:93–163

Krane SM (1977) Paget's disease of bone. Clin Orthop 127:24–36

Le Charpentier Y, Le Charpentier M, Forest M, Daudet-Monsac M, Lavenu-Vacher MC, Louvel A, Sedel L, Abelanet R (1977) Inclusions intranucléaires dans une tumeur osseuse à cellules giantes. Mis en évidence au microscope électronique. Nouv Presse Med 6:259–262

Lee WR (1967) Bone formation in Paget's disease: a quantitative microscopic study using tetracycline marks. J Bone Joint Surg [Br] 49:146–153

Lindsay JR (1976) Paget's disease and sensorineural deafness. Laryngoscope 86:1029–1042

McKenna RJ, Schwinn CP, Soonj KY, Higginbotham NL (1964) Osteogenic sarcoma arising in Paget's disease. Cancer 17:42–66

McKusick VA (1972) Heritable disorders of connective tissue. Mosby, St Louis

Meunier PJ, Coindre JM, Edouard CM, Arlot ME (1980) Bone histomorphometry in Paget's disease. Quantitative and dynamic analysis of Pagetic and non-Pagetic bone tissue. Arthritis Rheum 23:1095–1103

Milgram JW (1977) Radiographical and pathological assessment of the activity of Paget's disease of bone. Clin Orthop 127:43–54

Mills BG (1981) Comparison of the ultrastructure of a malignant tumor of the mandible containing giant cells with Paget's disease of bone. J Oral Pathol 10:203–215

Mills BG, Singer FR (1976) Nuclear inclusions in Paget's disease of bone. Science 194:201–202

Mills BG, Singer FR, Weiner LP, Holst PA (1980) Cell cultures from bone affected by Paget's disease. Arthritis Rheum 23:1115–1120

Mills BG, Singer FR, Weiner LP, Holst PA (1981) Immunohistological demonstration of respiratory syncytial viral antigens in Paget's disease of bone. Proc Natl Acad Sci USA 78:1209–1231

Mills BG, Stabile E, Holst PA, Graham C (1982) Antigens to two different viruses in Paget's disease of bone. J Dent Res 61:347

Mirra JM, Bauer FCH, Grant TT (1981) Giant cell tumor with viral-like intranuclear inclusions associated with Paget's disease. Clin Orthop 158:243–251

Morgan-Capner P, Robinson P, Clewley G, Darby A, Pattingale K (1981) Measles antibody in Paget's disease. Lancet II: 733

Nagent de Deuxchaisnes C, Krane SM (1964) Paget's disease of bone: clinical and metabolic observations. Medicine (Baltimore) 43: 233–266

Paget J (1877) On a form of chronic inflammation of bones (osteitis deformans). Med Chir Trans 60: 37–64

Poretta CA, Dahlin DC, Janes JM (1957) Sarcoma in Paget's disease of bone. J Bone Joint Surg [Am] 39: 1314–1329

Rebel A, Malkani K, Basle M (1974) Anomalies nucléaires des ostéoclastes de la maladie de Paget. Nouv Presse Med 3: 1299–1301

Rebel A, Basle M, Pouplard A, Malkani K, Filmon R, Lepatezour A (1980) Bone tissue in Paget's disease of bone. Ultrastructure and immunocytology. Arthritis Rheum 23: 1104–1114

Reich C, Brodsky AE (1948) Coexisting multiple myeloma and Paget's disease of bone treated with stilbamidine. J Bone Joint Surg [Am] 30: 642–646

Rhodes BA, Greyson ND, Hamilton CR, White RI, Garghiana FA, Wagner HM (1972) Absence of anatomic arteriovenous shunts in Paget's disease of bone. N Engl J Med 287: 686–689

Rosenbaum HD, Hanson DJ (1969) Geographic variation in the prevalence of Paget's disease of bone. Radiology 92: 959–963

Schajowicz F, Araujo ES, Berenstein M (1983) Sarcoma complicating Paget's disease of bone. A clinicopathological study of 62 cases. J Bone Joint Surg [Br] 65: 299–307

Schmidek HH (1977) Neurologic and neurosurgical sequelae of Paget's disease of bone. Clin Orthop 127: 70–77

Schmorl G (1932) Uber Ostitis deformans Paget. Virchows Arch [Pathol Anat] 283: 694–751

Schulz A, Delling G, Ringe JD, Ziegler R (1977) Morbus Paget des Knochens. Untersuchungen zur Ultrastrukter der Osteoclasten und ihrer Cytopathogenese. Virchows Arch [Pathol Anat] 376: 309–328

Schwinn CP, McKenna RJ (1973) The biologic behaviour of osteosarcoma. Proc Natl Cancer Conf 7: 925–939

Shannon FT, Hopkins JS (1977) Paget's sarcoma of the vertebral column with neurological complications. Acta Orthop Scand 48: 385–390

Simon L, Blotman F, Seignalet J, Claustre J (1975) Étiologie de la maladie osseuse de Paget. Rev Rheum 42: 535–544

Singer FR, Mills BG (1983) Evidence for a viral etiology of Paget's disease of bone. Clin Orthop 178: 245–251

Sofaer JA, Holloway SM, Amery AEH (1983) A family study of Paget's disease of bone. J Epidemiol Community Health 37: 226–231

Spjut HJ, Dorfman HD, Fechner RE, Ackerman LV (1971) Tumors of bone and cartilage. In: Atlas of tumor pathology (fascicle 5) Armed Forces Institute of Pathology, Washington DC

Storsteen KA, Jones JM (1954) Arteriography and vascular studies in Paget's disease of bone. J Am Med Sci 154: 472–474

Taurel J-P, Fages A, Amouroux J, de Sèze S, Kahn M-F (1973) Dégénerescence sarcomateuse d'une atteinte Pagétique de rachis cervical révélation par un syndrome de Pancoast et Tobias. Rev Rhum Mal Osteoartic 40: 145–148

Thompson JB, Patterson RH Jr, Parsons H (1970) Sarcomas of the calvaria: surgical experience with 14 patients. J Neurosurg 32: 534–538

Viola MV, Eilon G, Lazarus M (1982) Virus-like inclusions in osteosarcoma cells arising in Paget's disease. Lancet I: 848

Wellman HN, Schauwecker D, Robb JA, Khairi MR, Johnston CC (1977) Skeletal scintimaging and radiography in the diagnosis and management of Paget's disease. Clin Orthop 127: 55–62

Wick MR, McLeod RA, Siegal GP, Greditzer HG, Unni KK (1981) Sarcoma of bone complicating osteitis deformans (Paget's disease). Am J Surg Pathol 5: 47–59

Winfield J, Sutherland S (1981) Measles antibody in Paget's disease. Lancet I: 891

Woodhouse NJY (1972) Paget's disease of bone. Clin Endocrinol Metab 1: 125–141

Woodward HQ (1959) Long term studies of the blood chemistry in Paget's disease of bone. Cancer 12: 1226–1237

Chapter 7

Hyperostosis

Introduction

Hyperostosis is a term used to indicate an abnormal increase in the ossification of the skeleton, but not applicable to adaptive changes such as those in size and mass of bones related to increased mechanical work mentioned elsewhere (see Chap. 8, Physical activity). Osteosclerosis is, however, included with the term hyperostosis, being defined as an increase in bone density without alteration in the overall shape of the affected bone. Such a change is seen in renal osteodystrophy (Fig. 7.1) (see Chap. 5, Renal osteodystrophy). Osteosclerosis in relation to metastatic carcinoma, usually from the breast or prostate, is familiar, and the presence of appositional new bone about pre-existing trabeculae is easily recognised in biopsies submitted for the diagnosis of metastatic disease if the pathologist remembers the bone while looking at the bone marrow. Similar osteosclerosis may be present in association with myeloproliferative disorders, most notably myelosclerosis (Figs. 7.2, 7.3), and sufficient fibrosis of the marrow may occasionally occur in primary bone disease to cause depressed marrow function. New bone formation occurs in relation to inflammation in chronic osteomyelitis, and sclerosis around a focus of infection with development of a Brodie's abscess is discussed briefly elsewhere [see Chap. 10, Pathology of osteomyelitis; Chronic bone abscess (Brodie's abscess)]. Finally, Paget's disease of bone shows the radiological appearance of increased thickness and density of the affected parts of the skeleton and histologically shows evidence of excessive osteoblastic activity as well as increased bone resorption (see Chap. 6, Radiological appearances; Morbid anatomy and histopathology).

The aim of the present short chapter is to describe briefly a few other conditions which have not been included in other parts of this book. Some are common, some obscure and there are many others which cannot be included here.

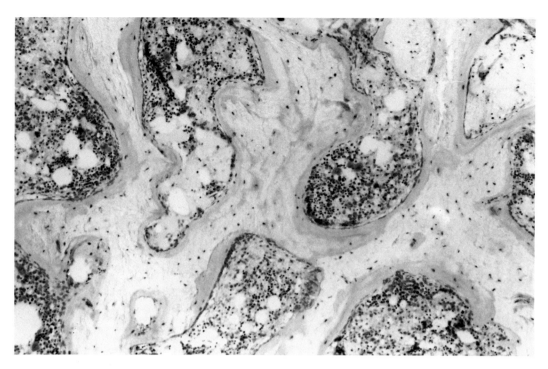

Fig. 7.1. Osteosclerosis in renal osteodystrophy. The amount of bone compared with that of total tissue is much greater than normal. There are wide osteoid seams with some active osteoblastic surfaces. (Methylmethacrylate, thionin × 250)

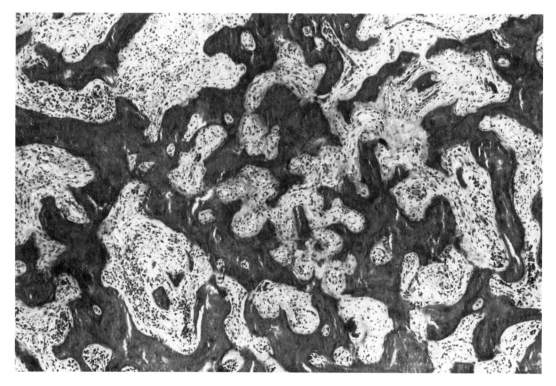

Fig. 7.2. Osteosclerosis occurring in association with myelofibrosis. (Methylmethacrylate, H&E × 250)

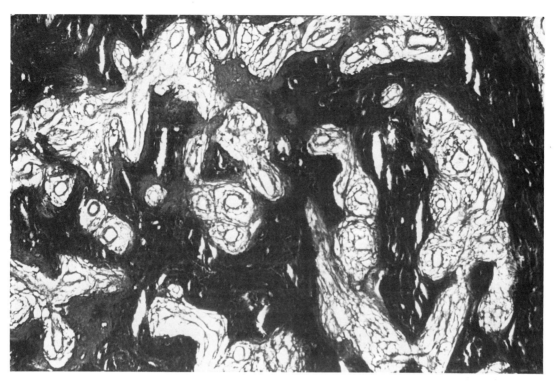

Fig. 7.3. Myelofibrosis with thickening of the adjacent bone trabeculae. The increased reticulin content of the bone marrow space is well marked (same case as Fig. 7.2). (Reticulin × 250)

Ankylosing hyperostosis of the spine (diffuse idiopathic skeletal hyperostosis)

An unusual type of ossification of the vertebral column in middle-aged and elderly patients was described by Forestier and Rotes-Querol (1950). The pathology of this condition has been described by Forestier and Lagier (1971), Vernon-Roberts and his colleagues (1974) and Revell and Pirie (1981), among others. Although initially considered a disorder of the thoracic spine, there is evidence that other levels of the spine are affected (Hukuda et al. 1981) and that spinal involvement is part of a generalised skeletal condition for which the term 'diffuse idiopathic skeletal hyperostosis' (DISH) has been used (Resnick et al. 1975; Resnick and Niwayana 1976). The main sites of hyperostosis apart from the spine are at points of ligament and tendon attachment to bone, for example the iliac crest (Fig. 7.4), ischial tuberosities, trochanters, linea aspera, calcaneus, patella, and as para-articular bony overgrowths, the development of which may interfere with the function of prosthetic joint replacements (Mazieres et al. 1981). Similar changes have been described in various animals ranging from fish through reptiles to mammals (but not birds; Lagier, 1979) and are reviewed by Desse et al. (1981).

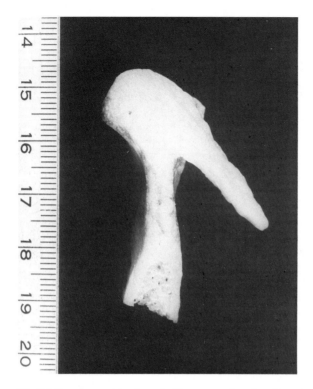

Fig. 7.4. Bony spur arising from the iliac crest at the point of attachment of a tendon (diffuse idiopathic skeletal hyperostosis)

In humans, the main spinal changes are to be found in the thoracic region, where there are typical bony overgrowths on the anterolateral surfaces of the vertebral bodies, mostly on the right side. The intervertebral discs are characteristically of normal thickness and the adjacent vertebral bodies may be joined by complete bony ridges across the disc margins (Fig. 7.5), or alternatively there may be bony outgrowths which extend from the margins of adjacent vertebral bodies to form parrot beak-like or so-called kissing osteophytes (Fig. 7.6). The overall naked eye appearance of the ossification resembles that which would be produced by the setting of melted wax flowing down the side of the vertebral column. Curiously, although there is marked hyperostosis of the edges of the vertebrae, the vertebral bodies themselves are osteoporotic, as has been shown by histomorphometry (Revell and Pirie 1981). Ankylosing hyperostosis is present in around 10% of all autopsies and must be differentiated pathologically from ankylosing spondylitis, the spinal changes of psoriatic arthritis and Reiter's syndrome, spondylosis deformans, fluorosis, ochronosis and acromegaly.

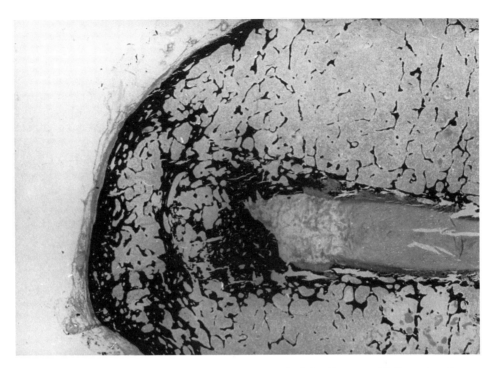

Fig. 7.5. Ankylosing hyperostosis of the spine (diffuse idiopathic skeletal hyperostosis). Formation of a complete bridge of sclerotic bone across the anterolateral margin of an intervertebral disc between two vertical bodies. This disc is normal in thickness. (Methylmethacrylate, von Kossa × 4)

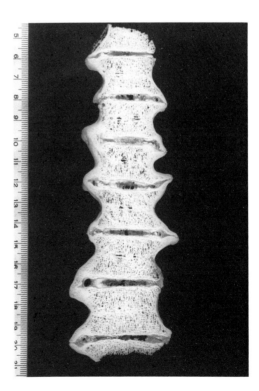

Fig. 7.6. Coronal slice of lower thoracic spine showing the presence of parrot-beak or kissing osteophytes and complete bony bridges across the disc margins. (Macerated specimen)

Hyperostosis frontalis interna

Hyperostosis frontalis interna is a common affection of the skull found to some degree or other in a little under half of post-menopausal women at autopsy and virtually never seen in males. There is abnormal thickening of the frontal bone, seen as increased radiopacity on the skull radiograph, in which the inner surface of the skull is irregular and knobbly. Macroscopic examination shows a bosselated outline to the inner surface of the front of the skull, which is due to the presence of numerous conjoined bony outgrowths (Figs. 7.7, 7.8) arising from the inner table, but converted to spongy bone on the deep aspect where attached to the underlying calvaria (Jaffe 1972). It is usually possible to discern the line of attachment by the pattern of residual bone (Collins 1966). Hyperostosis frontalis interna is associated with obesity and evidence of virilism, for example facial hirsuties, so that the question of a hormonal background to the disorder has been raised. Since the condition has minimal clinical significance, it seems doubtful that it will ever attract much attention in the way of deeper investigation. The appearance of similar outgrowths in pregnancy is mentioned briefly by Jaffe, who calls them 'pregnancy osteophytes'. They disappear at the end of pregnancy.

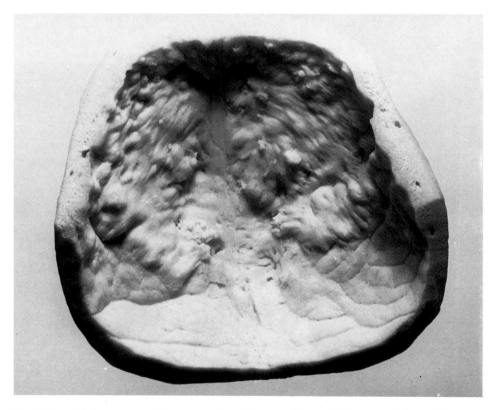

Fig. 7.7. Bosselated appearance of the inner surface of the front of the skull in hyperostosis frontalis interna

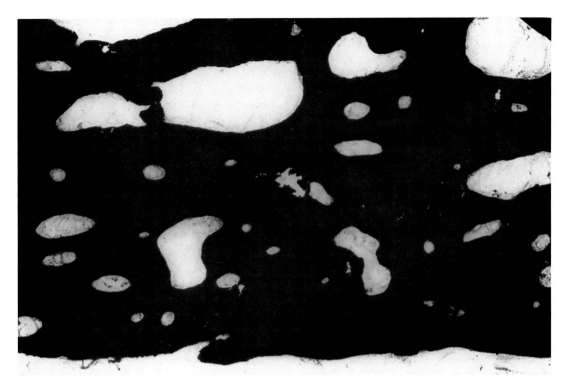

Fig. 7.8. Bone of greatly increased density from the inner aspect of the skull in hyperostosis frontalis interna. (Methylmethacrylate, von Kossa × 60)

Melorheostosis

Melorheostosis is a condition described originally by Leri (Leri and Joanny 1922), who derived its name from the Greek words meaning limb (*melos*) and flow or stream (*rheos*). The allusion to melting wax dropping down the side of a candle has already been made in connection with ankylosing hyperostosis of the spine, and this idea of flowing hyperostosis related to limb bones summarises the changes of melorheostosis. There are now numerous reports of the condition in the literature, and sources of references to these cases are to be found in the book by Beighton and Cremin (1980) and the review by Campbell et al. (1968), the latter also providing a description of further cases. Melorheostosis in children is considered separately by Younge et al. (1979).

This bone condition often presents in late childhood and, although it may be a chance radiographic finding, may cause skeletal pain and limb deformity, with development of discrepancies in lengths of limbs and secondary deformities like scoliosis and genu valgum. Pain is more of a feature in adults than in small children (Younge et al. 1979). The skin overlying the affected bone is thickened or indurated and there is erythema. Fibrous thickening of subcutaneous tissues and muscles and the development of contractures may occur.

Pathological fractures or malignant change in the involved bones have not been described. Results of laboratory tests, including those for serum calcium, phosphorus and alkaline phosphatase, have been within normal limits. The aetiology of the condition is unknown. There is no evidence of a familial or hereditary basis and the sexes appear to be affected equally frequently (Campbell et al. 1968).

Melorheostosis can affect any bone in the body; however, the skull, spine and ribs are least commonly and the long bones most frequently, involved. A single bone (monostotic) or limb (monomelic) may show changes, but there may be more widespread involvement affecting several limbs and bones, or skipping of the bones of one segment in an involved limb. Radiological examination shows thickening and increased density along the medullary (endosteal) surface of the affected bone with encroachment into the medullary cavity, and this pattern has been described by Younge et al. (1979) as a particular feature of childhood melorheostosis. The usual pattern of hyperostosis in adults is subperiosteal or extracortical. The morbid anatomical appearances have been described by Klümper and colleagues (1965) and showed thickening of cortical and trabecular bone, narrowing of the medullary space and the presence of islands of bone in the spongiosa in epiphyseal areas. There are well over 30 descriptions of histological features in separate cases in the literature, and references are available in Campbell et al. (1968). The histological appearances are those of hyperostotic bone and similar to those seen in other conditions like osteopoikilosis. There is membranous ossification and formation of thickened laminae of bone which may almost obliterate the Haversian systems of cortical bone. Osteoclastic activity is not marked, though it is present, and the formation of cartilage, when present, is confined to the end of the bones. The distribution of the osteosclerotic foci is the main point of differentiation from other conditions. Differentiation from osteopoikilosis has been discussed by Green et al. (1962), and this paper gives useful summary descriptions of both conditions.

Osteopoikilosis

Osteopoikilosis (Gk. *osteo+poikilos*, dappled, spotted + -*osis*, condition; spotted bones) is usually clinically silent and is a benign condition in which there are numerous sclerotic lesions in the bones discovered incidentally at radiological examination. There are descriptions of the radiology and pathology in books by Beighton and Cremin (1980) and Jaffe (1972), while a review of literature is provided by Szabo (1971). Skin changes are present in some cases and, although they are variable, the most common lesions are small lentil-sized firm yellowish nodules in the skin and subcutaneous tissue, regarded as analogous to dermatofibrosis lenticularis disseminata. Osteopoikilosis is inherited as an autosomal dominant condition but also occurs as sporadic cases. The lesions, once discovered, usually remain static, although increase in size and disappearance have both been described. The presence of osteosarcoma of the tibia in a subject of osteopoikilosis has been reported (Mindell et al. 1978), but this is the only case of its kind.

Radiological examination shows numerous discrete opacities measuring 5–50 mm in diameter, mainly in the epiphyseal and metaphyseal regions of affected limb bones, which are themselves normal in outline. The diaphysis is spared. Although the small bones of the wrist and ankle and the pelvis may be involved, the skull, mandible, spine and rib cage are not affected (Beighton and Cremin 1980). Gross morbid anatomical examination shows numerous small foci of compact bone within the cancellum, situated centrally in the epiphysis and peripherally in the metaphysis, according to Jaffe (1972), while histological examination shows discrete foci of compact bone in continuity with the trabecular bone of the medullary cavity. The appearances are illustrated by Jaffe (1972) and summarised in the review by Szabo (1971). Although osteopoikilosis has been considered of little clinical significance, there have been a few reports of coexistent abnormalities, which have included coarctation of the aorta, double ureter, endocrine abnormalities, arthritides, exostoses, facial and dental anomalies, including hare lip and cleft palate, as well as the skin abnormalities already mentioned (see Szabo 1971). Weisz (1982) has recently described a case of osteopoikilosis in which there was stenosis of the lumbar spinal canal.

Other sclerosing disorders of bone

There are several other well-recognised disorders of bone in which there is sclerosis, including osteopathia striata, endosteal hyperostosis, sclerosteosis and infantile cortical hyperostosis. These will be mentioned only briefly here, but further information can be obtained from sources such as the books by Beighton and Cremin (Beighton 1978; Beighton and Cremin 1980).

Osteopathia striata

'Osteopathia striata' is a term which may be used to describe the radiological appearance of bone striation which can be seen in various conditions including osteopetrosis, osteopoikilosis, melorheostosis, and even the effects of rubella and syphilis on the fetal skeleton. Some subjects with striated bone also have cranial sclerosis with increased head circumference, frontal bossing and hearing loss, and this condition may be considered separately as the osteopathia striata/cranial stenosis complex. Apart from sclerotic changes in the skull, there may be spinal deformity with scoliosis and lumbar spondylosis, fan-shaped striations in the iliac bones and vertical striations in the ends of long bones, most notably the lower and upper femur and upper tibia.

Endosteal hyperostosis

Endosteal hyperostosis is a condition divisible on genetic grounds into two (dominant and recessive) types, which are nevertheless difficult or impossible to differentiate on a clinical or radiological basis. There is progressive asymmetrical enlargement of the mandible, which starts in late childhood, with sclerosis of the skull and thickening of the cortex of the diaphyseal part of long bones as a result of endosteal hyperostosis. Intellect and habitus are normal and general health good. Cranial nerve involvement occurs more often in the recessive (van Buchen) form than in the dominant (Worth) form of the condition.

Sclerosteosis

Sclerosteosis was considered at the time of its first description to be a variant of osteopetrosis in which there was syndactyly (Truswell 1958). Mandibular prognathism and prominence of the frontal bone become obvious by the age of 5 years, and in adulthood the progression of the changes leads to severe facial deformity, dental malocclusion and proptosis. Children are taller than normal; adults may show gigantism. Most subjects have partial or total syndactyly of the second and third fingers. Seventh nerve palsy and deafness resulting from auditory nerve and middle ear encroachment occur, and optic nerve compression is present in varying degrees. The cranial cavity decreases in capacity because of thickening of the calvaria, headaches developing because of raised intracranial pressure. Death sometimes results from impaction of the medulla oblongata in the foramen magnum.

The hyperostosis, which can be seen radiologically in the skull, spine, ribs, scapulae, pelvis and limb bones, progresses until late in the third decade, when the condition no longer changes. The cortices of long bones are sclerotic but are undermodelled in the mid-shaft region, in contrast to endosteal hyperostosis in which normal diaphyseal narrowing of the bone outline occurs (Beighton et al. 1976). Only small numbers of cases of either condition have been described in the literature.

Infantile cortical hyperostosis

Infantile cortical hyperostosis (Caffey disease; Caffey 1946, 1957) is a condition which usually presents in the first few months of life and later completely regresses, although there is a rarer 'juvenile' form which has a longer time course. There is hyperostosis of the skull, limb girdles and limb bones and soft tissue swellings are also present together with pyrexia (leucocytosis) and a raised erythrocyte sedimentation rate. Subperiosteal enlargement of the cortices of long bones is asymmetrical and uneven within the same limb, while involvement of the scapula and clavicle is common and often one-sided. In the skull, the mandible has a thickened ground-glass appearance after about 3 weeks of involvement, but before this time overlying soft tissue swellings may obscure the radiographic changes.

The resolution of the bone changes as observed in radiographs occurs by gradual compaction and thinning of the hyperostotic bone as it becomes incorporated into the cortex and by the conversion of related cortex to more porous bone (Jaffe 1972). The result is that the marrow cavity is widened in the region of the lesion. Histological appearances of the bone vary with the stage of the disease. In the early stage, there is an acute inflammatory cell subperiosteal infiltrate with periosteal proliferation to form new bone. Related muscle and connective tissues are also inflamed. Later, the periosteum is thickened, fibrotic and has beneath it a layer of coarse bone trabeculae with vascular connective tissue in the intertrabecular spaces. The appearances are illustrated by Jaffe (1972). The aetiology of the condition is unknown, but infection, allergy, damage to the fetus and genetic factors have all been suggested.

Fluorosis

Prolonged exposure to fluoride results in its deposition in skeletal tissues with alterations in bone structure. Ingestion of fluoride may be due to industrial exposure or because of therapeutic administration, for example in the treatment of osteoporosis.

Industrial fluorosis has been reported as occurring in certain aluminium plants in Switzerland in which workers in electrolysis rooms with open furnaces are exposed to fluoride (Boillat et al. 1976; Baud et al. 1978), and advanced cases of the disease have been described in the cryolite industry (Möller and Gudjonsson 1932). Endemic fluorosis, caused by industrial exposure or water supplies with a high fluorine content, results in coarsening and thickening of bones seen at radiological examination. The changes occurring after administration of fluoride in osteoporosis are similar but less pronounced (Lagier 1978). Macroscopically, the skeleton is thickened in fluorosis, with the development of periosteal sleeves of new osseous tissue surrounding bones and ossification at ligament and tendon insertions (Singh et al. 1962; Aggarwal 1973; Weatherall and Weidmann 1959) with the formation of bony spurs. There is cancellisation of the cortex despite this new bone being deposited on the surface (Aggarwal 1973). Bridging across the edge of intervertebral discs, which are themselves normal in thickness, together with the development of exostosis, gives appearances which somewhat resemble diffuse idiopathic skeletal hyperostosis (see p. 171).

Light microscopic examination shows increased bone remodelling activity with increased trabecular bone volume, cortical porosity, osteoid volume and surface and osteoclastic resorptive activity (Rich et al. 1964; Faccini 1969; Faccini and Teotia 1974; Baud et al. 1978; Lagier 1978; Vigorita and Suda 1983). The bone may come to have a Pagetoid appearance (Lagier 1977; Fig. 7.9), although the surface of the trabeculae showing appositional new bone or osteoid may be smooth and not crenated at the cement lines, suggesting direct appositional new bone deposition without previous resorption (Vigorita and Suda 1983). Areas of unmineralised bone matrix within the bone trabeculae have been noted and termed 'osteoid lakes' by these authors. The periosteocytic lacunae become mottled or enlarged when seen in microradiographs and show evidence of periosteocytic osteolysis, according to Baud and Boivin (1978) and Baud et al. (1978).

The histological appearances present in fluorosis are non-specific, and ultimately diagnosis depends on demonstration of high bone fluoride content in the context of endemic disease (Baud et al. 1978).

There are increasing numbers of studies reporting the benefit of fluoride treatment in osteoporosis. Riggs et al. (1982) describe how significantly more effective the combination of fluoride, calcium and oestrogen was than any

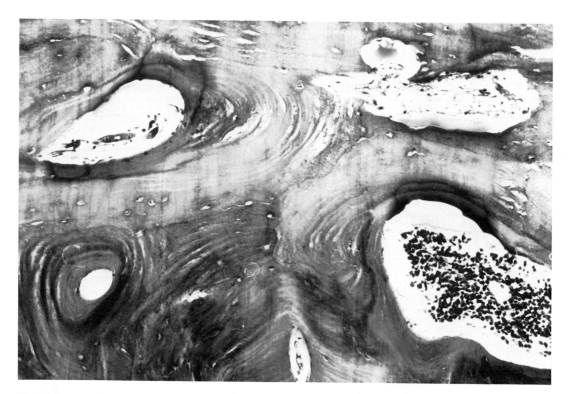

Fig. 7.9. Dense cortical bone of the tibia in fluorosis, showing Pagetoid appearance with numerous cement lines. (H&E × 160)

other treatment regimen in lowering the fracture rate among post-menopausal women. Quantitation of bone biopsies in osteoporotic patients treated with fluoride by Vigorita and Suda (1983) shows the differences described above, together with an increase in the number of enlarged osteocyte lacunae and the numbers of osteocytes. The significance of these changes and the existence of osteocytic osteolysis have been discussed elsewhere (see Chap. 1, Osteocytes).

Hypertrophic osteoarthropathy

Hypertrophic osteoarthropathy occurs in association with the same conditions as are related to clubbing of the fingers and toes. It is much less common than clubbing but usually associated with the latter, though this is not always the case. Hypertrophic osteoarthropathy is most often found in chronic pulmonary disease, carcinoma of the lung, pulmonary fibrosis, bronchiectasis and other lung diseases, but also occurs in congenital cyanotic heart disease, some cases of cirrhosis, chronic gastrointestinal disorders and (most recently described) cystic fibrosis (Ray and Fisher 1953; Jaffe 1972; Braude et al. 1984). Radiological examination shows cortical thickening caused by periosteal new bone formation, which is most pronounced in the mid-shaft region rather than towards the ends of the affected bones. The radius and ulna and the tibia and fibula are the most commonly affected long bones, followed by the femur, humerus and small bones of the wrist and ankle. The bones of the trunk are usually spared, but in advanced cases the clavicle, ribs, scapula and vertebrae may be affected (Ray and Fisher 1953). Histological studies show proliferative subperiosteal osteitis surrounding the shaft of the affected bone, with a predominance of lymphocytes and plasma cells, proliferation of both soft tissue and bone, the latter from the inner layer of the periosteum. The periosteal new bone is laid down in layers, which are at first separate from the original cortex but later less easy to distinguish. Deposition of new bone on the endosteal surface does not occur (Gall et al. 1951; Jaffe 1972).

References

Aggarwal ND (1973) Structure of human fluorotic bone. J Bone Joint Surg [Am] 55:331–334

Baud C-A, Boivin G (1978) Modifications of the perilacunar walls resulting from the effect of fluoride on osteocytic activity. Metab Bone Dis Relat Res 1:49–54

Baud C-A, Lagier R, Boivin G, Boillat M-A (1978) Value of the bone biopsy in the diagnosis of industrial fluorosis. Virchows Arch [A] 380:283–297

Beighton P (1978) Inherited disorders of the skeleton. Churchill Livingstone, Edinburgh

Beighton P, Cremin BJ (1980) Sclerosing bone dysplasias. Springer, Berlin Heidelberg New York, Chap 17

Beighton P, Cremin B, Hamersma H (1976) The radiology of sclerosteosis. Br J Radiol 49:934–939

Braude S, Kennedy H, Hodson M, Batten J (1984) Hypertrophic osteoarthropathy in cystic fibrosis. Br Med J 288:822–823

Boillat M-A, Baud C-A, Lagier R, Donath A, Dettwiler W, Courvoisier B (1976) Fluorose industrielle. Schweiz Med Wochenschr 106: 1842–1844

Caffey J (1946) Infantile cortical hyperostosis. J Pediatr 29:541–559

Caffey J (1957) Infantile cortical hyperostosis; a review of the clinical and radiographic features. Proc R Soc Med 50:347–354

Campbell CJ, Papademetriou T, Bonfiglio M (1968) Melorheostosis. J Bone Joint Surg [Am] 50:1281–1304

Collins DH (1966) Pathology of bone. Butterworths, London

Desse G, Meunier P-J, Peron M, Laroche J (1981) Hyperostose vertebrale chez l'animal. Rhumatologie 33:105–119

Faccini JM (1969) Fluoride and bone. Calcif Tissue Res 2:1–16

Faccini JM, Teotia SPS (1974) Histopathological assessment of endemic skeletal fluorosis. Calcif Tissue Res 16:45–57

Forestier J, Lagier R (1971) Ankylosing hyperostosis of the spine. Clin Orthop 74:65–83

Forestier J, Rotes-Querol J (1950) Senile ankylosing hyperostosis of the spine. Ann Rheum Dis 9:321–330

Gall EA, Bennett GA, Bauer W (1951) Generalized hypertrophic osteoarthropathy; a pathologic study of seven cases. Am J Pathol 27:349–381

Green AE, Ellswood WH, Collins JR (1962) Melorheostosis and osteopoikilosis: with review of literature. Am J Roentgenol Radium Ther Nucl Med 87:1096–1111

Hukuda S, Shichikawa K, Mochizuki T, Ogata M (1981) Cervical hyperostosic myelopathy and its surgical treatment. Rhumatologie 33:81–88

Jaffe HL (1972) Metabolic, degenerative and inflammatory diseases of bones and joints. Lea and Febiger, Philadelphia

Klümper A, Wendt M, Weller S, Plötner E (1965) Entwicklung einer Melorheostose. Fortschr Geb Roentgenstr Nuklearmed Erganzungsband 103:572–583

Lagier R (1978) Effects of fluorine on bone morphology. In: Courvoisier B, Donath A, Baud CA (eds) Fluoride and bone: 2nd symposium CEMO. Hans Huber, Berne, pp 32–42

Lagier R (1979) L'hyperostose vertebrale en pathologie comparée. Schweiz Med Wochenschr 109:410–411

Leri A, Joanny J (1922) Une affection non décrite des os: hyperostose 'en coulée' sur toute la longueur d'un membre ou mélorheostose. Bull Soc Med Hop Paris 46:1141–1145

Mazieres B, Jacqueline F, Depeyre M, Arlet J (1981) Coxopathies hyperostosignes. Rhumatologie 33:57–63

Mindell ER, Northup CS, Douglass HO (1978) Osteosarcoma associated with osteopoikilosis: case report. J Bone Joint Surg [Am] 60:406–408

Möller PF, Gudjonsson Ste U (1932) Massive fluorosis of bones and ligaments. Acta Radiol 13:269–294

Ray ES, Fisher HP (1953) Hypertrophic osteoarthropathy in pulmonary malignancies. Ann Intern Med 38:239–246

Resnick D, Niwayama G (1976) Radiographic and pathologic features of spinal involvement in diffuse idiopathic skeletal hyperostosis (DISH). Radiology 119:559–568

Resnick D, Shaul SR, Robins JM (1975) Diffuse idiopathic skeletal hyperostosis (DISH): Forestier's disease with extraspinal manifestations. Radiology 115:513–524

Revell PA, Pirie CJ (1981) The histopathology of ankylosing hyperostosis of the spine. Rhumatologie 33: 99–104

Rich C, Ensinck J, Ivanovich F (1964) The effects of sodium fluoride on calcium metabolism of subjects with metabolic bone disease. J Clin Invest 43:545–555

Riggs BL, Seeman E, Hodgson SF, Taves DR, O'Fallon WM (1982) Effect of the fluoride/calcium regimen on vertebral fracture occurrence in post-menopausal osteoporosis. N Engl J Med 306:446–450

Singh A, Dass R, Hayreh SS, Jolly SS (1962) Skeletal changes in endemic fluorosis. J Bone Joint Surg [Br] 44:806–815

Szabo AD (1971) Osteopoikilosis in a twin. Clin Orthop 79:156

Truswell AS (1958) Osteopetrosis with syndactyly. A morphological variant of Albers-Schönberg disease. J Bone Joint Surg [Br] 40:208–218

Vernon-Roberts B, Pirie CJ, Trenwith V (1974) Pathology of the dorsal spine in ankylosing hyperostosis. Ann Rheum Dis 33:281–288

Vigorita VJ, Suda MK (1983) The microscopic morphology of fluoride-induced bone. Clin Orthop 177:274–282

Weatherall JA, Weidmann SM (1959) The skeletal changes of chronic experimental fluorosis. J Pathol Bacteriol 78:233–241

Weisz GM (1982) Lumbar spinal stenosis in osteopoikilosis. Clin Orthop 166:89–92

Younge D, Drummond D, Herring J, Cruess RL (1979) Melorheostosis in children. J Bone Joint Surg [Br] 61:415–418

Chapter 8

Osteoporosis and Bone Atrophy

Introduction

Although there has been a fairly clear understanding of what is meant by 'osteoporosis' for many years, there is some potential for confusion with the terms currently in use. Collins (1966) considered osteoporosis to be a generalised form of atrophy of bone, while reserving the actual term 'bone atrophy' for a more localised process, such as might occur in a paralysed limb. The term 'localised osteoporosis' is, however, frequently used to describe the changes in disused limbs or around severely arthritic joints. Sissons (1955) defined osteoporosis as a structural change in bone in which the supporting tissue is reduced in amount while remaining highly mineralised, and McLean and Urist (1961) thought in terms of increased bone porosity. The current general definition is of a disorder in which there is a diminution of bone mass without detectable differences from normal in the relative proportions of mineralised and non-mineralised matrix (Figs. 8.1, 8.2). Many workers prefer to use the term 'osteopenia' to describe this state of affairs and to reserve 'osteoporosis' for those cases of osteopenia in which there is actual or potential mechanical failure of bone. There is no general agreement as to the definition of either term and no difference in meaning is implied in the following account, though this might entail a more loose use of words than many would prefer.

Pathological definitions of osteoporosis are couched in terms referring to bone morphometry and related measurements of trabecular bone volume. Such definitions, however, vary somewhat from author to author. The concept of 'critical bone mass' has been developed by Meunier, who considers that patients with a trabecular bone volume of 11% or less have osteoporosis, in that they are more likely to have vertebral fractures at or below this fracture threshold (Courpron et al. 1976; Meunier et al. 1979). Osteoporosis has also been defined as being present in those patients having a bone mass more than two standard deviations below the mean found in healthy young adults, while others define osteoporosis in a similar way, as occurring below one or two standard deviations of the mean, but use the mean of age- and sex-matched

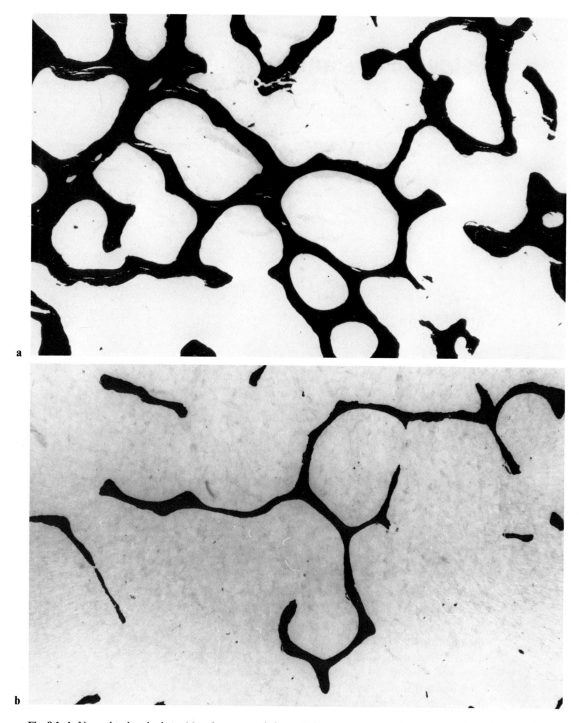

Fig. 8.1a,b. Normal trabecular bone (**a**) and osteoporotic bone (**b**) for comparison, the latter showing loss of some trabeculae and narrowing of others. Both photographs are reproduced at the same magnification. (Methylmethacrylate, von Kossa × 100)

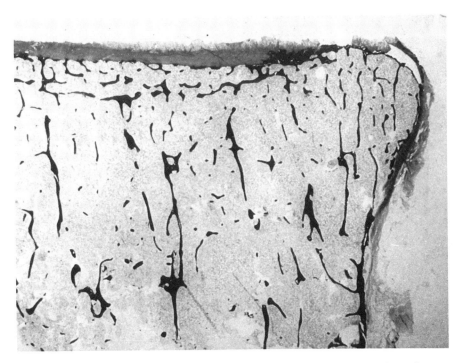

Fig. 8.2. Part of an osteoporotic vertebral body, showing relatively greater loss of horizontally arranged trabeculae compared with those which are vertically orientated. (Methylmethacrylate, von Kossa × 8)

controls. Various series have shown that trabecular bone volume in so-called normal bone gradually decreases with increasing age (see p. 99), so that, for example, the value for the iliac crest at age 60–69 is $15.3 \pm 4.6\%$, according to Courpron et al. (1980). Clearly, at this sort of age, a small but significant proportion of the so-called normal population will actually be at risk of vertebral fracture, osteopenic and/or osteoporotic depending on the definitions used. To some extent, disagreement as to whether osteoporosis is a heterogeneous group of disorders, an entity related to the process of ageing or the lower end of the normal range must result from differences in the definitions and concepts being used. It is important to remember that all present definitions of osteoporosis are arbitrary.

Clinical features

Osteoporosis affecting post-menopausal women and the elderly is the commonest form of generalised bone loss. Although the whole osteoporotic skeleton is at risk, certain bones have a particular tendency to fracture, namely the lower thoracic and upper lumbar vertebral bodies, the proximal femur (subcapital, intertrochanteric, subtrochanteric), the proximal humerus and the distal radius (Colles' fracture). Fractures of the forearm and hip almost invariably follow falls, whereas osteoporotic collapse of vertebrae apparently occurs spontaneously, although it can be stated that the location of these fractures is at that level of the spine which is subject to such everyday stresses as bending and lifting. Vertebral fractures usually cause pain which is localised to the fracture site and may be accompanied by spasm of the paraspinal muscles. Acute symptoms subside over a period of 6 weeks, and severe persistent pain for longer than this should call into question the diagnosis of an osteoporotic aetiology. Some patients have no history of back pain and the fractured vertebra is discovered as an incidental finding. Loss of height is greatest around the time of initial presentation (Dent and Watson 1966). Fracture of the long bones, most notably at the hip, occurs on average about 15 years later than vertebral compression fracture (Nagent de Deuxchaisnes 1983). This may be related to the fact that proportionally more of the femoral neck is composed of cortical bone compared with the vertebral body. There is gradual narrowing of cortical bone by a process of 'cancellisation' in osteoporosis. Colles' fracture increases in frequency only slightly with age in males (Alffram and Bauer 1962), and the sex incidence is about equal up to age 40, but this fracture is seven times more common in women than men after the age of 60 years (Nagent de Deuxchaisnes 1983). Since trauma, which is often relatively trivial by the standards of normal young adults, plays an important role in the fracturing of bones in osteoporosis, factors predisposing to falls in the elderly should perhaps also be taken into account. The elderly are much more likely to have vertebrobasilar insufficiency, cerebral ischaemic attacks, poor eyesight, joint disease and muscle weakness, all of which may predispose them to fall more frequently than younger members of the population.

Radiological signs of osteoporosis include increased radiolucency of the bones, prominence of vertically orientated trabeculae and of the bony end plates, asymmetrical biconcavity of the vertebral bodies and the presence of wedge and compression fractures (Fig. 8.3). Various methods of assessing ordinary radiographs for density have been used but are unreliable. The straight radiological diagnosis rests with the detection of the morphological changes of biconcavity, wedging and crush fractures. Quantitative assessment of vertebral body biconcavity is unreliable (Doyle et al. 1967).

The best non-invasive methods of evaluating bone mass comprise single photon absorptiometry using ^{125}I, with measurements being made over the distal radius, and the more expensive and sophisticated methods of dual photon absorptiometry of the spine and hips, neutron activation analysis of the axial skeleton and quantitative computerised axial tomography (Cameron and Sorenson 1963; Wahner et al. 1977; Wilson and Madsen 1977; Cann et al. 1980; Harrison et al. 1981). None of these methods is yet widely available.

Although it requires an invasive procedure, quantitation of bone biopsies provides a useful method of evaluating bone mass, expressed as trabecular bone volume for the cancellous bone (see p. 97). There is a good correlation between the trabecular bone volume of the iliac crest and that of the vertebral bodies (Meunier et al. 1973; see also p. 101), so that iliac crest biopsy is relevant to the detection of individuals at risk from vertebral fracture. Crush fractures of the spine are almost invariably associated with reduced trabecular bone volume assessed at the iliac crest (Boyce et al. 1978).

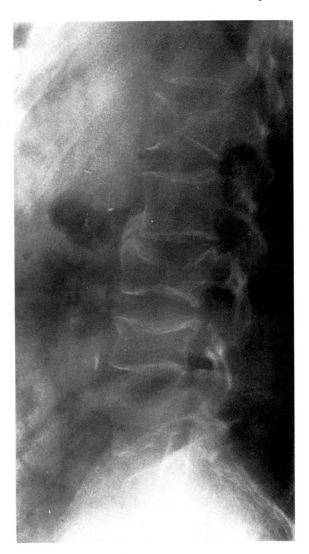

Fig. 8.3. Lumbar spine of an alcoholic with osteoporosis, showing collapse of vertebral bodies

Involutional osteoporosis

'Involutional osteoporosis' describes a condition related to the ageing process and/or the decline in sex hormone production, and the term excludes all other causes of osteoporosis like Cushing's disease, hyperthyroidism, diabetes mellitus and immobilisation. Clinically, osteoporosis of this type presents two particular problems in old age, namely collapse of vertebrae and fractures of the limb bones, notably of the neck of the femur and distal radius (see p. 185). It has been shown by morphometry that the amount of bone diminishes with age (see p. 99), that this loss of bone begins earlier and is more rapid in women compared with men, and that it probably has its onset at the time of the menopause in women (Newton-John and Morgan 1970). Bone mass shows a normal distribution at any particular age and the standard deviation is similar, even though the mean decreases with age.

Epidemiological studies have shown that pathological fractures in osteoporotic individuals occur most particularly in white females (Smith and Rizek 1966). Significantly less pathological fractures occur in blacks than in whites (Moldawer et al. 1965; Nordin 1966; Smith and Rizek 1966; Dent et al. 1968; Engh et al. 1968; Solomon 1979), and vertebral compression fractures also occur much less frequently in blacks compared with whites (Boukhris and Becker 1973).

The gradual loss of bone from the skeleton with age has already been described elsewhere in this volume (see p. 99). This process begins in early adult life and progresses so that the average white female loses 47% of her vertebral bone mass, as measured by dual photon absorptiometry of the spine (Riggs et al. 1981), a figure which coincides with the percentage loss of bone from the iliac crest assessed by histomorphometry over the age range 25–85 years. Loss of bone mass from the limb bones occurs from the sixth decade onwards with such a rapid decline that the average female loses 39% of the bone of her distal radius (Riggs et al. 1981).

Principal aetiological factors

Involutional or post-menopausal osteoporosis is almost certainly not a single disease entity but the result of any one of or a combination of different pathogenetic mechanisms, including cessation of ovarian activity, altered calcium metabolism, changes in hormones regulating bone turnover and dietary factors.

Hormonal effects

The role of decreased gonadal function in the development of osteoporosis is strongly suggested, since physiological decline in ovarian activity or oophorectomy result in increased serum calcium and phosphorus levels and increased urinary calcium/creatinine ratios (Young and Nordin 1967). Oestradiol and oestrone levels are low in both osteoporotic and post-menopausal women, but oestrone levels are much lower in the former than the latter (Crilly et al. 1979). There is a reduction in intestinal absorption of calcium with increasing age (Avioli et al. 1965; Bullamore et al. 1970; Gallagher et al. 1979), and this is even greater in osteoporotic compared with non-osteoporotic post-menopausal women (Kinney et al. 1966; Gallagher et al. 1973). Studies of calcium balance in normal perimenopausal women by Heaney and colleagues (1978a) showed that the menopause led to decreased calcium absorption and increased urinary calcium excretion and that this could be corrected by oestrogen treatment. Improvement in calcium balance in both normal and osteoporotic post-menopausal women with oestrogen therapy has been shown by various workers, including Lafferty et al. (1964), Gallagher et al. (1973), Gallagher and Nordin (1975) and Heaney et al. (1978a), and post-oophorectomy or post-menopausal bone loss is also prevented by oestrogen administration (Aitken et al. 1973; Meema et al. 1975; Lindsay et al. 1976; Horsman et al. 1977; Recker et al. 1977). Patients with osteoporosis have decreased calcium absorption (Lafferty et al. 1964; Gallagher et al. 1973; Gallagher and Nordin 1975; Gallagher et al. 1979), so that prevention of bone loss with oestrogens must be mediated either by altered calcium metabolism or inhibition of bone resorption.

Gallagher et al. (1980a) measured the serum levels of vitamin D metabolites in osteoporotic women treated with oestrogen and showed an increase in 1,25(OH)$_2$D compared with controls. The coincidental improvement in calcium absorption was similar to that produced by administration of 1,25(OH)$_2$D to other osteoporotic women. Since immunoreactive parathyroid hormone levels also increased after oestrogen treatment, it was concluded that the enhanced calcium absorption was due to increased 1,25(OH)$_2$D produced by stimulation of renal 1α-hydroxylase by parathyroid hormone. Caniggia et al. (1970) also demonstrated a significant increase in calcium absorption in osteoporotic women given oestrogen/progestogen treatment. The effects on bone resorption have been demonstrated by Riggs et al. (1969) and Heaney et al. (1978b), among others. The latter authors showed that bone remodelling increases slightly but significantly after the menopause, that resorptive activity predominates and that low doses of oestrogen prevent these post-menopausal changes.

Changes in vitamin D and parathyroid hormone levels after the menopause and in osteoporotic patients have already been alluded to above. Some investigators have found normal vitamin D levels in osteoporosis, while others have found low levels (Nagent de Deuxchaisnes 1983). Vitamin D metabolism appears to be normal (Davies et al. 1977; Lawoyin et al. 1980). Normal parathyroid hormone levels in osteoporosis have been recorded (Riggs et al. 1973; Bouillon et al. 1979), although subpopulations having raised levels of the hormone also occur (Teitelbaum et al. 1976; Gallagher et al. 1980b). The possible role of changes in calcitonin levels in osteoporosis is difficult to determine. Calcitonin inhibits osteoclastic activity and its absence may therefore result in bone loss. Possible links with osteoporosis are suggested by the finding that plasma levels of immunoreactive calcitonin are lower in women than men and that responses of immunoreactive calcitonin to calcium may decrease with age (Heath and Sizemore 1977; Deftos et al. 1980). There is not agreement, however, on whether calcitonin levels are decreased in osteoporosis (Franchimont and Heynen 1976; Cundy et al. 1978; Milhaud et al. 1978; Chesnut et al. 1980).

Calcium metabolism

The possible role of decreased calcium absorption has been discussed briefly above. Other calcium balance studies have been concerned with the effects of differing calcium intake. Studies of perimenopausal women on normal self-selected diets by Heaney et al. (1977, 1978b) showed that this group had an average calcium intake below the US recommended daily allowance, that they were in negative calcium balance and that there was a positive correlation between calcium intake and calcium balance. A greater calcium intake was required after the menopause than before in order to stay in calcium balance, the higher calcium requirement being considered as due partly to altered intestinal calcium absorption, partly to less effective conservation of calcium by the kidney, the latter point being previously stressed by Bhandarkar and Nordin (1962). The importance of adequate calcium intake is also suggested by a world-wide study in which the lowest fracture frequency was found in Finland, where calcium intake was highest (Nordin 1966), and by similar results obtained in Puerto Rico and Yugoslavia, where those with the lowest fracture rates have the highest calcium intakes (Smith and Rizek 1966; Matkovic et al. 1979). Not only do calcium requirements increase with age, but average calcium intake has been shown to decrease with age (Avioli 1981; Draper and Scythes 1981). A further relevant finding is that lactose deficiency is present in a significantly higher proportion of patients with post-menopausal osteoporosis compared with controls and that the former have significantly lower intakes of both lactose and calcium (Newcomer et al. 1978). Lactose deficiency itself decreases calcium absorption (Condon et al. 1970).

A high protein diet induces calciuria and brings about negative calcium balance (Heaney and Recker 1982), the calciuric effect most likely being related to increased production of organic acids (Whiting and Draper 1980). Other possible but poorly understood factors include high caffeine intake, which increases urinary calcium levels (Heaney and Recker 1982) and alcoholism, in which bone mass is reduced (Fig. 8.3) and calcium intake is usually below the recommended daily allowance (Saville 1965; Nilsson and Westlin 1973). Alcohol inhibits intestinal absorption of calcium (Krawitt 1973, 1974).

Mast cells

A further area of interest in osteoporosis is the possible role of mast cells and their products in bone resorption. Recently, Fallon and colleagues (1983) have reported the presence of greater numbers of mast cells in the bone marrow of post-menopausal osteoporotic patients than in normals. Increased numbers of marrow mast cells had previously been reported in osteoporosis associated with ageing (Frame and Nixon 1968) and in osteitis fibrosa cystica occurring as part of renal osteodystrophy (Peart and Ellis 1975; Fig. 8.4); while

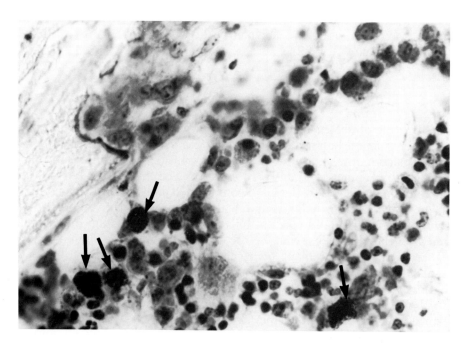

Fig. 8.4. Mast cells (*arrows*) adjacent to an area of osteoclastic resorption. (Thionin × 400)

generalised osteopenia occurs in some cases of systemic mastocytosis (Fallon et al. 1981). Increased numbers of osteoclasts with accompanying osteolysis have been noted near bone lesions in systemic mastocytosis (Brunning et al. 1983), and there is a localised form of mast cell accumulation in the bone marrow, which is also accompanied by osteoporosis (te Velde et al. 1978). Urist and McLean (1957) noted the accumulation of mast cells in the bone of calcium-deficient rats. Mast cells contain heparin and other vasoactive substances and it is of interest that osteoporosis and the development of fractures have been described in patients receiving long-term heparin treatment (Griffith et al. 1965; Jaffe and Willis 1965).

Physical activity

Although most considerations of the mechanisms involved in the development of osteoporosis have been concerned with hormonal and metabolic changes, and thus related to the calcium homeostatic function of bone, the effects of physical activity and the relationship of bone changes to the mechanical support role of the skeleton must also be considered. This aspect has been highlighted recently by Lanyon and Rubin (1983). Athletes, long-distance runners, ballet dancers and weight lifters have all been shown to have higher than average bone mass (Nilsson and Westlin 1971; Dalen and Olssen 1974; Aloia et al. 1978a; Nilsson et al. 1978). Nilsson and Westlin (1971) also compared healthy men who exercised regularly with those who did essentially no exercise but were matched for weight, height and age. The femoral bone mineral content was significantly higher in the former, suggesting that even moderate physical exercise may increase bone mass. The effects of prolonged immobilisation and weightlessness will be considered separately (see this chapter, Immobilisation osteoporosis), but it is apparent that physical activity should also be brought into the equation of possible factors in age-related osteoporosis.

Histomorphometry

There are several different theoretical mechanisms by which loss of bone with increasing age may occur (Table 8.1), and various quantitative studies of bone histology have attempted to answer questions relating to the mode of bone loss.

Trabecular bone volume is low by definition in osteoporosis, and osteoid volume expressed in absolute terms is also decreased, merely because of its relationship to trabecular bone volume (Nagent de Deuxchaisnes 1983). Rela-

Table 8.1. Theoretical possibilities for loss of bone with increasing age

1. Resorption and formation both remain constant, with ageing
2. Resorption increases, formation remains constant
3. Resorption remains constant, formation decreases
4. Resorption and formation both decrease, but unequally
5. Resorption and formation both increase, but unequally
6. Resorption increases, formation decreases

tive osteoid volume has been found to be no different from normal (Whyte et al. 1982; Nagent de Deuxchaisnes 1983). However, examination of osteoid seam widths and surface measurements of bone provide evidence that osteoporosis has a heterogeneous histological appearance. The width of osteoid seams has been shown to be decreased (Schenk and Merz 1969; Parfitt et al. 1981; Nagent de Deuxchaisnes 1983) and so considered as showing evidence of an abnormality of osteoblastic function.

Changes in mineralisation rate, as judged by a double tetracycline label, show a decreased rate in involutional osteoporosis (Meunier et al. 1979) and are therefore evidence for a decrease in osteoblastic activity in the form of reduced lifespan of these cells (Darby and Meunier 1981). Age-related changes in protein synthetic activity are almost certainly present in other cell types, for example skin fibroblasts (Hayflick 1976), so that osteoporotic patients have been shown to have thin, transparent skin (McConkey et al. 1963; Ng et al. 1984) resulting from a decrease in dermal collagen (Leong and Balasubramaniam 1978). Resorptive activity has not been shown to be increased in osteoporosis by Schenk and Merz (1969) and Meunier et al. (1979), although Nordin et al. (1981) found evidence of increased resorption. Care is required in interpretation of results relating to formation and resorption surfaces in osteoporosis, where the decreased trabecular bone volume results in a decrease in absolute trabecular bone surface (Darby 1981). Evidence has been presented for different subgroups within the population of osteoporotic patients. Meunier and his colleagues (1981, 1983) showed that one-third of 157 cases had high remodelling activity, while Whyte and his co-workers (1982) were also able to divide their smaller series of untreated osteoporotic women into active and inactive remodelling groups. Those with active remodelling osteoporosis had significantly higher values for percentage osteoblastic osteoid surface, osteoclastic resorbing surface and mean osteoid seam width, as well as increases in osteoclast counts and percentage total resorbing surface, which did not, however, reach statistical significance. Meunier and his colleagues (1983) measured calcification rate using double tetracycline labelling. Since there was no significant change in calcification rate with age and sex found in a previous study (Meunier et al. 1979), they deduced that when osteoid seam thickness is normal, collagen synthesis by osteoblasts and mineralisation of osteoid occur at the same rate, so that calcification rate is equivalent to osteoblastic apposition rate. Tetracycline labelling was available in 109 cases, of which 21% showed calcification rate more than two standard deviations below the normal mean, 48% showed no detectable abnormality of appositional rate or remodelling surfaces, and the remainder had either high remodelling osteoporosis (31%) or high remodelling with osteoblastic depression (5%).

An interesting approach to the consideration of pathogenetic mechanisms has been taken by Courpron and other members of the French group (Courpron et al. 1980; Meunier et al. 1983). Bone resorption and subsequent formation are considered to be coupled in the remodelling process. Examination of the trabecular surfaces of bone reveals areas of past remodelling at what have been called 'bone basic structural units' (BSU) (Fig. 8.5). The thickness of the bone set down in previous resorption lacunae, that is from the cement line to the nearby trabecular surface has been called the 'mean wall thickness' and has been measured in osteoporosis (Lips et al. 1978; Courpron et al. 1980). In males aged 18–82 years (mean 47.9 years) the mean wall thickness was

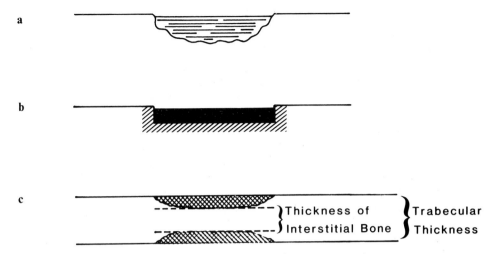

Fig. 8.5a–c. Diagram of basic structural unit. **a** As it might appear on microscopy, showing post-resorption lacuna which has become filled with new bone (*shaded*) in the normal remodelling process. **b** Schematic representation of basic structural unit, showing how the subsequently formed new bone (*black*) may not fully fill the defect resulting from previous resorption. **c** Measurement of thickness of interstitial bone by measuring trabecular thickness and mean wall thickness. The mean depth of the *shaded* or *black area* in **a, b** and **c** is the mean wall thickness in each case

50.2 ± 8.7 µm and in females aged 19–90 years (mean 55.6 years) the value was 59 ± 9.1 µm. Both sexes showed negative correlation of mean wall thickness with age and this single fact indicates that only mechanisms 3, 4 and 6 in Table 8.1 can be responsible for age-related bone loss. Distinction between these possibilities was made by the further simple technique of measuring mean trabecular bone thickness, from which it is possible to obtain an estimate of the thickness of the interstitial bone (Fig. 8.5). Mechanisms 3 and 6 should result in a gradual decrease in the thickness of interstitial bone, while if mechanism 4 were responsible for bone loss, interstitial bone would increase with increasing age. The French group have presented evidence for progressive increase in the thickness of interstitial bone, so that age-related osteopenia may be due to decreased resorption and formation, the latter decreased to a greater extent. Darby and Meunier (1981) found that both the mean wall thickness and the timespan of the osteoblastic formation period were lower in osteoporotic patients without remodelling abnormalities than in age- and sex-matched controls.

Osteoporosis in the young

Osteoporosis is rare in childhood and when it occurs it is important to exclude Cushing's syndrome, osteogenesis imperfecta, homocystinuria, Turner's syndrome, malabsorption disease and immobilisation. There is a small group of children who have an osteoporosis of obscure aetiology called 'idiopathic juvenile osteoporosis' (Dent and Friedman 1965; Dent 1977). This condition is self limiting and with onset before puberty; it affects previously healthy children, who show growth arrest, loss of stature, joint pain, fractures of vertebrae and of long bones. It is important to exclude other possible causes of vertebral collapse such as the presence of leukaemic deposits, as well as the generalised diseases listed above. Useful reviews of cases of idiopathic juvenile osteoporosis in the literature are by Teotia et al. (1979) and Smith (1980). A characteristic radiological appearance is that of osteoporotic areas in the metaphyses of long bones, for which the term 'neo-osseous osteoporosis' has been used to denote involvement of newly formed bone at this site. While the most obvious skeletal changes seem to occur in the growing parts of the skeleton, bone histology is confined largely to the iliac crest. Quantitative microradiography has shown normal bone formation and increased bone resorption (Jowsey and Johnson 1972), but the necessity to distinguish between increased resorption and failure of subsequent bone formation in resorbed areas has been pointed out by Smith (1979), who subsequently considered that there was a failure of bone formation (Smith 1980). The results of biochemical investigation in idiopathic juvenile osteoporosis are confusing, most values being normal, although Jowsey and Johnson (1972) found raised plasma alkaline phosphatase and urinary hydroxyproline levels in some of their cases. References are available in the papers by Teotia and his colleagues (1979) and by Smith (1979). Interpretation is made all the more difficult because of changes which occur normally at the time of the prepubertal growth spurt. The most important differential diagnosis is from osteogenesis imperfecta (Smith 1980; Smith and Sykes 1983). Brenton and Dent (1976) stated that the long bones were of normal width in idiopathic juvenile osteoporosis, that the cortex might be thinned and that metaphyseal fractures were common. The onset of osteogenesis imperfecta is usually much earlier in life; the children have blue sclerae and abnormalities of collagen.

It is worthwhile to separate juvenile osteoporosis from idiopathic bone loss occurring in adults before the age of 50 years. There are occasional reports of such idiopathic osteoporosis in young adults (Jackson 1958; Bordier et al. 1973), and a group of five male patients with osteoporosis and hypercalciuria has been described recently by Perry et al. (1982). No abnormalities were found in thyroxine, cortisol, testosterone or vitamin D levels, and parathyroid hormone levels were normal. No cause for osteoporosis was identified. Histomorphometry showed evidence of an increased rate of bone formation. A further interesting case report by Stevenson et al. (1982) described severe osteoporosis after puberty in a young man found to have calcitonin deficiency and an increased remodelling rate on bone biopsy.

Immobilisation osteoporosis

Disuse or immobilisation osteoporosis is the loss of bone mass which results from muscular inactivity or reduced weightbearing and may affect the whole or part of the skeleton. Donaldson et al. (1970) showed a 4.2% loss of bone in volunteers after prolonged bed rest for an 8-month period. Sustained weightlessness during space flight is also well recognised as resulting in bone loss (Mack and LaChance 1967; Lutwak et al. 1969; Morey and Baylink 1978; Whedon et al. 1976; Tilton et al. 1980). Astronauts lose 4 g calcium per month during space flight, according to Whedon et al. (1976), and Tilton and his colleagues (1980) demonstrated a 5% long-term loss of bone mineral content from the os calcis, proportional to the length of flight of the Skylab mission.

Hypercalcaemia and hypercalciuria occur with prolonged immobilisation, for example in patients with post-traumatic spinal cord lesions (Minaire et al. 1974), and the changes may be sufficiently marked to be life threatening. There may also be increased parathyroid hormone secretion (Lerman et al. 1977).

The role of continuing mechanical forces in the maintenance of bone mass has already been mentioned (see p. 191). Modification of involutional bone loss by exercise has been reported (Aloia et al. 1978b). Changes in bone mass relating to physical activity also affect individual bones, and it is such examples which particularly point to the importance of mechanical effects.

The cortical thickness of the humerus of male tennis players is greater on the playing side compared with the non-playing side (Jones et al. 1977), and the bone mineral content of the distal femur is increased in weightlifters, throwers, runners and soccer players, but not in swimmers (Nilsson and Westlin 1971). The effects of immobilisation have been studied in dogs by the use of plaster casts by Uhthoff and Jaworski (1978), whose radiomorphometry and histomorphometry studies suggested different mechanisms might be involved in bone loss according to age, younger animals losing subperiosteal bone while older ones showed endosteal resorption (Uhthoff and Jaworski 1978; Jaworski et al. 1980). References to other animal studies are available in these two papers. As well as loss of bone in limbs immobilised in plaster casts (Nilssen 1966), osteopenia occurs in paralysed limbs (Heaney 1962). Loss of muscle may also affect growth in the paralysed limb, the shortening of lower limbs in a series of adult poliomyelitis victims being related to muscle strength in a study by Stinchfield et al. (1949).

The pathogenetic mechanisms in immobilisation osteopenia may be more complicated than they first appear. Minaire et al. (1974) showed a 33% reduction in trabecular bone volume over a 25-week period followed by stabilisation at a lower plateau level. Immobilisation caused an early increase in trabecular osteoclastic resorption surfaces, depression of osteoblastic activity and thinning of the cortices, with a new steady state being reached later. Alterations in parathyroid hormone secretion have already been mentioned. Changes in piezoelectricity may play a role, and bone loss in an immobilised limb has been prevented by application of electrical forces (Martin and Gutmann 1978). The loss of bone with disuse, as in other forms of osteoporosis, affects trabecular bone, but if immobilisation is prolonged there is progression to cortical atrophy with conversion of cortical to cancellous bone.

Corticosteroid-induced osteopenia

High-circulating levels of adrenocorticosteroids result in loss of bone mass whether they are due to adrenal disease or therapeutic administration. The latter is relatively common, patients with iatrogenic disease having a high risk of developing such sequelae as vertebral collapse. Loss of both cortical and trabecular bone occurs and is demonstrable in bones such as ribs and pelvis as well as in the spine. Fractures may occur from a month to several years after the commencement of treatment and are increasingly likely with increasing time, although there is no information available about whether the risk continues to accumulate or reaches a constant level. The amount of bone loss has been shown to increase in proportion to the length of therapy (Hahn et al. 1974; Caniggia et al. 1981).

Various studies have shown results in broad agreement, although there are differences. There is evidence of decreased intestinal absorption of calcium, raised serum parathyroid hormone levels and decreased metaphyseal bone mass, together with histomorphometric evidence of decreased bone formation and increased numbers of osteoclasts (Jowsey and Riggs 1970; Gallagher et al. 1973; Fucik et al. 1975; Klein et al. 1977; Bressot et al. 1979; Hahn et al. 1979, 1981). It seems likely that there is some degree of hyperparathyroidism, resulting as a response to altered intestinal calcium and phosphate absorption. High-dose corticosteroid treatment induces calcium malabsorption, and this is associated with slightly raised plasma levels of $1,25(OH)_2D$ (Hahn et al. 1981). The effect may be a direct one on transmucosal calcium transport (Hahn et al. 1981) or due to a dose-related abnormality in vitamin D metabolism (Klein et al. 1977). Further details of the effects of glucocorticoids on calcium metabolism are available elsewhere (Crilly et al. 1983; Gennari et al. 1983).

Increased bone resorption found with moderate doses of steroids may be related to increased parathyroid activity, or possibly a direct effect on osteoclasts. Parathyroidectomy abolishes the osteoclastic response of bone to glucocorticoids in animals (Jee et al. 1970). Apart from changes in osteoclast numbers and the amount of resorptive activity, examination of bone turnover and histomorphometric studies have shown that glucocorticoids reduce osteoblastic activity in bone and the rate of mineralisation is decreased, as determined by double tetracycline labelling, so that diminished bone formation appears to play a significant part in the development of osteopenia (Klein et al. 1965; Epker 1970; Bressot et al. 1979).

The administration of glucocorticoids to children has growth inhibiting effects because of the influence on the skeleton. These have been described by Maassen (1952) and Sissons and Hadfield (1955).

Localised bone loss

Local osteoporosis in relation to joints affected by chronic rheumatoid arthritis is well recognised. It develops over a period of months or years and could be considered as a form of disuse atrophy. The question of generalised bone disease in rheumatoid arthritis has been considered by various workers (Maddison and Bacon 1974; Kennedy and Lindsay 1977; Bird 1979; O'Driscoll and O'Driscoll 1980; Ng et al. 1984). While evidence was presented in these papers for either osteomalacia or hyperparathyroidism in rheumatoid disease, we were able only to find osteoporosis (Ng et al. 1984).

A further form of local bone loss is Sudeck's bone atrophy, a painful post-traumatic atrophy of bone which is poorly described and little understood. This is a clinical syndrome, not a pathological entity, and comprises deep-seated pain at the site of an injury, together with local rarefaction of the bones in the area and with changes in the temperature, colour and texture of the overlying skin in some cases.

Disappearing bone disease

Disappearing bone disease is a rare condition of bone in which there is spontaneous and massive osteolysis, the affected bone literally vanishing on radiological examination. This is not osteoporosis. Histological examination shows the presence of numerous thin-walled vessels within the interosseous spaces of both cortical and lamellar bone. Bone is lost in relation to these vessels and replaced by fibrous tissue. A relationship to haemangioma of bone seems likely. Enzyme histochemistry shows the presence of strongly positive acid phosphatase and leucine aminopeptidase staining in perivascular cells, and few osteoclasts are visualised removing bone.

References

Aitken JM, Hart DM, Lindsay R (1973) Oestrogen replacement therapy for prevention of osteoporosis after oophorectomy. Br Med J 3:515–518

Alffram PA, Bauer GCH (1962) Epidemiology of fracture of the forearm. J Bone Joint Surg [Am] 44:105–114

Aloia JF, Cohn SH, Babu T, Abesamis C, Kalici N, Ellis K (1978a) Skeletal mass and body composition in marathon runners. Metabolism 27:1793–1796

Aloia JF, Stanton HC, Ostumi JA, Cane R, Ellis K (1978b) Prevention of involutional bone loss by exercise. Ann Intern Med 89:356–358

Avioli LV (1981) Post-menopausal osteoporosis: prevention versus cure. Fed Proc 40:2418–2422

Avioli LV, McDonald JE, Lee SW (1965) The influence of age on the intestinal absorption of 47-Ca in post menopausal osteoporosis. J Clin Invest 44:1960–1967

Bhandarkar SD, Nordin BEC (1962) Effect of low-calcium diet on urinary calcium in osteoporosis. Br Med J I:145–147

Bird HA (1979) Bone biopsy in the investigation of bone pain and fractures. Rheumatol Rehabil 18:38–42

Bordier PHJ, Miravet L, Hioco D (1973) Young adult osteoporosis. Clin Endocrinol Metab 2:272–292

Bouillon R, Geusens P, Dequeker J, De Moor P (1979) Parathyroid function in primary osteoporosis. Clin Sci 57:167–171

Boukhris R, Becker KL (1973) The inter-relationship between vertebral fractures and osteoporosis. Clin Orthop 90:209–216

Boyce BF, Courpron P, Meunier PJ (1978) Parathyroid function in primary osteoporosis. Metab Bone Dis Relat Res 1:35–38

Brenton DP, Dent CE (1976) Idiopathic juvenile osteoporosis. In: Bickel H, Stern J (eds) Inborn errors of calcium and bone metabolism. MTP Press, Lancaster, pp 222–238

Bressot C, Meunier PJ, Chapuy MC, Lejeune E, Edouard C, Darby AJ (1979) Histomorphometric profile, pathophysiology and reversibility of corticosteroid-induced osteoporosis. Metab Bone Dis Relat Res 1:303–311

Brunning RO, Parkin JL, McKenna RW, Risdall R, Rosai J (1983) Systemic mastocytosis. Extra-cutaneous manifestations. Am J Surg Pathol 7:425–438

Bullamore JR, Gallagher JC, Wilkinson R, Nordin BEC, Marshall DH (1970) Effect of age on calcium absorption. Lancet II:535–537

Cameron JR, Sorenson J (1963) Measurement of bone mineral in vivo: an improved method. Science 142:230–232

Caniggia A, Gennari C, Borrelo G (1970) Intestinal absorption of calcium-47 after treatment with oral oestrogen-gestogens in senile osteoporosis. Br Med J 4:30–32

Caniggia A, Nuti R, Lore F, Vattimo A (1981) Pathophysiology of the adverse effects of glucoactive corticosteroids on calcium metabolism in man. J Steroid Biochem 15:153–161

Cann CE, Genant HK, Ettinger B, Gordon GS (1980) Spinal mineral loss in oophorectomized women. JAMA 244:2056–2059

Chesnut CH III, Baylink DJ, Sisom K, Nelp WB, Roos BA (1980) Basal plasma immunoreactive calcitonin in post-menopausal osteoporosis. Metabolism 20:559–562

Collins DH (1966) The pathology of bone. Butterworths, London

Condon JR, Nassim JR, Hilbe A, Millard EJC, Stainthorpe EM (1970) Calcium and phosphorus metabolism in relation to lactose tolerance. Lancet I:1027–1029

Courpron P, Meunier P, Bressot C, Giroux JM (1976) Amount of bone in iliac crest biopsy. In: Meunier PJ (ed) Bone histomorphometry. 2nd international workshop. Armour Montagu, Paris, pp 39–53

Courpron P, Lepire P, Arlot M, Lips M, Meunier PJ (1980) Mechanisms underlying the reduction in age of the mean wall thickness of trabecular basic structure unit (BSU) of human iliac bone. In: Jee WSS, Parfitt AM (eds) Bone histomorphometry. 3rd international workshop. Metab Bone Dis Relat Res 2(Suppl):323–329

Crilly R, Horsman A, Marshall DH, Nordin BEC (1979) Prevalence, pathogenesis and treatment of post-menopausal osteoporosis. Aust NZ J Med 9:24–30

Crilly RG, Marshall DH, Horsman A, Nordin BEC, Peacock M (1983) Corticosteroid osteoporosis. In: Dixon A St J, Russell RGG, Stamp TCB (eds) Osteoporosis. A multidisciplinary problem. International Congress and Symposium Series No 55. Academic Press and Royal Society of Medicine, London, pp 153–158

Cundy T, Heynen G, Ackroyd C, Kissin M, Kirby R, Kanis JA (1978) Plasma-calcitonin in women. Lancet II:158–159

Dalen N, Olssen KE (1974) Bone mineral content and physical activity. Acta Orthop Scand 45:170–174

Darby AJ (1981) Bone formation and resorption in post-menopausal osteoporosis. Lancet II:536

Darby AJ, Meunier PJ (1981) Mean wall thickness and formation periods of trabecular bone packets in idiopathic osteoporosis. Calcif Tissue Int 33:199–204

Davies M, Mawer EB, Adams PH (1977) Vitamin D metabolism and the response to 1,25-dihydroxycholecalciferol in osteoporosis. J Clin Endocrinol Metab 45:199–208

Deftos LJ, Weisman MH, Williams GW, Karpf DB, Frumar AM, Davidson BJ, Parthemore JG, Judd HL (1980) Influence of age and sex on plasma calcitonin in human beings. N Engl J Med 302:1351–1353

Dent CE (1977) Osteoporosis in childhood. Postgrad Med J 53:450–456

Dent CE, Friedman M (1965) Idiopathic juvenile osteoporosis. Q J Med 34:177–210

Dent CE, Watson L (1966) Osteoporosis. Postgrad Med J 42(Suppl):583–608

Dent CE, Engelbrecht HE, Godfrey RC (1968) Osteoporosis of lumbar vertebrae and calcification of abdominal aorta in women living in Durban. Br Med J 4:76–79

Donaldson CL, Hulley SB, Vogel JM, Hattner RS, Bayers JH, McMillian DE (1970) Effect of prolonged bed rest on bone mineral. Metabolism 19:1071–1084

Doyle FH, Gutteridge DH, Joplin GF, Fraser R (1967) An assessment of radiological criteria used in the studies of spinal osteoporosis. Br J Radiol 40:241–250

Draper HH, Scythes CA (1981) Calcium, phosphorus and osteoporosis. Fed Proc 40:2434–2438

Engh G, Bollet AJ, Hardin G, Parson W (1968) Epidemiology of osteoporosis. II Incidence of hip fractures in mental institutions. J Bone Joint Surg [Am] 50:557–562

Epker BN (1970) Studies on bone turnover and balance in the rabbit. I Effects of hydrocortisone. Clin Orthop 72:315–326

Fallon MD, Whyte MP, Teitelbaum SL (1981) Systemic mastocytosis associated with generalised osteopenia: histopathological characterization of the skeletal lesion using undecalcified bone from two patients. Human Pathol 12:813–820

Fallon MD, Whyte MP, Craig RB, Teitelbaum SL (1983) Mast cell proliferation in postmenopausal osteoporosis. Calcif Tissue Int 35:29–31

Frame B, Nixon RK (1968) Bone marrow mast cells in osteoporosis of aging. N Engl J Med 279:626–630

Franchimont P, Heynen G (1976) Parathormone and calcitonin radioimmunoassay in various medical and osteoarticular disorders. Masson, Paris

Fucik RF, Kukreja SC, Hargis GK (1975) Effect of glucocorticoids on function of the parathyroid glands in man. J Clin Endocrinol Metab 40:152–155

Gallagher JC, Nordin BEC (1975) Effects of oestrogen and progestogen therapy on calcium metabolism in post menopausal women. Front Horm Res 3:150–176

Gallagher JC, Aaron J, Horsman A, Wilkinson R, Nordin BEC (1973) Corticosteroid osteoporosis. Clin Endocrinol (Oxf) 2:355–368

Gallagher JC, Aaron J, Horsman A, Marshall DH, Wilkinson R, Nordin BEC (1973) The crush fracture syndrome in post-menopausal women. Clin Endocrinol Metab 2:293–315

Gallagher JC, Riggs BL, Eisman J, Hamstra A, Arnaud SB, DeLuca HF (1979) Intestinal calcium absorption and serum vitamin D metabolites in normal subjects and osteoporotic patients. J Clin Invest 64:729–736

Gallagher JC, Riggs BL, DeLuca HF (1980a) Effect of estrogen on calcium absorption and serum vitamin D metabolites in postmenopausal osteoporosis. J Clin Endocrinol Metab 51:1359–1364

Gallagher JC, Riggs BL, Jerpbak CM, Arnaud CD (1980b) The effect of age on serum immunoreactive parathyroid hormone in normal and osteoporotic women. J Lab Clin Med 95:373–385

Gennari C, Bernini M, Nardi P, Fusi L, Francini G, Nami R, Montagnani M, Imsimbo B, Avioli LV (1983) Glucocorticoids: radiocalcium and radiophosphate absorption in man. In: Dixon A St J, Russell RGG, Stamp TCB (eds) Osteoporosis. A multidisciplinary problem. International Congress and Symposium Series No 55. Academic Press and Royal Society of Medicine, London, pp 75–80

Griffith GC, Nichols, G, Asher JD, Flanagan B (1965) Heparin in osteoporosis. JAMA 193:85–88

Hahn TJ, Boisseau VC, Avioli LV (1974) Effect of chronic corticosteroid administration on diaphyseal and metaphyseal bone mass. J Clin Endocrinol Metab 39:274–282

Hahn TJ, Halstead LR, Teitelbaum SL, Hahn BH (1979) Altered mineral metabolism in glucocorticoid-induced osteopenia. Effect of 25-hydroxyvitamin D administration. J Clin Invest 64:655–665

Hahn TJ, Halstead LR, Baran DT (1981) Effects of short term glucocorticoid administration on intestinal calcium absorption and circulating vitamin D metabolite concentrations in man. J Clin Endocrinol Metab 52:111–115

Harrison JE, McNeill KG, Sturtridge WC, Bailey TA, Murray TM, Williams C, Tam C, Fornasier V (1981) Three-year changes in bone mineral mass of post-menopausal osteoporotic patients based on neutron activation analysis of the central third of the skeleton. J Clin Endocrinol Metab 52:751–758

Hayflick L (1976) The cell biology of human aging. N Engl J Med 295:1302–1308

Heaney RP (1962) Radiocalcium metabolism in disuse osteoporosis in man. Am J Med 33:188–200

Heaney RP, Recker RR (1982) Effects of nitrogen, phosphomased caffeine on calcium balance in women. J Lab Clin Med 99:46–55

Heaney RP, Recker RR, Saville PD (1977) Calcium balance and calcium requirements in middle-aged women. Am J Clin Nutr 30:1603–1611

Heaney RP, Recker RR, Saville PD (1978a) Menopausal changes in calcium balance performance. J Lab Clin Med 92:953–963

Heaney RP, Recker RR, Saville PD (1978b) Menopausal changes in bone remodelling. J Lab Clin Med 92:964–970

Heath H III, Sizemore GW (1977) Plasma calcitonin in normal man: differences between men and women. J Clin Invest 60:1135–1140

Horsman A, Nordin BEC, Gallagher JC, Kirby PA, Milner RM, Simpson M (1977) Observations of sequential changes in bone mass in postmenopausal women; a controlled trial of oestrogen and calcium therapy. Calcif Tissue Res 22:217–224

Jackson WPU (1958) Osteoporosis of unknown cause in younger people. Idiopathic osteoporosis. J Bone Joint Surg [Br] 40:420–441

Jaffe MD, Willis PW (1965) Multiple fractures associated with long-term sodium heparin therapy. JAMA 193:152–154

Jaworski ZFG, Leskove-Kiar M, Uthoff HK (1980) Effect of long term immobilisation on the pattern of bone loss in older dogs. J Bone Joint Surg [Br] 62:104–110

Jee WSS, Park HZ, Roberts WE (1970) Corticosteroid and bone. Am J Anat 129:477–481

Jones HH, Priest JD, Haynes WC, Trichenor CC, Nogel DA (1977) Humoral hypertrophy in response to exercise. J Bone Joint Surg [Am] 59:204–208

Jowsey J, Johnson KA (1972) Juvenile osteoporosis. Bone findings in seven patients. J Pediatr 81:511–517

Jowsey J, Riggs BL (1970) Bone formation in hypercorticolism. Acta Endocrinol (Copenh) 63:21–28

Kennedy AC, Lindsay R (1977) Bone involvement in rheumatoid arthritis. Clin Rheum Dis 3:403–420

Kinney VR, Tauxe WN, Dearing WH (1966) Isotopic tracer studies of intestinal calcium absorption. J Lab Clin Med 66:187–203

Klein M, Villanueva AR, Frost HM (1965) A quantitative histological study of rib from eighteen patients treated with adrenal cortical steroids. Acta Orthop Scand 35:171–184

Klein RG, Arnaud SB, Gallagher JC, DeLuca HF, Riggs BL (1977) Intestinal calcium absorption in exogenous hypercorticolism. Role of 25-hydroxyvitamin D and corticosteroid dose. J Clin Invest 60:253–259

Krawitt EL (1973) Ethanol inhibits intestinal calcium transport in rats. Nature 243:88–89

Krawitt EL (1974) Effect of acute ethanol administration on duodenal calcium transport. Proc Soc Exp Biol Med 146:406–408

Lafferty FW, Spencer GE, Pearson OH (1964) Effects of androgens, estrogens and high calcium intakes on bone formation and resorption in osteoporosis. Am J Med 36:514–528

Lanyon LE, Rubin CT (1983) Regulation of bone mass in response to physical activity. In: Dixon A St J, Russell RGG, Stamp TCB (eds) Osteoporosis. A multidisciplinary problem. International Congress and Symposium Series No 55. Academic Press and Royal Society of Medicine, London, pp 51–61

Lawoyin S, Zerwekh JE, Glass K, Pak CYC (1980) Ability of 25-hydroxyvitamin D3 therapy to augment serum 1,25- and 24,25-dihydroxy-vitamin D in postmenopausal osteoporosis. J Clin Endocrinol Metab 50:593–596

Leong AS, Balasubramaniam P (1978) The estimation of dermal collagen in osteoporotic patients by a histomorphometric method. Pathology 10:365–371

Lerman S, Canterbury JM, Reiss E (1977) Parathyroid hormone and the hypercalcaemia of immobilization. J Clin Endocrinol Metab 45:425–428

Lindsay R, Aitken JM, Anderson JB, Hart DM, MacDonald EB, Clarke AC (1976) Long term prevention of postmenopausal osteoporosis by oestrogen. Lancet I:1038–1042

Lips P, Courpron P, Meunier PJ (1978) Mean wall thickness of trabecular bone pockets in the human iliac crest: changes with age. Calcif Tissue Res 26:13–17

Lutwak L, Whedon GD, LaChance PA (1969) Mineral, electrolyte and nitrogen balance studies of the Gemini VII fourteen-day orbital space flight. J Clin Endocrinol Metab 29:1140–1156

Maassen AP (1952) The effect of desoxycorticosterone acetate (Doca) on body-growth and ossification. Acta Endocrinol (Copenh) 9:291–296

Mack PB, LaChance PC (1967) Effects of recumbency and space flight on bone density. Am J Clin Nutr 20:1194–1205

Maddison PJ, Bacon PA (1974) Vitamin D deficiency, spontaneous fractures and osteopenia in rheumatoid arthritis. Br Med J 4:433–435

Martin RB, Gutman W (1978) The effect of electric fields on osteoporosis of disuse. Calcif Tissue Res 25:23–27

Matkovic V, Kosteial K, Simonovic I, Buzina R, Brodarec A, Nordin BEC (1979) Bone status and fracture rates in two regions of Yugoslavia. Am J Clin Nutr 32:540–549

McConkey B, Fraser GB, Bligh AS, Whiteley H (1963) Transparent skin and osteoporosis. Lancet I:693–695

McLean FC, Urist MR (1961) Bone: an introduction to the physiology of skeletal tissue, 2nd edn. University of Chicago Press, Chicago

Meema S, Bunker ML, Meema HE (1975) Preventive effect of estrogen on postmenopausal bone loss. A follow up study. Arch Intern Med 135:1436–1440

Meunier P, Courpron P, Edouard C, Bernard J, Bringuier J, Vignon G (1973) Physiological senile involutional and pathological rarefaction of bone: quantitative and comparative histological data. Clin Endocrinol Metab 2:239–256

Meunier PJ, Courpron P, Edouard C, Alexandre C, Bressot C, Lips P, Boyce BF (1979) Bone histomorphometry in osteoporotic states. In: Barzel US (ed) Osteoporosis II. Grune and Stratton, New York, pp 27–47

Meunier PJ, Sellami S, Briancon D, Edouard C (1981) Histological heterogeneity of apparently idiopathic osteoporosis. In: DeLuca HF, Frost HM, Jee WSS, Johnson CC Jr, Parfitt AM (eds) Osteoporosis. Recent advances in pathogenesis and treatment. University Park Press, Baltimore, pp 293–301

Meunier PJ, Briancon D, Sellami S, Edouard C, Chavassieux P, Arlot P (1983) Dynamic bone histomorphometry in primary osteoporosis. In: Dixon A St J, Russell RGG, Stamp TCB (eds) Osteoporosis. A multidisciplinary problem. International Congress and Symposium Series No 55. Academic Press and Royal Society of Medicine, London, pp 67–73

Milhaud G, Benezech-Lefrevre M, Moukhtar MS (1978) Deficiency of calcitonin in age related osteoporosis. Biomedicine 29:272–276

Minaire P, Meunier P, Edouard C, Bernard J, Courpron P, Bourret J (1974) Quantitative histological data on disuse osteoporosis. Calcif Tissue Res 17:57–73

Moldawer M, Zimmerman SJ, Collins LC (1965) Incidence of osteoporosis in elderly whites and elderly negroes. JAMA 194:859–862

Morey ER, Baylink DJ (1978) Inhibition of bone formation during space flight. Science 201:1138–1341

Nagent de Deuxchaisnes C (1983) The pathogenesis and treatment of involutional osteoporosis. In: Dixon A St J, Russell RGG, Stamp TCB (eds) Osteoporosis: A multidisciplinary problem. International Congress and Symposium Series No 55. Academic Press and Royal Society of Medicine, London, pp 291–333

Newcomer AD, Hodgson SF, McGill DB, Thomas PJ (1978) Lactose deficiency: prevalence in osteoporosis. Ann Intern Med 89:218–220

Newton-John HF, Morgan DB (1970) The loss of bone with age, osteoporosis and fractures. Clin Orthop 71:229–252

Ng KC, Revell PA, Beer M, Boucher BJ, Cohen RD, Currey HLF (1984) The incidence of metabolic bone disease, rheumatoid arthritis and osteoarthritis. Ann Rheum Dis 43:370–377

Nilsson BE (1966) Post-traumatic osteopenia. A quantitative study of the bone mineral mass in the femur following fracture of the tibia in man using americum-241 as a photon source. Acta Orthop Scand 37(91):1–55

Nilsson BE, Westlin NE (1971) Bone density in athletes. Clin Orthop 77:179–182

Nilsson BE, Westlin NE (1973) Changes in bone mass in alcoholics. Clin Orthop 90:229–232

Nilsson BE, Anderson SM, Havdrup T, Westlin NE (1978) Ballet-dancing and weightlifting—effects on BMC. Am J Roentgenol Radium Ther Nucl Med 131:541–542

Nordin BEC (1966) International patterns of osteoporosis. Clin Orthop 45:17–30

Nordin BEC, Aaron J, Spear R, Crilly RG (1981) Bone formation and resorption as the determinants of trabecular bone volume in postmenopausal osteoporosis. Lancet II:277–279

O'Driscoll S, O'Driscoll M (1980) Osteomalacia in rheumatoid arthritis. Ann Rheum Dis 39:1–6

Parfitt AM, Mathews C, Rao D, Frame B, Kleerekoper M, Villanueva AR (1981) Impaired osteoblast function in metabolic bone disease. In: DeLuca HF, Frost HM, Jee WSS, Johnson CC Jr, Parfitt AM (eds) Osteoporosis: recent advances in pathogenesis and treatment. University Park Press, Baltimore, pp 321–330

Peart KM, Ellis HA (1975) Quantitative observations on iliac bone marrow mast cells in chronic renal failure. J Clin Pathol 28:947–955

Perry HM, Fallon MD, Bergfeld M, Teitelbaum SL, Avioli LV (1982) Osteoporosis in young men: a syndrome of hypercalciuria and accelerated bone turnover. Arch Intern Med 142:1295–1298

Recker RR, Saville PD, Heaney RP (1977) Effect of estrogens and calcium carbonate on bone loss in post-menopausal women. Ann Intern Med 87:649–655

Riggs BL, Jowsey J, Kelly PJ, Jones JD, Maher FT (1969) Effect of sex hormones on bone in primary osteoporosis. J Clin Invest 48:1065–1072

Riggs BL, Arnaud CD, Jowsey J, Goldsmith RS, Kelly PJ (1973) Parathyroid function in primary osteoporosis. Clin Invest 52:181–184

Riggs BL, Wahner HW, Dunn WL, Mazess RB, Offord KP, Melton LJ III (1981) Differential changes in bone mineral density of the appendicular and axial skeleton with aging. J Clin Invest 67:328–335

Saville PD (1965) Changes in bone mass with age and alcoholism. J Bone Joint Surg [Am] 47:492–499

Schenk RK, Merz WA (1969) Histologisch-morphometrische Untersuchungen über Altersatrophie und senile Osteoporose in der Spongiosa des Beckenkammes. Dtsch Med Wochenschr 94:206–208

Sissons HA (1955) The structural pathology of osteoporosis. Proc R Soc Med 48:566–578

Sissons HA, Hadfield GJ (1955) The influence of cortisone on the structure and growth of bone. J Anat 89:69–78

Smith R (1979) Idiopathic juvenile osteoporosis. Am J Dis Child 133:889–891

Smith R (1980) Idiopathic osteoporosis in the young. J Bone Joint Surg [Br] 62:417–427

Smith R, Sykes BC (1983) Osteogenesis imperfecta and idiopathic juvenile osteoporosis. In: Dixon A St J, Russell RGG, Stamp TCB (eds) Osteoporosis. A multidisciplinary problem. International Congress and Symposium Series No 55. Academic Press and Royal Society of Medicine, London, pp 133–135

Smith RW Jr, Rizek J (1966) Epidemiologic studies of osteoporosis in women of Puerto Rico and South Eastern Michigan with special reference to age, race, national origin and to other related or associated findings. Clin Orthop 45:31–48

Solomon L (1979) Bone density in ageing Caucasian and African populations. Lancet II:1326–1330

Stevenson JC, White MG, Joplin GF, MacIntyre I (1982) Osteoporosis and calcitonin deficiency. Br Med J 285:1010–1011

Stinchfield AJ, Reidy JA, Barr JS (1949) Prediction of unequal growth of lower extremities in anterior poliomyelitis. J Bone Joint Surg [Am] 31:478–486

Teitelbaum SL, Rosenberg EM, Richardson CA, Avioli LV (1976) Histological studies of bone from normo-calcemic postmenopausal osteoporotic patients with increased circulating parathyroid hormone. J Clin Endocrinol Metab 42:537–543

Teotia M, Teotia SPS, Singh RK (1979) Idiopathic juvenile osteoporosis. Am J Dis Child 133:894–900

te Velde J, Vismans FJFE, Leenheers-Binnendijk L, Voz CJ, Smeenk D, Bijvoet OLM (1978) The eosinophilic fibrohistiocytic lesion of the bone marrow. A mastocellular lesion in bone disease. Virchows Arch [A] 377:277–285

Tilton FE, Degioanni TTC, Schneider VS (1980) Long term follow-up of Skylab bone demineralization. Aviat Space Environ Med 51:1209–1213

Urist MR, McLean FC (1957) Accumulation of mast cells in endosteum of bone of calcium-deficient rats. Arch Pathol 63:239–251

Uthoff HK, Jaworski ZFG (1978) Bone loss in response to long-term immobilisation. J Bone Joint Surg [Br] 60:420–429

Wahner HW, Riggs BL, Beabout JW (1977) Diagnosis of osteoporosis: usefulness of photon absorptiometry at the radius. J Nucl Med 18:432–437

Whedon GD, Lutwak L, Rambaut P, Whittle M, Leach C, Reid J, Smith M (1976) Effect of weightlessness on mineral metabolism: metabolic studies on Skylab orbital space flights. Calcif Tissue Res 21(Suppl):423–430

Whiting SJ, Draper HH (1980) The role of sulfate in the calciuria of high protein diets in adult rats. J Nutr 110:212–222

Whyte MP, Bergfeld MA, Murphy WA, Avioli LV, Teitelbaum SL (1982) Postmenopausal osteoporosis. A heterogeneous disorder as assessed by histomorphometric analysis of iliac crest bone from untreated patients. Am J Med 72:193–202

Wilson CR, Madsen M (1977) Dichromatic absorptiometry of vertebral bone mineral content. Invest Radiol 12:180–184

Young MM, Nordin BEC (1967) Effect of natural and artificial menopause on plasma and urinary calcium and phosphorus. Lancet II:118–120

Chapter 9

Necrosis and Healing in Bone

Introduction

This chapter deals with what may seem a miscellany of conditions. Nevertheless, there are some relevant cross-correlations to be made with respect to the pathological processes, for example the appearances of bone necrosis and subsequent healing in relation to fractures, bone grafts and that of fragments of bone broken away at the time of trauma or joint replacement surgery. The following account will deal with the broad areas of fractures, bone grafts, reactions to prostheses and avascular necrosis, with a short section on electrical effects in bone.

Fractures and fracture healing

Fractures occur when bone is broken by mechanical forces. It is not relevant to give a detailed description here of the many different types of fracture which may occur in various bones, some of which have time-honoured eponyms (e.g. Colles' fracture). One approach to fracture classification is to be found in the article by Johner and Wruhs (1983), which specifically deals with tibial fractures and gives details of the type of trauma most often associated with a particular type of break. In their study in Switzerland, they found that a simple spiral fracture of the shaft of the tibia, for example, was caused by skiing accidents or falls in the home or street in two-thirds of cases, while transverse fractures, although also occurring with skiing, were associated with motorcycle or footballing accidents in young men (Johner and Wruhs 1983). It is not possible to enter into the detail given even by these authors, who describe the different effects of torsion, bending, compression and low- and high-speed impacts. Further information of a more specialist orthopaedic nature is available in large textbooks such as that of Watson-Jones (1982a,b), and perusal of the orthopaedic literature will reveal recent specialist articles, such as those relating to the tibia (Heppenstall 1983; Patzakis et al. 1983a,b; Waddell and Reardon 1983) and distal femur (Healy and Brookes 1983).

Many of the terms used in describing fractures are self evident, but a few will be mentioned here. A simple closed fracture is one which occurs within the tissues without exposure of the bone or breaking of the related skin surface. When skin and soft tissue injuries occur so that a piece of fractured bone is likely to be exposed to the external environment, then a fracture is considered to be an 'open fracture' (compound fracture). The distinction between closed and open lesions is important in orthopaedic management. Open fractures have a higher infection rate than closed fractures (see Johner and Wruhs 1983, and orthopaedic textbooks), and the rate of infection increases with increasing severity of soft tissue damage (Gustilo and Anderson 1976; Clancey and Hansen 1978). A 'comminuted' fracture is one which has become shattered into several small fragments. Other specialist types of fracture need not be described here but include impacted and crush fractures and those extending to articular surfaces—all features of importance to the orthopaedic surgeon.

The factors influencing the treatment, prognosis and anatomical result of healing in fractures include the mechanism of the accident causing the trauma, the presence of comminution, soft tissue injury and displacement of the fractured bone ends. Recent references to these factors are available in Johner and Wruhs (1983). The complications of fracture healing include delayed union and non-union, which have been defined in various ways, for example lack of radiological union within 4 months and 8 months respectively (Johner and Wruhs 1983). Such attempts at separation would seem arbitrary, and the author prefers the approach of McKibbin (1982), who uses 'failure of union' to embrace both delayed and non-union of fractures.

Detailed descriptions of the healing of fractures are available in standard texbooks of histology and general pathology and are based on experimental transverse breaks of tubular bones of rodents, since this is the only way in which the sequence of events may be studied systematically. A classic description is that by Ham and Harris (1971), while further accounts include McKibbin (1978). From time to time, the histopathologist has the opportunity to study human fractures, either at autopsy or in those cases with failure of union which finally come to amputation. The sequence of changes is outlined here.

The initial event is the severing of vessels as well as the separation of bone, so that blood is present between the bone ends. This may be confined within the periosteum or spread further afield into the surrounding soft tissues, which may themselves be lacerated. There is also a serofibrinous exudate formed as part of the acute inflammatory reaction to tissue damage. Fibrous, fatty and haemopoietic tissue all die as a result of the direct physical trauma of the injury and because of the loss of blood supply. Detached fragments of bone become necrotic and there is a variable degree of cell death in the fractured ends still in continuity with the main bone, although the classic appearance of empty osteocyte lacunae is not seen until at least 7 days after the cells die (see p. 226). The process of acute inflammation at the fracture site continues for 24–48 h with exudation and migration of polymorphonuclears at first, followed by macrophages; the process then passes into the repair phase, in which there is granulation tissue formation with the proliferation of small blood vessels and migration of fibroblasts into the area. The rate at which subsequent development of fibrous tissue between the bone ends occurs depends on local conditions, but under optimal conditions there is fibrous union by around 2 weeks. While this repair is taking place, there is also removal of fragments of dead bone by osteoclasts. The conversion of this reparative granulation tissue to hard tissue is that of callus formation (L. *callum*, hard (skin); Fig. 9.1). A potential cause of confusion arises over the different types of callus described. External callus is the mass of ossifying fibrous tissue outside the bone at the fracture site, while internal callus is the same sort of tissue present between and within the bone ends, and primary callus is the term used to describe the newly formed primitive (woven) bone formed initially.

There has been debate about whether the cells forming this new bone are derived from pre-existing osteoblastic cells on the endosteal and periosteal surfaces or whether the cells are derived locally by induction of tissue fibroblasts into osteoblasts. Almost certainly, both mechanisms occur at the same time, as is apparent from the presence of both appositional new bone formation around existing living, and dead (Fig. 9.2) bone and lace-like bone formation *de novo* in fibrous tissue. The primary callus comes to bridge the gap between the bone ends completely and is composed of woven bone (Fig. 9.3). Resorption of this primitive bone and the formation of lamellar bone marks the development of secondary callus, which leads to the formation of a firm bony fusion across the fracture site. Subsequent remodelling takes place under such influences as mechanical loading with weight bearing and resumption of normal activity. The presence of small islands of cartilage within the callus is interpreted by some as evidence of movement of the imperfectly immobilised fractured bone ends, but others have related it to the presence of avascular conditions locally (Collins 1966). Whatever the explanation, small amounts of chondroid tissue often may be seen within the callus of a healing fracture.

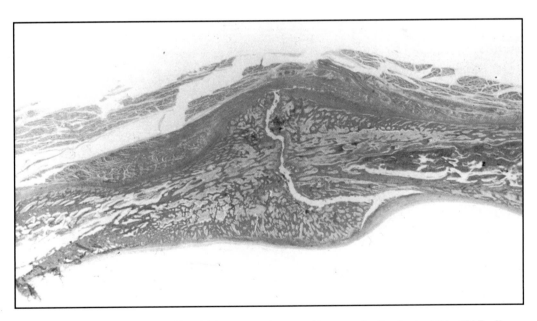

Fig. 9.1. Fracture of a rib, showing callus with bone expansion caused by external callus clearly visible. (H&E × 8)

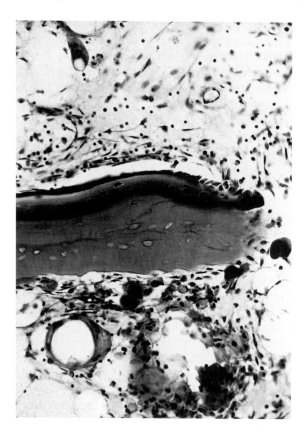

Fig. 9.2. Fragment of dead trabecular bone at a fracture site, showing appositional new bone formation. (H&E × 200)

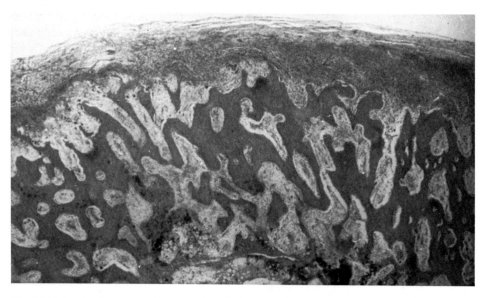

Fig. 9.3. External callus composed of woven bone in fibrous tissue. (H&E × 60)

Sometimes the pathologist may be asked to give some idea as to the age of a fracture, and a useful guide to the timing of the process under optimal conditions is that given by Collins (1966) and summarised in Table 9.1. There is obviously considerable variability from bone to bone and with age. Ellis (1958) showed that immobilisation for more than 12 weeks was never necessary under the age of 16 years, whereas older subjects required 15 weeks and some of them were delayed over 20 weeks. The severity of the fracture together with the degree of separation of the fragments also affect the rate of healing (Ellis 1958; Johner and Wruhs 1983).

Table 9.1. Timetable for fracture healing (after Collins 1966)

12 h	Blood clot and exudate between fragments
24 h	Acute inflammation with migration of polymorphonuclears and macrophages
48 h	Formation of granulation tissue
5 days	Earliest new bone formation
7 days	Empty osteocyte lacunae in remaining dead fragments
3 weeks	Fibrous union; some primary callus
6 weeks	Periosteal shell of external callus; complete meshwork of woven bone
After 6 weeks	Progressive formation of secondary callus and subsequent remodelling

Factors affecting the healing of fractures

The various factors affecting the healing of a fracture need not be dealt with in great detail here since accounts are available in specialist orthopaedic text-books. The type of fracture (Urist et al. 1954), its site and method of treatment are all important aspects to be taken into consideration. Healing is considered to occur in much the same way as the natural process of fracture repair with closed methods of treatment (i.e. treatment without deliberate exposure and internal fixation of the fracture site), by the use of splints with or without traction or plaster casts. The purpose of this external fixation is to preserve length and alignment in addition to obtaining some degree of immobilisation. It is likely that some minute degree of movement is required to stimulate callus formation mechanically, but excessive movement, that is inadequate immobilisation, affects healing adversely. The actual size of the gap to be bridged in the healing process is also important, as are such factors as loss of blood supply and coexistent infection. The interposition of soft tissue, muscle and large fragments of dead bone are further impediments to the repair of fractures.

The influence of internal fixation devices on callus formation should be borne in mind. Many devices act as a means of holding the bone ends together, and the healing process is much like that associated with external fixation, with the formation of external callus. The repair process is, however, modified when methods of secure fixation and rigid immobilisation are used. This was first noted radiologically by Danis (1949), when he found that rather than formation of callus the fracture line just disappeared gradually. This minimal callus formation with secure fixation has also been noted by Blockley (1956) and Hicks (1961). It was subsequently shown histologically by Schenk and Willenegger (1967) that there was revascularisation of bone, including Haversian systems, together with formation of woven bone in the small space between the bone ends. The presence of the implant itself gives rise to further pathological questions, one of which concerns altered mechanical properties, because those forces which would normally be at work on the healing bone are carried by the implant (Tonino et al. 1976), so that there is the possibility of the development of local bone atrophy and subsequent refracture. Intramedullary fixation is less rigid, seldom suppresses external callus formation, and is followed by a process more like that occurring naturally. It does, however, suffer from the disadvantages of the increased likelihood of infection after open methods of fixation, as already mentioned, and of the potential damage done to the viability of the bone by interference with the medullary blood supply. The appearance of bone in relation to surgical implants is described later in this chapter (see Reactions of bone adjacent to joint prostheses and other implants).

Failure of union

The factors involved in a case where a fracture has failed to unite satisfactorily are described above. No attempt will be made to separate such terms as 'delayed union', 'non-union' or 'mal-union' here. The pathological findings in fractures which had not healed were described by Urist et al. (1954). An increase in separation of the fractured bone ends of more than 0.5 cm increased

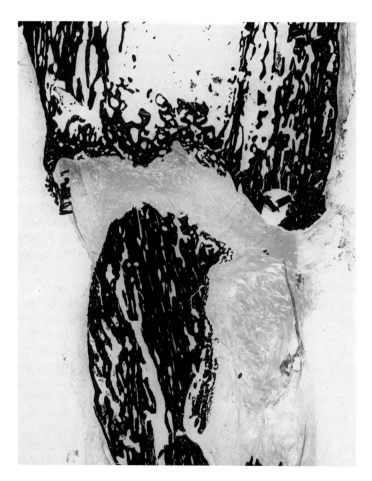

Fig. 9.4. Failure of union of a fractured tibia with well-formed fibrous tissue between the bone ends at the site of the fracture. (von Kossa × 10)

the healing time to between 12 and 18 months, and a gap of over 1 cm took even longer. Slowly healing lesions showed the enclosure of the fracture line in a spindle-shaped collection of fibrous tissue from 4 to 6 months after injury. The endosteal surfaces away from the fracture line showed new bone formation, while the bone ends were covered in hyaline and fibrocartilage. The centre of the intervening connective tissue contained amorphous fibrinoid material, associated with which there was sometimes a local accumulation of mucinous fluid, the early stage in the formation of a pseudarthrosis. Between 6 months and 2 years, the bone ends were capped with cartilage and from 2 to 5 years there was a mature pseudarthrosis, with expansion of the fractured bone ends, dense cortical and cancellous bone related to a cartilaginous joint surface and a cavity containing viscous fluid. Examples of fractures showing non-union are shown in Figs. 9.4 and 9.5, the latter illustrating the development of a joint-like space though not an established pseudarthrosis.

Pathological fractures

A pathological fracture has been described as a fracture occurring after injury so trivial that its force would not break normal healthy bone (Collins 1966). The author would prefer to shift the emphasis of this definition and say that a pathological fracture is one occurring in diseased bone, thereby removing the inference that trivial injury is responsible, since clearly the trauma could also be of the same order as for ordinary fractures. A list of many of the conditions in which pathological fractures may occur is given in Table 9.2. Most of these have been described elsewhere in this book and only certain particular points will be brought out here.

Firstly, although vitamin lack is not a factor in Europe and North America, nutritional deficiency is still a cause of deformity and fracture in parts of Africa and Asia. There is also little doubt that unrecognised vitamin C deficiency short of clinical scurvy is a cause of slow union of fractures (Watson-Jones 1982b). Rickets and osteomalacia usually appear in lists of conditions in which pathological fractures occur. It is necessary to distinguish true fractures from the pseudofractures or Looser's zones which occur in vitamin D-deficient individuals (see p. 124). Incomplete cracks may occur on the convex side of the bent long bones in rickets, and trivial injury may convert these to complete fractures (Fig. 9.6).

The significance of the loss of bone has been discussed in the chapter on osteoporosis, which includes the concept of a fracture threshold (see Chap. 8, Introduction; Involutional osteoporosis). Corticosteroids are a potent cause of bone loss and important in the consideration of vertebral crush fractures, which are frequently sustained during trivial incidents. Local osteoporosis may occur with disuse, and such atrophy of bone may result in a second (pathological) fracture following sustained recumbency of a patient with a pre-existing complicated fracture or severe trauma. According to Nilsson and Westlin (1974), fracture of the distal end of the forearm was related to a reduction in bone mineral content in women, but bone mineral content was also found to be significantly reduced in children, in whom fractures were caused by low energy trauma (Landin and Nilsson 1983), suggesting that endogenous factors

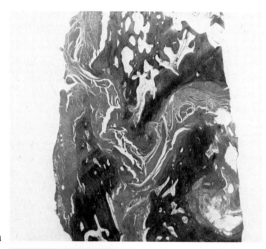

a

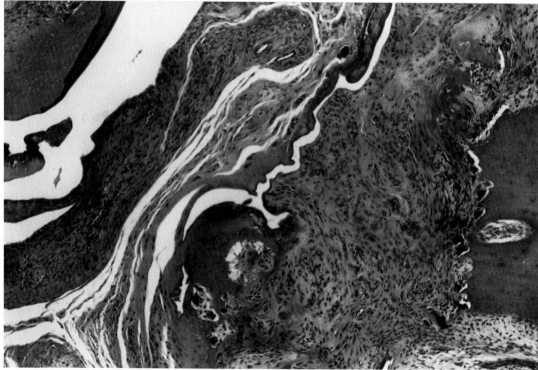

b

Fig. 9.5. a Failure of union of a fracture, showing the presence of cleft-like spaces in the fibrous tissue between the irregularly shaped bone ends. (Azan × 16)
b Higher power view of region of cleft seen in **a**, showing that this is partly lined by cells resembling synovial intimal cells. Note osteoclastic resorption of bone fragment (*right*). (H&E × 80)

Fig. 9.6. Fractured rib in rachitic bone caused by Fanconi syndrome, showing poorly mineralised bone between the fracture ends. (von Kossa × 10)

Table 9.2. Conditions in which there may be pathological fracture of bone

1. *Developmental and biochemical disorders:*
   a) Osteogenesis imperfecta
   b) Osteopetrosis
   c) Enchondromatosis
   d) Gaucher's disease
2. *Hormonal and metabolic disorders:*
   a) Hyperparathyroidism
   b) Cushing's syndrome; corticosteroid therapy
   c) Vitamin C deficiency; vitamin D deficiency
3. *Bone atrophy:*
   a) Generalised osteoporosis (N.B. corticosteroids)
   b) Disuse osteoporosis
4. *Paget's disease of bone*
5. *Infection and infestation:*
   a) Osteomyelitis (pyogenic, tuberculosis)
   b) Syphilis
   c) Hydatid disease
6. *Neoplasms of bone:*
   a) Benign, primary (chondroma, chondroblastoma, chondromyxoid fibroma, haemangioma, giant cell tumour)
   b) Malignant, primary (osteosarcoma, giant cell tumour, fibrosarcoma, malignant fibrous histocytoma, Ewing's sarcoma, multiple myeloma)
   c) Malignant, secondary (carcinoma of breast, lung, kidney, prostate, thyroid)
7. *Cysts and tumour-like lesions:*
   a) Solitary bone cyst
   b) Aneurysmal bone cyst
   c) Fibro-osseus dysplasia
   d) Histocytosis X
8. *Neurological disorders:*
   a) Tables dorsalis
   b) Syringomyelia
   c) Diabetic neuropathy
9. *Surgical*—previous orthopaedic procedures (screws, cement, prostheses, biopsy)

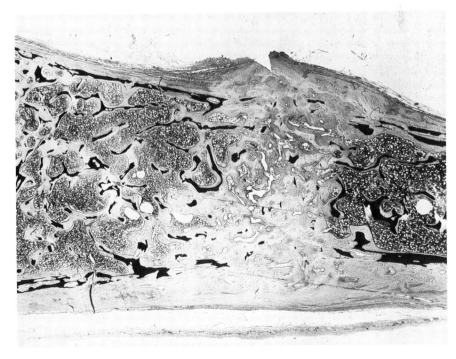

Fig. 9.6.

may even play a role in the apparently normal young person. These cases could not be defined as pathological fractures in the present sense but they give rise to an interesting philosophical question about the normality of bone in the light of more sophisticated investigative methods.

Pathological fracture through bone of increased density occurs in osteopetrosis and Paget's disease, the latter being one of the commoner causes of pathological fracture in the elderly (see p. 150).

The list of tumour and tumour-like conditions in which there may be pathological fractures is fairly long. Metastatic carcinoma is by far the most frequent neoplastic cause. Bone secondaries may occur from almost any primary site, but those particularly prone to osseous spread are breast, lung, kidney, prostate and thyroid. Skeletal secondaries of carcinoma are often widespread and developed in the terminal stages of the disease, but this is not always the case.

A familiar problem to the pathologist interested in bone tumours is the differential diagnosis of the solitary metastatic lesion, which may even sometimes resemble a primary bone tumour on histological examination, for example a predominantly spindle-celled metastasis from a renal carcinoma. An osteolytic lesion in the mid-shaft of a long bone of a patient in the appropriate 'cancer age group' should lead to suspicion of secondary disease, as should an apparently clean transverse fracture at this site seen on the radiograph (Fig. 9.7). Biopsy of such an osteolytic lesion may itself precipitate a fracture. The

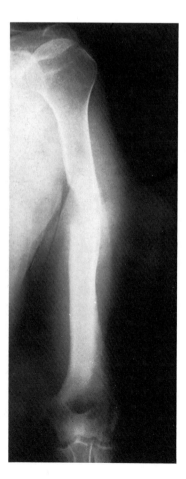

Fig. 9.7. Transverse fracture in the mid-shaft of the humerus, caused by metastatic carcinoma

presence of osteosclerosis in relation to metastatic carcinoma of breast or prostate does not make pathological fracture less likely. Fracture healing in metastatic bone disease has most recently been studied by Gainor and Buchert (1983). Bony healing was observed in 67% of fractures associated with multiple myeloma, 44% of those associated with renal carcinoma and 37% of those associated with secondary breast carcinoma. No bone repair was seen in relation to secondary carcinoma of the lung, but then none of the patients lived for more than 6 months after fracture. A total dose of radiotherapy of up to 3000 rad did not inhibit callus formation, and internal fixation improved the rate of fracture union as compared with external immobilization.

Primary malignant bone tumours in which there may be pathological fracture are listed in Table 9.2. Whether or not an osteosarcoma will be a site of fracture must depend partly on the degree to which the tumour is a sclerotic or destructive and lytic lesion. A pathological fracture through an osteosarcoma is illustrated in Fig. 9.8. Giant cell tumours have been classified under both benign and malignant (see p. 286) and for this reason are included twice in Table 9.2. Pathological fracture may sometimes be the presenting feature in chondrosarcoma, fibrosarcoma, malignant fibrous histiocytoma and sarcoma in Paget's disease, whatever the particular tumour type. Bone weakened by benign tumours and tumour-like conditions may also fracture. Further details may be obtained in Watson-Jones (1982b).

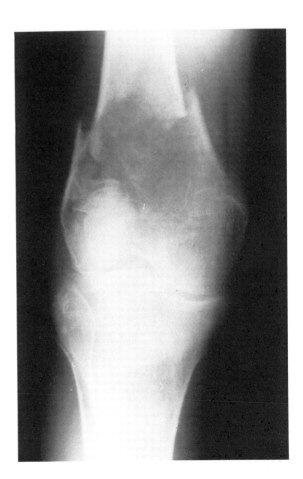

Fig. 9.8. Osteosarcoma. Pathological fracture through a large osteolytic lesion in the lower metaphysis of the femur of a 20-year-old man

Tabes dorsalis and syringomyelia are conditions which give rise to a neurological deficit in the legs and arms. Loss of joint position sense and of the sensation of pain give rise to the severe joint damage seen in the neuropathic joint, but the patient may also fracture bones and have markedly comminuted fractures with little or no pain. Union of fractures or elective arthrodeses is usually slow and toleration of metal implants poor where there is neurotrophic disturbance of bone (Watson-Jones 1982b).

Modern orthopaedic surgery includes the use of various implants made of a variety of different materials. Unsupported screw holes expose bone to the hazard of pathological fracture (Brooks et al. 1970), and resorption of bone by the cellular reaction in relation to bone cement or wear debris is a potential cause of weakening of bone and fracture (see this chapter, Reaction of osseous tissue adjacent to bone cement; Wear debris and the implant bed). Removal of cortical bone when performing a biopsy or treating osteomyelitis may also result in a predisposition to fracture.

Stress or fatigue fractures

A fatigue (or stress) fracture occurs in normal bone as a result of accumulated stress and is analogous with fatigue failure in such materials as metals, in which repeated application of the same stress results in fracture. The most familiar lesion of this type is the so-called march fracture of the metatarsal, which occurs in soldiers on long route marches and in others making unaccustomed long walks. Such fractures occur in the distal part of the second metatarsal bone. Although there may be some pain, the patient may first complain of a swelling, which coincides with the development of callus at the site of the fracture, and local tenderness.

The sites of other fatigue fractures, together with the activity or occupation often associated with their development, are shown in Table 9.3. Apart from march fractures, military recruits may also suffer stress fractures of the calcaneus, the fibula and femur. Stress fractures of the upper fibula occur in association with repeated jumping and landing with the knees flexed, so that this is a lesion also occurring in parachutists (Burrows 1948). Athletes get stress fractures at different sites depending on their type of activity. Track athletes, cross-country runners and marathon runners develop tenderness, swelling and radiological evidence of localised bone sclerosis of the lower fibula at the site of the fracture. Athletes and ballet dancers get stress fractures of the tibia,

Table 9.3. Sites of fatigue fractures and often associated categories or occupations of patients

Site	Occupation/category
March fracture of (2nd) metatarsal	Military recruits, long-distance walkers
Calcaneus	Military recruits, athletes
Lower fibula	Middle-aged women; track, cross-country and marathon runners
Upper fibula	Military recruits, parachutists
Tibia	Ballet dancers, athletes
Femur	Military recruits

but not in the same places; in the former they occur in the posteromedial aspect of the lower tibia, while in the latter the anterior part of the middle third of the bone is affected (Burrows 1956; Devas 1958, 1980). Stress fractures of the upper tibia, with associated local pain, increased warmth and radiological changes, may give rise to the clinical suspicion of osteomyelitis or even sarcoma (Devas 1980). Fatigue fractures in the upper limb, ribs and clavicle have been reported in association with such occupations as clay-pigeon shooting and forking farm manure (Kitchin 1948; Boyer 1975). Further examples of such curiosities are given in Watson-Jones (1982b).

Bone grafts

Bone grafts have been used in orthopaedics for over 60 years. During this period the following techniques have all been used in varying degrees:

Autograft—bone removed from one site and implanted elsewhere in the same patient
Allograft or *homograft*—bone from one human implanted in another
Xenograft or *heterograft*—animal bone implanted in a human

Autografts have found greatest favour over recent years, but the use of allografts has been moderately successful, even though long-term follow-up shows a high incidence of failure of union and fatigue fracture. A comprehensive review by Buchhardt (1983) gives a good source of references to the subject of bone grafting.

A long-standing question arises over the viability of grafted bone and the origin of the osteogenic cells within the graft, so that it has been suggested that the term 'implant' might be more appropriate than graft. The incorporation of a graft into the skeleton is almost certainly a result of activity both by viable osteoblasts and progenitor cells within the graft bone and of cells in the recipient bone, although the relative contribution of these different cells is uncertain (Siffert 1955; Heslop et al. 1960; Arora and Laskin 1964; Collins 1966; Ray 1972; Albrektsson 1980; Buchhardt 1983). Death of osteocytes in the grafted bone will result through loss of blood supply in much the same way as occurs with small detached fragments in fractures. The source of potential cells from the graft depends partly on the type of graft, whether cortical or cancellous, but there is evidence for a contribution being made by cells from the periosteum, cortex, endosteal surface and bone marrow (Urist and McLean 1952; Tonna and Cronkite 1961; Arora and Laskin 1964; King 1976; Gray and Elves 1979). Some light has been thrown on the question as to whether cells of the graft, recipient tissue, or both, play a role in healing by Elves and Pratt (1975), using strontium labelling of rat bone. They were able to show that although histological examination could not detect different phases of activity, radio-labelling demonstrated two distinct peaks of osteogenesis after implantation of grafts in rats. The first phase occurred during the first 3 weeks with intact grafts, was absent from non-viable irradiated grafts, but present when bone marrow elements had been removed from the graft, suggesting that endosteal cells were a major component in early osteogenesis. The second phase occurred after 8 weeks and had a major host tissue component.

Undoubtedly, whatever the proportion of graft cells surviving, and the degree of response from the recipient tissue, a vital factor is the continued vascularity and viability of the recipient site and the proliferation of cells from this source. The term 'creeping substitution' was introduced many years ago and is still used by some orthopaedic surgeons to describe the gradual replacement of the old necrotic bone of the graft by new viable bone. The actual process of repair around bone autografts is, however, little different from that seen in a healing fracture. A good critique of the concept of 'creeping substitution' is given by Glimcher and Kenzora (1979a).

At first, the graft is the site of inflammation, with the development of vascular granulation tissue between and around the fragments of dead bone. This is followed by an increase in osteoclastic activity in the graft. Cancellous bone grafts are rapidly revascularised and soon show deposition of appositional new bone by osteoblasts upon the scaffolding of the dead bone chips of the graft (Urist and McLean, 1952). At the same time, there may be new woven bone formation in the vascular fibrous tissue between the graft fragments (Fig. 9.9). Vascularisation of cortical grafts is slower, and even after considerable lengths of time they contain both dead and living bone, in contrast to cancellous bone grafts, which eventually become more or less completely repaired with replacement by living bone. Details relating to the mechanical strength of dead as against living bone and to the strength of grafts are available in Enneking et al. (1975) and Buchhardt (1983).

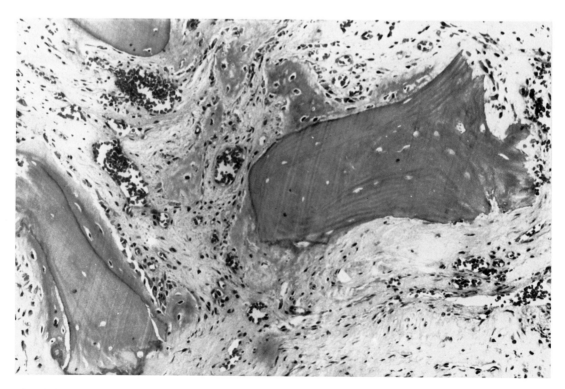

Fig. 9.9. Appositional new bone formation around fragments of dead bone in a healing bone graft. There is vascular fibrous tissue between the graft fragments. (H&E × 400)

Surgical reconstruction may require supplies of bone over and above those reasonably obtained from the patient himself as an autograft. While various synthetic materials can be used to restore defects, these are not as satisfactory as bone since they never become incorporated and converted to bone. For this reason, the possibility of using allografts and xenografts has been explored. As soon as foreign bone is introduced, however, the whole question of histocompatibility becomes relevant. A good review and source of references to this and the different alternatives to bone autografts is available in the review by Buchhardt (1983). Bone is immunogenic and the major source of differences in histocompatibility is considered to be the bone marrow, although bone matrix may also contribute.

The tissue response to a bone allograft is different from that of an autograft, although much of the background information relates to animal studies and the use of predominantly cortical bone. Vascularisation and new bone formation are less marked in allografts, which show more resorptive activity than autografts. At first, the cellular response is like that seen with an autograft, but between 2 weeks and 2 months, lymphocytes predominate and the graft eventually becomes surrounded by fibrous tissue (Bonfiglio and Jetter 1972). Soon after grafting, small vessels near the implant may be surrounded by inflammatory cells and their lumens become occluded (Nisbet et al. 1960; Zeiss et al. 1960). The implant undergoes necrosis because of vascular insufficiency, and any secondary new bone formation on the scaffolding of the graft is less successful than with an autograft (Buchhardt 1983).

Reactions of bone adjacent to joint prostheses and other implants

Prosthetic joint replacement is extensively practised in developed countries, mainly for rheumatoid arthritis and osteoarthrosis, although implants are also used in the treatment of fractured neck of femur and, most recently, to allow local excision of some bone tumours in preference to amputation. In addition, various plates, screws and nails have been used for many years in orthopaedics. While there is an ever-expanding number of different materials being tried, with various ways of fixing implants to the skeleton, the most common implant materials are metals (stainless steel, cobalt-chrome alloy) and plastics (polyethylene, polyester, polyformaldehyde), together with acrylics ('bone cements'). The changes in tissues adjacent to joint prostheses have been described in reviews by Willert (1973), Vernon-Roberts and Freeman (1976) and Revell (1982). The following account will deal with the appearances of bone adjacent to prostheses fixed with bone cement, those where there is direct contact of the implant with bone and the effects of excess wear debris on the interface between implant and bone.

Pathological examination of bone related to implants

The histopathologist may receive bone related to an implant either at the time of surgical revision or at autopsy, and his function is slightly different in these two circumstances. In the former case, exclusion of infection, for example by the use of frozen sections of any available soft tissue (Mirra et al. 1976), and determination of the amount of wear debris are important considerations. Microbiological examination is vital where infection is suspected. Autopsies of cases having an indwelling prosthesis give a unique opportunity for the examination of the reactions around well-functioning implants.

Special problems arise in the examination of bone having an implant firmly attached to it. Polymethylmethacrylate bone cement is readily removed by immersing the fixed specimen in a solvent such as acetone. Metal and/or polyethylene may be sectioned while still attached to bone by using a water-cooled circular saw with a diamond-impregnated steel or carborundum wheel (Revell 1982).

Reaction of osseous tissue adjacent to bone cement

Many joint prostheses currently in use are fixed to the skeleton with bone cement, which is pressed into the implant bed while still in a soft doughy state. The outline of the interface between bone and cement may be smooth or, more often, comprise a series of nobbly projections which interdigitate with the trabecular bone (Fig. 9.10; Willert et al. 1974). The ultrastructural changes at the bone–cement interface are described by Linder and Hansson (1983). Necrosis of bone and bone marrow occurs for a distance of 3–5 mm adjacent to the cement as a result of the destruction of the local blood supply at implantation, the heat generated by polymerisation of the polymethylmethacrylate cement dough and the toxicity of unpolymerised methylmethacrylate monomer diffusing from the cement, as well as the effects of reaming during preparation of the implant bed. In the first 2 or 3 weeks after implantation, there is a layer of necrotic tissue and fibrin adjacent to the bone cement. For a period of several months after this, there is gradual repair of tissue damage with demarcation of dead bone and bone marrow by a zone of reactive hyperaemia, phagocytosis of necrotic tissue, proliferation of small vessels and fibrous replacement of the necrotic bone marrow. Where there is revascularisation, appositional new bone is formed around dead trabeculae. The cement and bone are always separated by a fibrous tissue membrane (Fig. 9.10) although this is sometimes attenuated. Careful examination of the interface reveals the presence of macrophages and multinucleate giant cells on the cement side of this membrane (Revell 1982). There continues to be evidence of remodelling of bone with osteoclastic and osteoblastic activity on the trabecular surfaces adjacent to the implant, even when the prosthesis is healed into place. Reorganisation of the bone around the prosthesis occurs in accordance with Wolff's law (Wolff 1892), changes in structure corresponding to altered physical requirements. Trabeculae are formed parallel to the cemented surface and come to encircle the stem of the femoral component in the case of a hip

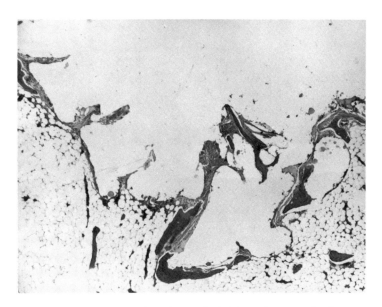

Fig. 9.10. Bone-cement interface of a prosthetic joint replacement, showing irregular nobbly projections of cement (*top*) extending between trabeculae and into marrow space. Cement is separated from the tissues by a fibrous membrane. (H&E × 100)

prosthesis. Chondroid metaplasia may occur in the fibrous tissue between bone and cement, but is seen more frequently where fixation is without cement (see below). The development of a malignant fibrous histiocytoma adjacent to a cemented hip prosthesis has recently been reported (Bago-Granell et al. 1984).

Direct contact of bone with implant material

The use of prostheses designed to be fixed directly to the skeleton avoids the problems of cement-related bone death and the tissue reactions described above. Cementless arthroplasty of the hip has been reviewed recently by Morscher (1983). The author has had the opportunity to examine bone adjacent to polyethylene tibial plateaux of knee prostheses at different times after implantation (Blaha et al. 1982; Revell 1982). In the first 3 weeks after implantation, there are fragments of necrotic trabeculae and otherwise intact living and dead bone right up to the polyethylene implant surface, as a result of the surgical preparation of the bone to receive the implant (Fig. 9.11). Granulation tissue formation and healing occur along exactly the same lines as already described in relation to fractures and bone grafts (see pp. 204, 216). Appositional new bone is formed around living and dead trabeculae and there is also new woven bone formation in the intertrabecular spaces (Fig. 9.12). The longterm result seen in prostheses up to 3 years after implantation is the formation of horizontally disposed bridges of bone between the pre-existing vertical trabeculae of the upper tibia to form a bony plateau. This bone is separated from polyethylene by a layer of fibrous tissue in which there is usually abundant chondroid metaplasia (Fig. 9.13; Blaha et al. 1982; Revell 1982). Exactly the same appearances have been observed by the author at the interface with a metal tibial component of a Toronto knee prosthesis, and the examination

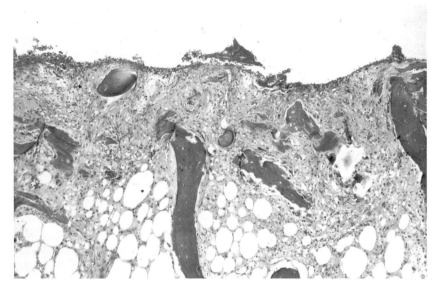

Fig. 9.11. Upper end of tibia adjacent to an uncemented polyethylene prosthetic component, 3 weeks after implantation, showing fragmented bone trabeculae in fibrous tissue. (H&E × 120)

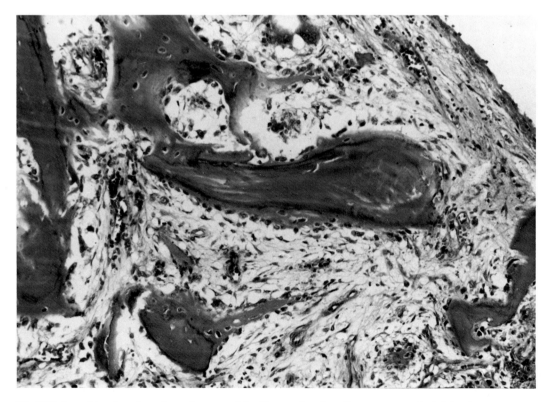

Fig. 9.12. Appositional new bone formation around dead bone trabeculae adjacent to a prosthetic joint. (H&E × 500)

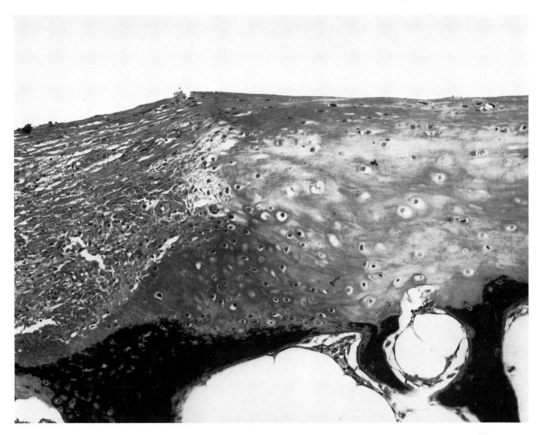

Fig. 9.13. Uncemented polyethylene-bone interface, showing separation of prosthesis (*top*) and bone (*bottom*) by a fibrous tissue layer in which there is formation of cartilaginous tissue. (Azan × 500)

of osseous tissue related to flanged pegs, polyethylene screws and metal pegs shows similar appearances (Revell 1982; unpublished personal observations). The appearances of bone in relation to metal screws and nails have been described by Collins (1953), Hickman et al. (1958), Revell (1982) and Freeman et al. (1982) (Fig. 9.14). The screw or nail becomes surrounded by a fibrous membrane, outside which is living and dead bone with new bone remodelled to encase the implant circumferentially (Fig. 9.15). The tissue reaction at the interface between bone and titanium has been described at the ultrastructural level by Linder et al. (1983).

The tissue reactions to other types of implant material cannot all be included here. Reactions to ceramics are described by Rhinelander et al. (1971), Griss et al. (1974) and others, including Revell (1982). The question of whether bone growth occurs into appropriately designed prostheses has been studied by various workers; for example Salzer et al. (1976) claimed success in demonstrating growth of bone into ceramic implants. The author's personal experience suggests that no bone growth occurs into holes in an implant unless they have been previously packed with bone chips (Freeman et al. 1983). Further details with respect to bone growth into porous implants is available in Morscher (1983).

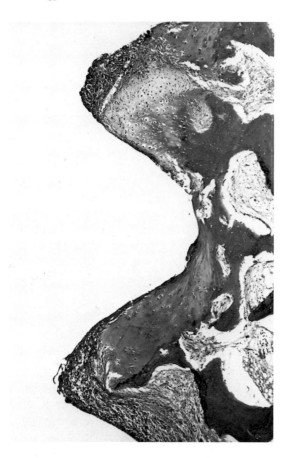

Fig. 9.14. Bone adjacent to a polyethylene screw showing outline of screw thread and a combination of fibrous and chondroid tissue at the interface. (H&E × 120)

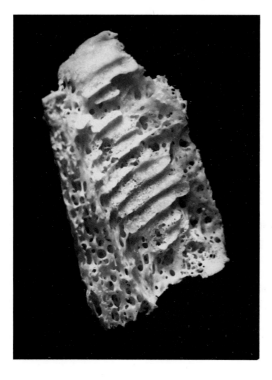

Fig. 9.15. Macerated specimen of bone adjacent to a flanged polyethylene peg, showing ridges of remodelled bone, which encased the peg circumferentially

Wear debris and the implant bed

Particulate debris may be formed at the articulating surfaces of the implant for reasons which are discussed elsewhere (Vernon-Roberts and Freeman 1976; Willert and Semlitsch 1976; Willert 1977; Revell et al. 1978; Revell 1982). Production of excess debris overloads the phagocytic defence mechanisms of the synovial cavity, and there is extension of the cellular reaction into the region between implant and bone. Details of the tissue reactions to metal, polyethylene, other plastics, ceramic, silicone and bone cement are available in the sources mentioned above. The exact response varies with the type of debris, so that, for example, small metal and polyethylene particles excite a macrophage response, while multinucleate giant cells are seen in relation to larger flakes of polyethylene and beaded cement polymer not incorporated into the main block or spilled at the time of implantation. Whatever the source of macrophage and giant cell response, one of its most significant effects is the resorption of bone at the implant bed with resultant loosening of the prosthesis (Fig. 9.16; see also Revell 1982).

Necrosis of bone

Death of bone is mentioned elsewhere in this book in relation to Gaucher's disease (see Fig. 9.19), fractures, bone grafting, sickle cell disease and osteomyelitis (see pp. 75, 204, 216, 239, 241). 'Avascular necrosis of the femoral head' is the term used in those cases where the bone is deprived of its blood supply by virtue of a fracture of the neck of the femur. This is the most common

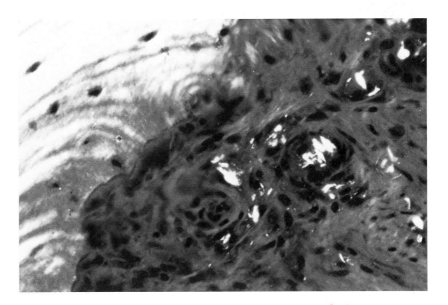

Fig. 9.16. Effect of the cellular reaction to wear debris on bone. Macrophage and giant cells containing birefringent polyethylene wear debris, with resorption of related bone (*top left*). Methylmethacrylate, thionin × 600)

cause of femoral head necrosis, and the features have been described by Catto (1965a), Herndon and Aufranc (1972) and Glimcher and Kenzora (1979a,c). Several authors have tried to correlate the amount of necrosis with the severity and type of fracture (Smith 1959; Banks 1962; Brown and Abrami 1964; Barnes 1967; Massie 1973; Barnes et al. 1976), while others have examined the effects of orthopaedic treatment including fracture reduction and the use of internal fixation devices (Jacobs 1978). A prospective review of 1500 subcapital femoral head fractures has shown that 24% are asymptomatic (Barnes et al. 1976). Estimates of the interval of time between fracture and evidence of femoral head necrosis vary, with radiographic changes rarely being seen before 6 months but usually apparent within 2 years (Catto 1965a; Garden 1971; Massie 1973; Jacobs 1978). Some cases of femoral neck fracture apparently successfully treated by internal fixation may undergo collapse of part of the femoral head after an interval of time; the term 'late segmental collapse', is then applicable, because the change results from collapse of already necrotic bone subjected to the long-term effect of weightbearing (Catto 1965b).

Death of bone occurs other than after fracture of the neck of the femur and is then called 'idiopathic (primary) necrosis'. The most frequent site for this type of aseptic bone necrosis is also the femoral head (Fig. 9.17), although the humerus and the tibia or radius may sometimes be affected. Non-traumatic bone death of this kind may be associated with various factors, as shown in

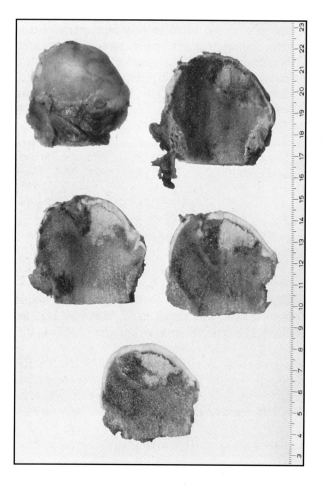

Fig. 9.17. Cross sections of femoral head show a zone of subchondral bone necrosis which is clearly delineated from the normal bone

Table 9.4. Non-traumatic 'idiopathic' bone necrosis: associations and related conditions

Alcoholism
Caisson disease (tunnelling, diving, high altitude)
Corticosteroid treatment and Cushing's disease
Gaucher's disease
Haemoglobinopathies (sickle cell disease)
Hyperlipidaemia
Hyperuricaemia and gout
Iron overload
Immunosuppressive agents
Non-steroid anti-inflammatory drugs
Polycythaemia
Radiation
Renal transplantation

Occasionally occurs in other generalised conditions—rheumatoid arthritis, systemic lupus erythematosus, diabetes mellitus, liver disease, pancreatitis and others.

Table 9.4. There are several excellent reviews on the subject so that an outline need only be given here (Herndon and Aufranc 1972; Glimcher and Kenzora 1979a,b,c; Jacobs 1978). More than one association may be present in any individual patient, and separation of causative factors may be extremely difficult. Many of those with rheumatoid arthritis, systemic lupus erythematosus or a renal transplant may have received steroids, immunosuppressive and/or non-steroidal anti-inflammatory drugs. Jacobs (1978) found hyperuricaemia, pancreatitis, steroid usage, sickle cell disease and diabetes in alcoholics with femoral head necrosis. Detailed figures for the incidence of these associations are available in the reviews already mentioned. Nearly all cases with pancreatitis are alcoholics (Herndon and Aufranc 1972; Jacobs 1978), but this is not apparently true of liver disease, since Jacobs reported the presence of various types of liver disease unrelated to either alcohol or steroids. Further details about bone necrosis after renal transplantation (Aichroth et al. 1971; Evarts and Phalen 1971; Harrington et al. 1971), in relation to steroids (Fisher and Bickel 1971; Solomon 1973; Cruess et al. 1975), non-steroidal anti-inflammatory drugs (Solomon 1973), and caisson disease (Fig. 9.18; Calder 1982) are available elsewhere. Although the conditions in which bone necrosis occurs are well recognised, the aetiopathogenesis is unknown. Factors which may contribute are changes in vessels and thrombotic or embolic phenomena, including coagulation abnormalities, fat embolism, the aggregation of sickle cells in osseous vessels and the gradual compression of these vessels by Gaucher's cells (Boettcher et al. 1970; Herndon and Aufranc 1972; Glimcher and Kenzora 1979c).

Radiographic evidence of bone necrosis is visible only some time after the initiating event. Increased radiodensity of the femoral head becomes apparent from about 6 months after femoral neck fracture and is thought to be due to revascularisation with new bone formation occurring in the healing process. The development of a subchondral 'crescenteric' line of radiolucency is a definitive sign resulting from collapse of necrotic bone in the load-bearing area of the femoral head.

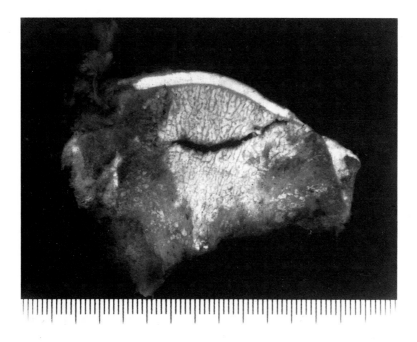

Fig. 9.18. Caisson disease. Separation of necrotic area of bone in the femoral head

Idiopathic (primary) bone necrosis shows no distinctive radiological change initially and the femoral head has a normal outline. Subsequently, a crescenteric line may develop, and in the course of time a wedge-shaped area of radio-density may be seen in the superior part of the femoral head with the broader part of its outline placed towards the articular surface. The appearances of a slice of bone from the femoral head are shown in Fig. 9.19. The significance of the radiological appearances in relation to the histological changes are discussed by Catto (1965a) and Glimcher and Kenzora (1979a,b,c).

The pathological features of bone necrosis may be considered from the point of view of the recognition of bone as being dead and that of the distribution of changes in a particular disease. The earliest histological change is seen after a few days when there is necrosis of haemopoietic cells, fat and related vessels. The hallmark of bone death is the loss of osteocytes (Fig. 9.20). Changes amounting to loss of nuclear staining may be detected within a few days, but the presence of empty osteocyte lacunae throughout trabeculae is rarely seen until 14 days after fracture and is not complete until 3 or 4 weeks in uncrushed parts of the bone away from the femoral neck fracture (Catto 1965a). The subsequent repair reaction is characterised by the replacement of the dead intertrabecular tissue by fibroblasts forming fibrous tissue, proliferating capil-laries and collections of foamy macrophages. After revascularisation, osteoblasts form new bone upon the necrotic trabeculae in a way similar to that seen in ordinary fracture repair. There may be some new woven bone formed in the intertrabecular spaces near the fracture site. Some of the necrotic bone may undergo osteoclastic resorption.

The particular appearances following partial or total necrosis of the femoral head and the healing process seen at the fractured femoral neck have been described by Catto (1965a). Revascularisation was confined to a wedge-shaped

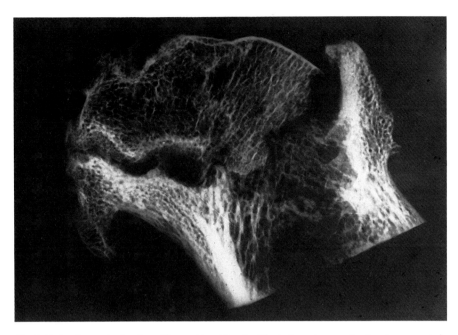

Fig. 9.19. Radiograph of a slice of femoral head involved by ischaemic necrosis, showing separated ischaemic fragment with sclerosis of adjacent bone. Histological examination showed the presence of Gaucher's cells in the interosseous spaces in this specimen. (× 2.5)

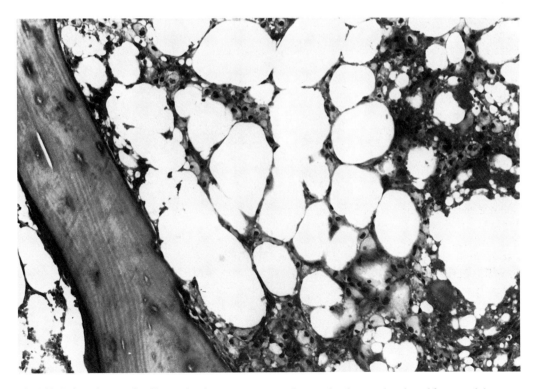

Fig. 9.20. Ischaemic necrosis of bone, showing empty osteocyte lacunae in a bone trabecula and fat necrosis in the marrow space with large coalescent fat spaces and foamy macrophages. (H&E × 400)

area near the fovea in most cases, while in a few there was progress towards union of the fracture with vessel proliferation from the femoral neck and callus formation about the fracture. The features of the femoral head in primary necrosis are indistinguishable, no matter what the associated condition. Under these circumstances, an area of bone and bone marrow necrosis is seen which is usually larger than that suspected on radiological examination. The border between necrotic and revascularised bone is marked by a band of dense fibrous tissue (Figs. 9.21, 9.22). There is deposition of new bone upon the dead bone adjacent to this fibrous tissue on the viable side of the interface and this gives rise to sclerosis of the region as seen on radiographs. Examination of subchondral fractures which have given rise to the radiological crescent sign shows that the fracture line may pass through the subchondral bone and articular cartilage to give a relatively loose osteochondral fragment. The development of degenerative joint disease (osteoarthritis) in the hip joint deformed by ischaemic necrosis is described in the review articles already quoted. A rare complication is the presence of a tumour at the site of bone necrosis (Furey et al. 1960; Dorfman et al. 1966; Mirra et al. 1974; Heselson et al. 1983).

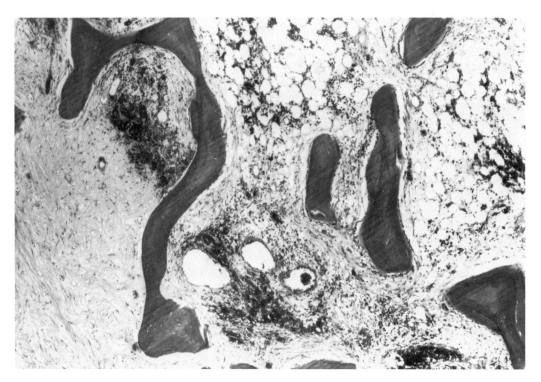

Fig. 9.21. Boundary between fibrous tissue containing necrotic bone and surviving bone with appositional new bone formation (*right*). (H&E × 240)

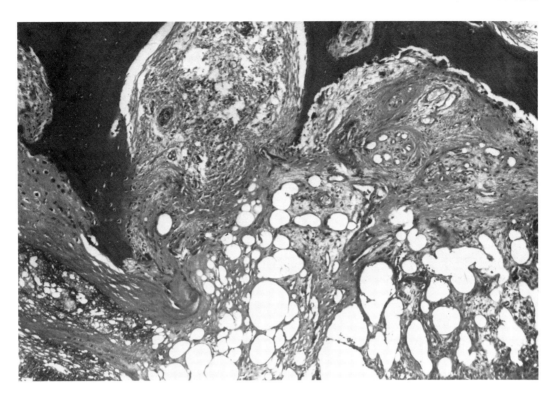

Fig. 9.22. Margin of an area of ischaemic necrosis of the femoral head, showing well-developed fibrous tissue containing small vessels. There is resorption of necrotic bone by osteoclasts (*top right*) and formation of new bone and chondroid tissue adjacent to other dead bone (*top left*). (H&E × 75)

Perthes disease (Legg–Calve–Perthes disease)

Perthes disease affects the femoral head during childhood and is due to alteration in the blood supply, which results in partial or total necrosis of the epiphysis with its ossification centre. Boys are affected about four times more frequently than girls and the age of onset is usually between 5 and 9 years. Radiologically, the affected femoral head shows an area of radiolucency some months after onset with such symptoms as intermittent pain and limping after exertion. There are indistinct similarities to ischaemic necrosis of the femoral head in adults. The site of necrosis is in the anterosuperior segment like that in adult idiopathic bone necrosis (Ferguson 1975). It has been suggested that destruction of the growth plate restricts the blood flow to the epiphyseal ossification centre (Ponseti and Cotton 1961). The shape of the femoral head remains normal for some time after the initial episode of necrosis, but subsequently there is subchondral collapse, which results in a flattened mushroom-shaped profile to the femoral head. The development of this deformity is considered to result from the effects of weight bearing by Ferguson (1975), but evidence has been presented that the femoral head is subjected to several episodes of infarction in Perthes disease by Inoue et al. (1976), who believed that these were responsible for deformation by disturbing growth.

Effects of electrical stimulation on healing in bone

The application of electrical stimuli to bone as a means of stimulating growth, repair and healing arises from the discovery of endogenous electrical signals in bone. There are two main types of electrical effect in bone, and different methods of applying electricity in clinical practice also give rise to a variety of electrical effects. There is a considerable literature on both endogenous electrical signals and the effects of the exogenous application of electricity, so that the following is but the briefest outline of a few points. Black (1984) and Pollack (1984) have provided recent reviews dealing respectively with these two main aspects.

Endogenous electrical signals in bone

Bioelectric effects in bone came to attention with the demonstration by Fukada and Yasuda (1957) of the piezoelectric properties of this tissue. 'Piezoelectricity' is the term used to describe the occurrence of electrical potentials in a material when stress or external forces are applied to it. The potentials arise by charge separation in materials lacking a centre of symmetry, the stress-induced orientation of dipoles and the stress-induced formation of dipoles in the material. There is, however, a second type of electrical effect in tissues, known as the 'electrokinetic phenomena'. These occur at the interface of a solid with a fluid which contains ions, and involve the intersection between ions adsorbed onto the surface of the solid, so that in the presence of pressure in the fluid there is a tangential motion along a 'slip plane' in the fluid which results in an electrical current, the 'electrical convection current'. The relative contribution of these two types of electrical effect in bone is not known. More details of the effects with a source of literature may be found in Pollack (1984).

Bioelectric potentials in bone have been reported by various workers (Friedenberg and Brighton 1966; Friedenberg and Smith 1969; Friedenberg et al. 1971, 1973; Lake et al. 1979; Stern and Yageya 1980). Electrical potentials are recorded from the surface of bone in vivo without the application of stress and potential differences by the use of two separated electrodes. Measurements on long bones indicate that the potentials are several millivolts in amplitude, that the diaphysis is more positive than the metaphyseal parts of the bone and that the cortex is electropositive relative to the medullary cavity. It has been demonstrated that bioelectric potentials in bone are dependent on cell viability, but not on innervation, and that these decrease in amplitude near bone damage, while there is significant electronegativity at the site of a fracture or bone growth. When a long bone is subjected to bending forces along its length, the concave surface is under maximum compression and is electronegative, while the convex surface is under maximum tension and shows electropositivity (Bassett and Becker 1962; Shamos et al. 1963). Bioelectric potentials do not require the application of stress, and no unequivocal experiment has been performed to determine the physiological significance of endogenous electrical signals in bone (Pollack 1984). It is tempting, however, to speculate that positive electrical effects on the convex side and electronegativity on the concave side may contribute to the stimulation or effectiveness of osteoclastic and osteoblastic activity at these two respective sites.

Bone response to exogenous electrical stimuli

Electrical stimulation of bone has been used in the treatment of fractures, limb inequality in children and osteoporosis. The actual physical effect depends on the nature of the system used to stimulate the skeleton, there being three distinctive types:

1. Faradic, in which electrodes are placed directly in the tissue
2. Capacitive, where external electrodes are placed on the limb to be stimulated
3. Inductive, in which a coil is placed externally so that its axis passes through the area to be stimulated

Each of these systems produces different conditions in the tissues. Faradic systems have characteristic focal fields with high local potential gradients, while capacitive systems produce relatively low voltage gradients, and inductive methods give magnetic fields with potential fields as a secondary effect. It is important when considering the effects of electrical stimulation on healing processes to be aware of which particular method is being used. All three methods have been used in the study of bone defects and fracture healing in experimental animals and stimulatory effects have been claimed (Black 1984). Bioelectric stimulation of fractures showing non-union has also been used in humans, with claims of varying degrees of success using a variety of methods (Becker et al. 1977; Bassett et al. 1977, 1981; Krempen and Silver 1981; Sedel et al. 1982; Heppenstall 1983; see also Black 1984).

References

Aichroth P, Branfoot AR, Huskisson EC, Loughridge LW (1971) Destructive joint changes following kidney transplantation. J Bone Joint Surg [Br] 53:488–494

Albrektsson T (1980) The healing of autologous bone grafts after varying degrees of surgical trauma. J Bone Joint Surg [Br] 62:403–410

Arora BK, Laskin DM (1964) Sex chromatin as a cellular label of osteogenesis of bone grafts. J Bone Joint Surg [Am] 46:1269–1276

Bago-Granell J, Aguirre-Canyadel M, Nardi J, Tallada N (1984) Malignant fibrous histiocytoma of bone at the site of a total hip arthroplasty. J Bone Joint Surg [Br] 66:38–40

Banks HH (1962) Factors influencing the result in fractures of the femoral neck. J Bone Joint Surg [Am] 44:931–964

Barnes R (1967) Fracture of the neck of the femur. J Bone Joint Surg [Br] 49:607–617

Barnes R, Brown JT, Garden RS, Nicoll FA (1976) Subcapital fracture of the femur, a prospective review. J Bone Joint Surg [Br] 58:2–24

Bassett CAL, Becker RO (1962) Generation of electrical potentials in bone in response to mechanical stress. Science 137:1063–1064

Bassett CAL, Pilla AA, Pawluk RJ (1977) A non-operative salvage of surgically resistant pseudoarthrosis and non-unions by pulsating electromagnetic fields. Clin Orthop 124:128–143

Bassett CAL, Mitchell BS, Gaston SR (1981) Treatment of ununited tibial diaphyseal fractures with pulsating electromagnetic field. J Bone Joint Surg [Am] 63:511–523

Becker RO, Spadara JA, Marino AA (1977) Clinical experiences with low intensity direct current stimulation of bone growth. Clin Orthop 124:75–83

Black J (1984) Tissue response to exogenous electromagnetic signals. Orthop Clin North Am 15:15–31

Blaha JD, Insler HP, Freeman MAR, Revell PA, Todd RC (1982) The fixation of proximal tibial polyethylene prosthesis without cement. J Bone Joint Surg [Br] 64:326–335

Blockley NJ (1956) The value of rigid fixation in the treatment of fractures of the adult tibial shaft. J Bone Joint Surg [Br] 38:518–527

Boettcher WG, Bonfiglio M, Hamilton H, Sheets R, Smith K (1970) Non-traumatic necrosis of the femoral head. Part 1. Relation of altered hemostasis to etiology. J Bone Joint Surg [Am] 52:312–321

Bonfiglio M, Jeter WS (1972) Immunological responses to bone. Clin Orthop 87:19–27

Boyer DW (1975) Trapshooter's shoulder; stress fracture of the coracoid process. J Bone Joint Surg [Am] 57:862

Brooks DB, Burnstein AH, Frankel V (1970) The biomechanics of torsional fractures. The stress concentration of a drill hole. J Bone Joint Surg [Am] 52:507–514

Brown JT, Abrami G (1964) Transcervical femoral fracture. A review of 195 patients treated by sliding nail-plate fixation. J Bone Joint Surg [Br] 46:648–663

Buchhardt H (1983) The biology of bone graft repair. Clin Orthop 174:28–42

Burrows HJ (1948) Fatigue fractures of the fibula. J Bone Joint Surg [Br] 30:266–279

Burrows HJ (1956) Fatigue infraction of the middle tibia in ballet dancers. J Bone Joint Surg [Br] 38:83–94

Calder IM (1982) Bone and joint disease in workers exposed to hyperbaric conditions. In: Berry CL (ed) Bone and joint disease. Springer, Berlin Heidelberg New York, pp 103–122 (Current topics in pathology, vol 71)

Catto M (1965a) A histologic study of avascular necrosis of the femoral head after transcervical fracture. J Bone Joint Surg [Br] 47:749–776

Catto M (1965b) The histologic appearance of late segmental collapse of the femoral head after transcervical fracture. J Bone Joint Surg [Br] 47:777–791

Clancey GJ, Hansen ST (1978) Open fractures of the tibia. J Bone Joint Surg [Am] 60:118–122

Collins DH (1953) Structural changes around nails and screws in human bones. J Pathol Bacteriol 85:109–121

Collins DH (1966) The pathology of bone. Butterworths, London

Cruess RL, Ross D, Crawshaw E (1975) The etiology of steroid-induced avascular necrosis of bone. A laboratory and clinical study. Clin Orthop 113:178–183

Danis (1949) Theorie et pratique de l'osteosynthese. Masson et Cie, Paris

Devas MB (1958) Stress fractures in the tibia in athletes or 'shin soreness'. J Bone Joint Surg [Br] 40:227–239

Devas MB (1980) Stress fractures in athletes. Medisport 2:227–230

Dorfman HD, Norman A, Wolff H (1966) Fibrosarcoma complicating bone infarction in a caisson worker. J Bone Joint Surg [Am] 48:528–532

Ellis H (1958) The speed of healing after fracture of the tibial shaft. J Bone Joint Surg [Br] 40:42–46

Elves MW, Pratt LM (1975) The pattern of new bone formation in isografts of bone. Acta Orthop Scand 46:549–560

Enneking WF, Burchhardt H, Puhl JJ, Piotrowski G (1975) Physical and biological aspects of repair in dog cortical bone transplants. J Bone Joint Surg [Am] 57:237–252

Evarts CM, Phalen GS (1971) Osseous avascular necrosis associated with renal transplantation. Clin Orthop 78:330–335

Ferguson AB (1975) The pathology of Legg–Perthes disease and its comparison with aseptic necrosis. Clin Orthop 106:7–18

Fisher DE, Bickel WH (1971) Corticosteroid-induced avascular necrosis. J Bone Joint Surg [Am] 53:859–873

Freeman MAR, Bradley GW, Revell PA (1982) Observations upon the interface between bone and polymethylmethacrylate cement. J Bone Joint Surg [Br] 64:489–493

Freeman MAR, McLeod H, Revell PA (1983) Bone ingrowth and graft incorporation in polythene pegs in man. Trans Orthop Res Soc 8:133

Friedenberg ZB, Brighton CT (1966) Bioelectric potentials in bone. J Bone Joint Surg [Am] 48:915–923

Friedenberg ZB, Smith HG (1969) Electrical potentials in intact and fractured tibia. Clin Orthop 63:222–225

Friedenberg ZB, Dyer RH, Brighton CT (1971) Electro-osteograms of long bones of immature rabbits. J Dent Res 50:635–639

Friedenberg ZB, Harlow MC, Heppenstall RB, Brighton CT (1973) The cellular origin of bioelectric potentials in bone. Calcif Tissue Res 13:53–62

Fukada E, Yasuda I (1957) On the piezo-electric effect of bone. J Phys Soc Jpn 10:1158–1169

Furey JG, Ferrer-Torellis M, Reagan JW (1960) Fibrosarcoma arising at the site of bone infarcts. J Bone Joint Surg [Am] 42:802–810

Gainor BJ, Buchert P (1983) Fracture healing in metastatic bone disease. Clin Orthop 178:297–302

Garden RS (1971) Malreduction and avascular necrosis in subcapital fractures of the femur. J Bone Joint Surg [Br] 53:183–197

Glimcher MJ, Kenzora JE (1979a) The biology of osteonecrosis of the human femoral head and its clinical implications. I Tissue biology. Clin Orthop 138:284–309

Glimcher MJ, Kenzora JE (1979b) The biology of osteonecrosis of the human femoral head and its clinical implications. II The pathological changes in the femoral head as an organ and the hip. Clin Orthop 139:283–312

Glimcher MJ, Kenzora JE (1979c) The biology of osteonecrosis of the human femoral head and its clinical implications. III Discussion of etiology and genesis of the pathological sequelae: comments on treatment. Clin Orthop 140:273–312

Gray JC, Elves MW (1979) Early osteogenesis in compact bone isografts: a quantitative study of the contributions of the different graft cells. Calcif Tissue Int 29:225–237

Griss P, Krempien B, von Andrian-Werburg HF, Heimke G, Fleiner R, Diehm T (1974) Experimental analysis of ceramic-tissue interactions. A morphologic, fluorescenceoptic and radiographic study on dense alumina oxide ceramic in various animals. J Biomed Mater Res 5:39–48

Gustilo RB, Anderson JT (1976) Prevention of infection in the treatment of one thousand and twenty five open fractures of long bones. J Bone Joint Surg [Am] 58:453–458

Ham AW, Harris WR (1971) Repair and transplantation of bone. In: Bourne GH (ed) The biochemistry and physiology of bone, 2nd edn, vol 3. Academic, New York, pp 337–399

Harrington KD, Murray WR, Kountz SL, Belzer FO (1971) Avascular necrosis after renal transplantation. J Bone Joint Surg [Am] 53:203–215

Hartley JB (1942) Fatigue fractures of the tibia. Br J Surg 30:9–14

Healy WL, Brooker AF (1983) Distal femoral fractures. Comparisons of open and closed methods of treatment. Clin Orthop 174:166–171

Heppenstall RB (1983) Constant direct current treatment for established non-union of the tibia. Clin Orthop 178:180–184

Herndon JH, Aufranc OE (1972) Avascular necrosis of the femoral head in the adult. A review of its incidence in a variety of conditions. Clin Orthop 86:43–62

Heselson NG, Price SK, Mills EED, Conway SSM, Marks RK (1983) Two malignant fibrous histiocytomas in bone infarcts. J Bone Joint Surg [Am] 65:1166–1171

Heslop BF, Zeiss IM, Nisbet NW (1960) Studies on transference of bone. I A comparison of autologous and homologous bone implants with reference to osteocyte survival, osteogenesis and host reaction. Br J Exp Pathol 41:269–287

Hickman J, Clarke EGC, Jennings AR (1958) Structural changes in bone associated with metallic implants. J Bone Joint Surg [Br] 40:799–803

Hicks JH (1961) Fracture of the forearm treated with rigid fixation. J Bone Joint Surg [Br] 43:680–687

Inoue A, Freeman MAR, Vernon-Roberts B, Muzuno S (1976) The pathogenesis of Perthe's disease. J Bone Joint Surg [Br] 58:453–461

Jacobs B (1978) Epidemiology of traumatic and non-traumatic osteonecrosis. Clin Orthop 130:51–67

Johner R, Wruhs O (1983) Classification of tibial shaft fractures and correlation with results after rigid internal fixation. Clin Orthop 178:7–25

King KF (1976) Periosteal pedicle grafting in dogs. J Bone Joint Surg [Br] 58:117–121

Kitchin JD (1948) Fatigue fractures of the ulna. J Bone Joint Surg [Br] 30:622–623

Krempen JF, Silver RA (1981) External electromagnetic fields in the treatment of non-unions of bones. Orthop Rev 10:33–39

Lake FT, Solomon G, Davis RW, Pace N, Morgan JR (1979) Bioelectric potentials associated with the growing deer antler. Clin Orthop 142:237–243

Landin L, Nilsson BE (1983) Bone mineral content in children with fractures. Clin Orthop 178:292–296

Linder L, Hansson H-A (1983) Ultrastructural aspects of the interface between bone and cement in man. J Bone Joint Surg [Br] 65:646–649

Linder L, Albrektsson T, Brancemark, P-I, Hansson H-A, Ivarsson B, Jönsson U, Lundström J (1983) Electron microscopic analysis of the bone titanium interface. Acta Orthop Scand 54:45–52

McKibbin B (1978) The biology of fracture healing in long bones. J Bone Joint Surg [Br] 60:149–162

McKibbin B (1982) Repair of fractures. In: Wilson JN (ed) Watson-Jones' Fractures and joint injury, 6th edn, vol 1. Churchill Livingstone, Edinburgh pp 15–28

Massie WK (1973) Treatment of femoral neck fractures emphasising long term follow up and observations on aseptic necrosis. Clin Orthop 92:16–62

Mirra JM, Bullough PG, Marcove RC, Jacobs B, Huvos AG (1974) Malignant fibrous histiocytomas and osteosarcoma in association with bone infarcts. J Bone Joint Surg [Am] 56:932–940

Mirra JM, Amstutz HC, Matos M, Gold R (1976) The pathology of the joint tissues and its clinical relevance in prosthesis failure. Clin Orthop 117:221–240

Morscher EW (1983) Cementless total hip arthroplasty. Clin Orthop 181:79–91

Nilsson BE, Westlin N (1974) The bone mineral content in the forearm in women with Colles' fracture. Acta Orthop Scand 45:836–844

Nisbet NW, Heslop BF, Zeiss IM (1960) Studies on transference of bone. III Manifestations of immunological tolerance to implants of homologous cortical bone in rats. Br J Exp Pathol 41:443–451

Patzakis MJ, Wilkins J, Moore TM (1983a) Use of antibiotics in open tibial fractures. Clin Orthop 178:31–35

Patzakis MJ, Wilkins J, Moore TM (1983b) Considerations in reducing the infection rate in open tibial fractures. Clin Orthop 178:36–41

Pollack SR (1984) Bioelectrical properties of bone. Endogenous electrical signals. Orthop Clin North Am 15:3–14

Ponseti IV, Cotton RL (1961) Legg–Calve–Perthes disease—pathogenesis and evolution. J Bone Joint Surg [Am] 43:261–274

Ray RD (1972) Vascularization of bone grafts and implants. Clin Orthop 87:43–48

Revell PA (1982) Tissue reactions to joint prostheses and the products of wear and corrosion. In: Berry CL (ed) Bone and joint disease. Springer, Berlin Heidelberg New York, pp 73–101 (Current topics in pathology, vol 71)

Revell PA, Weightman B, Freeman MAR, Vernon-Roberts B (1978) The production and biology of polyethylene wear debris. Arch Orthop Trauma Surg 91:167–181

Rhinelander FW, Rouweyha M, Milner JC (1971) Microvascular and histogenic responses to implantation of a porous ceramic in bone. J Biomed Mater Res 5:81–112

Salzer M, Locke H, Plenk H, Punzet G, Stärk N, Zweymüller K (1976) Experience in bioceramic prostheses of the hip. In: Shaldach H, Hohmann D (eds) Advances in artificial hip and knee joint technology. Springer, Berlin Heidelberg New York, pp 459–474

Schenk R, Willenegger H (1967) Morphological findings in primary fracture healing. Symp Biol Hungarica 8:75–86

Sedel L, Christel P, Duriez J, Duriez R, Evrard J, Ficat C, Cauchoix J, Witwoet J (1982) Results of non-unions treatment by pulsed electromagnetic field stimulation. Acta Orthop Scand 53(196):81–91

Shamos MH, Lavine LS, Shamos MI (1963) Piezoelectric effects in bone. Nature 197:81

Siffert RS (1955) Experimental bone transplants. J Bone Joint Surg [Am] 37:742–758

Smith FB (1959) Effects of rotary and valgus malposition on blood supply to femoral head. J Bone Joint Surg [Am] 41:800–815

Solomon L (1973) Drug-induced arthropathy and necrosis of the femoral head. J Bone Joint Surg [Br] 55:246–261

Stern LL, Yageya J (1980) Bioelectric potentials after fracture of the tibia in rats. Acta Orthop Scand 51:601–608

Tonino AJ, Davidson CL, Klopper PJ, Lindau LA (1976) Protection from stress in bone and its effects. J Bone Joint Surg [Br] 58:107–113

Tonna EA, Cronkite EP (1961) Cellular response to fracture studied with tritiated thymidine. J Bone Joint Surg [Am] 43:352–362

Urist MR, McLean FC (1952) Osteogenetic potency and new-bone formation by induction in transplants to the anterior chamber of the eye. J Bone Joint Surg [Am] 34:443–476

Urist MR, Mazet R, McLean FC (1954) The pathogenesis and treatment of delayed union and non-union. A survey of eighty-five ununited fractures of the shaft of the tibia and one hundred control cases with similar injuries. J Bone Joint Surg [Am] 36:931–968

Vernon-Roberts B, Freeman MAR (1976) Morphological and analytical studies of the tissues adjacent to joint prostheses: investigation into the causes of loosening of prostheses. In: Shadach M, Hohmann DD (eds) Advances in artificial hip and knee joint technology. Springer, Berlin Heidelberg New York, pp 148–186

Waddell JP, Reardon GP (1983) Complications of tibial shaft fractures. Clin Orthop 178:173–178

Watson-Jones' Fractures and joint injury, 6th edn, vol 1 (1982a) Wilson JN (ed) Churchill Livingstone, Edinburgh

Watson-Jones' Fractures and joint injury, 6th edn, vol 2 (1982b) Wilson JN (ed) Churchill Livingstone, Edinburgh

Willert H-G (1973) Tissue reactions around joint implants and bone cement. In: Chapchal G (ed) Arthroplasty of the hip. Thieme, Stuttgart, pp 11–21

Willert HG (1977) Reactions of the articular capsule to wear products of artificial joint prostheses. J Biomed Mater Res 11:157–164

Willert HG, Semlitsch M (1976) Tissue reactions to plastic and metallic wear products of joint endoprostheses. In: Geschwerd N, Debrunner HH (eds) Total hip prosthesis. Huber, Bern, pp 205–239

Willert HG, Ludwig J, Semlitsch M (1974) Reaction of bone to methacrylate after hip arthroplasty. J Bone Joint Surg [Am] 58:1368–1382

Wolff J (1892) Das Gesetz der Transformation der Knochen. Hirschwold, Berlin

Zeiss IM, Nisbet NW, Heslop BF (1960) Studies on transference of bone. II Vascularization of autologous and homologous implants of cortical bone in rats. Br J Exp Pathol 41:345–363

Chapter 10

Infection of bone

Introduction

Infection of bone is usually bacterial, although fungal and viral diseases occasionally affect the skeleton, as do parasite infestations. The following account will deal mainly with bacterial osteomyelitis, and the other forms of infection will be discussed more briefly.

Pyogenic infection of bone is usually blood borne and occurs more often during a bacteraemia than a septicaemia. The organisms lodge in the bone marrow tissues, where an acute inflammatory reaction develops, hence the name 'ostoemyelitis'. The site of infection and the type of organism vary a little with the age and type of the subject. The majority of cases of osteomyelitis are due to staphylococcal infection and this will serve as the model for the pathological appearances described later (see this chapter, Pathology of osteomyelitis).

Osteomyelitis in children

Osteomyelitis caused by *Staphylococcus aureus* infection is most frequent in the age range 3–15 years, though it does also occur in babies and infants. The other organisms which may cause childhood bone infection are *Streptococcus pyogenes*, *Strep. pneumoniae* and *Haemophilus influenzae*, all of which tend to affect babies and very young children. The results recorded by Fink et al. (1977) for a series of cases are summarised in Table 10.1. Neonatal osteomyelitis is most frequently caused by group B streptococci, *Staph. aureus* and *Escherichia coli* (Edwards et al. 1978; Fox and Sprunt 1978) and there may be multiple bone involvement (Waldvogel and Vasey 1980). Important predisposing factors in neonatal osteomyelitis are pre-eclampsia, caesarean

Table 10.1. Causative organisms in childhood osteomyelitis (after Fink et al. 1977)

Organism	Age	Percentage of cases affected
Staphylococcus aureus	Nearly 70% aged between 2 and 10 years	59
Streptococci	70% of cases aged less than 5 years	9
Staphylococcus epidermidis	70% of cases aged less than 2 years	4
Haemophilus influenzae	80% of cases aged less than 2 years	3
Pseudomonas aeruginosa		2
Others (*Salmonella*)		8 (1)
Organism unknown		15

section, premature rupture of membranes and local infections resulting from invasive procedures like catheterisation of umbilical vessels in the perinatal period (Lim et al. 1977; Waldvogel and Vasey 1980). Almost any bone may become infected in children, but the common sites are in the lower limb, with 75% of cases occurring in the femur or tibia at their proximal or distal ends. The lumbar region is the most frequent site of haematogenous infection of the vertebral column. Abscess formation occurs as the organisms lodge in the bone marrow of the metaphyseal region of the long bones, and there is death and fragmentation of related bone trabeculae (Fig. 10.1).

Haematogenous osteomyelitis may involve the pelvic bones of children when abnormalities in gait, pain on abduction of the hip or even abdominal pain may be the clinical presentations (Edwards et al. 1978). Gram-negative organisms are becoming recognised more frequently in bone infections, and, although most cases occur in adults, infections with anaerobic organisms have also been described in children (Ogden and Light 1979).

Adult osteomyelitis

Adults with osteomyelitis tend to be in the age group of 50 years and over with illnesses like diabetes mellitus or malignant disease and have foci of infection elsewhere like boils, abscesses or urinary tract and respiratory infections (Garcia and Grantham 1960; Stone and Bonfiglio 1963; Waldvogel et al. 1970). *Staph. aureus* is the commonest organism, as in the case of childhood osteomyelitis (Waldvogel et al. 1970). There has been increasing awareness over recent years of the frequency of vertebral osteomyelitis in adults, and the results of eight series of cases are summarised by Waldvogel and Vasey (1980). Briefly, between 60% and 100% of vertebral osteomyelitis occurred in adults as distinct from children, and the commonest organism was *Staph. aureus*, which affected 48%–75% of cases. Enterobacteria formed another important group in the causation of adult vertebral osteomyelitis. The adults varied in age from the mid forties to the early sixties, though they were mostly aged around 60 years. The lumbar spine was most commonly affected, followed by the thoracic spine (Waldvogel and Vasey 1980).

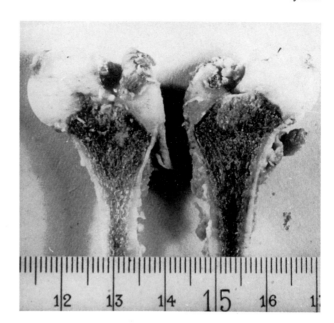

Fig. 10.1. Osteomyelitis in the metaphysis of a 4-year-old child, showing area of dead bone (*grey area*)

The organisms typically lodge near the bone end plate of the vertebral body and most frequently involve two such adjacent plates together with the intervening intervertebral disc (Fig. 10.2). Posterior extension of the inflammatory process has led to the development of a paraplegia in a significant number of cases.

There is now some interest in the question as to the extent to which anaerobic bacteria may be responsible for osteomyelitis, though detailed studies of the incidence of such infections in bone are lacking. Raff and Melo (1978) have presented 8 cases and reviewed a further 193 from the literature. They recognised distinct clinical syndromes caused by anaerobic osteomyelitis and related these to the anatomical sites of involvement. The long bones were the site in 40% of cases and the skull and facial bones were involved in a further 26.5%. Other sites were the foot, hand, sacrum and pelvis, spine and clavicle, in that order of frequency. Previous fracture was a prominent predisposing factor (nearly 50% of cases), while diabetes mellitus ($\pm$11%) and human bites ($\pm$9%) were the next most common accompaniments. *Bacteroides* species were by far the most common organisms, and the authors give a full list of all the other bacteria isolated. Aerobic organisms were also recovered in a large minority of the cases, with *Staph. aureus* and streptococci most frequent. In some cases, there was no history of previous trauma, bone disease or other predisposing factor and no apparent focus which could have given rise to a bacteraemia. Positive blood cultures at the time of osteomyelitis were rare. The gastrointestinal tract is considered the commonest site from which anaerobic bacteraemia might originate (McHenry et al. 1961; Bornstein et al. 1964; Felner and Dowell 1971; Chow and Guze 1974).

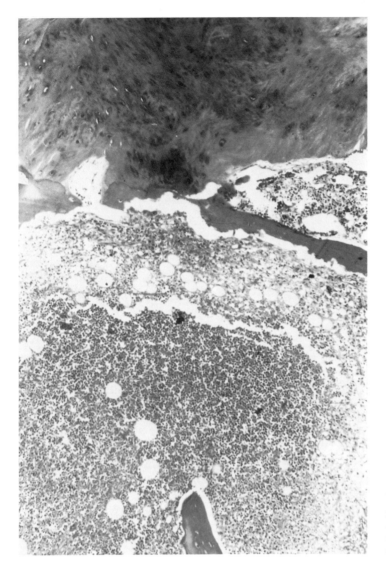

Fig. 10.2. Osteomyelitis of vertebral body, showing extension of inflammatory infiltrate destroying the subchondral bone plate and extending into the intervertebral disc (*top*). (H&E × 80)

Osteomyelitis in drug addicts

It is worthwhile separating osteomyelitis occurring in drug addicts from that occurring in the general adult population. Osteomyelitis in heroin addicts presents, as might perhaps be expected, at a much younger age. Roca and Yoshikawa (1979) reviewed the literature in English and combined these cases with their own to present the features of 123 cases. The vertebral column was the most common site of osteomyelitis (53% of all cases) and the lumbar region predominated. Other frequent sites were the pelvis, especially the sacroiliac joints, the sternal region (mostly sternoclavicular) and the extremities, which formed 17% of cases. The organisms responsible were different from those in non-addicts, aerobic gram-negative bacilli being predominant. The single most common pathogen was *Pseudomonas aeruginosa*, which alone or in combination with other organisms was isolated from 78% of all cases. *Staph.*

aureus was next most common (9%), and other organisms included streptococci, *Enterobacter, Klebsiella* and *Serratia*. The reason for the predominance of pseudomonas infections in the osteomyelitis of drug addicts is unknown. The use of contaminated equipment and self innoculation of organisms during the process of 'fixing up' are usually considered important.

Osteomyelitis and haemoglobinopathy: salmonella infection

Osteomyelitis caused by salmonella infection is rare. When it does occur it is frequently in patients having sickle cell anaemia (SS-haemoglobinopathy or SC-haemoglobinopathy; Golding et al. 1959; Ortiz-Neu et al. 1978; Adeyokunnu and Hendrickse 1980). In the series of 37 patients with salmonella osteomyelitis presented by Ortiz-Neu et al. (1978), only 14 had haemoglobinopathy (12 SS-disease, 2 SC-disease). Ten of these were aged under 20 years. Previous trauma or surgery were features in many of the cases not associated with sickle cell disease, while three further cases had received steroid treatment for connective tissue disease. The femur was the commonest site both in the whole group and in those with haemoglobinopathy. Other bones involved in the sickle cell group were the tibia, fibula, humerus, clavicle, vertebrae and ankle. In the larger series of specifically childhood cases of salmonella osteomyelitis in Nigeria 90% were HbS homozygotes and 6% were heterozygous for HbS (Adeyokunna and Hendrickse 1980). Osteomyelitis affected multiple sites in most patients; the small bones of the hands and feet were more commonly affected in the very young (less than 2 years old), while long bones in the limbs were involved in older children.

Differentiation of salmonella osteomyelitis from aseptic necrosis of bone in sickle cell disease may present considerable diagnostic difficulty, especially since pain, local inflammation and pyrexia may accompany the latter. The radiological changes in the early stages of salmonella osteomyelitis may also be indistinguishable from aseptic necrosis of bone.

Osteomyelitis caused by direct spread of organisms

Haematogenous spread of organisms to the bones is by far the commonest form of osteomyelitis. However, it will be apparent from the above account that cases also occur in which direct spread of organisms from an adjacent focus of infection is the method of bone involvement. Such a mechanism holds true in cases following middle ear infection, dental sepsis, sinusitis, cellulitis of the face, fractures, other traumatic injuries and surgical procedures. A relatively recent development is the use of prostheses for joint replacement; infection under these circumstances presents a serious local problem necessitating removal of the implant (Hunter and Dandy 1977). Direct infection in the perioperative period is considered to be responsible for early infections and attention has been paid to operating room facilities, including the use of ultra-clean air (Charnley and Eftekhar 1969; Charnley 1972; Freeman et al. 1977). Of a large series of cases of infected prostheses reported by Hunter and Dandy (1977) 50% were clinically apparent within 1 month of operation. However, 6% of their cases showed evidence of being due to haematogenous spread of infection, and there are other well-authenticated cases of implants becoming infected by this means, often a long time after initial surgery (Mallory 1973; Hall 1974; Artz et al. 1975; Cruess et al. 1975). *Staph. aureus* and *Staph. albus* (*epidermidis*) were the commonest gram-positive organisms in the series reported by Hunter and Dandy (1977), while *E. coli* was a prominent gram-negative pathogen.

Radiological appearances of osteomyelitis

The bone changes associated with infection are local destruction and reactive new bone formation and these are seen radiologically as lytic lesions and areas of increased bone density. Unfortunately, there may be some delay between onset of significant bone infection and appearance of radiological changes. No lytic changes are visible until between 30% and 50% of bone mineral has been removed and mineralisation of newly formed osteoid proceeds at the rate of 1 μm/day (Waldvogel et al. 1970), so that radiographic signs of osteomyelitis do not appear for 7–10 days.

Lytic lesions and periosteal elevation appear almost simultaneously, while bone sclerosis usually indicates disease which has been present for more than 1 month. For reasons which may be related to bone kinetics, radiological evidence of healing may also be delayed, and there may even be worsening of the radiographic appearance while there is clinical improvement (Waldvogel et al. 1970).

Difficulties in the interpretation of radiographs have led to the use of radio-isotope bone scanning techniques with technetium-99m (^{99m}Tc) and gallium-67 (^{67}Ga). Such methods are useful in the early detection of bone infection (Letts et al. 1975; Treves et al. 1976) and have been demonstrated to be effective in animal models of osteomyelitis (Deysine et al. 1976; Rinsky et al. 1977). Limitations of the method include the occasional negative bone scan in the presence of bacteriologically and histologically proven osteomyelitis, which may be explained by impaired blood supply or infarction of the infected bone. Technetium scanning also does not permit discrimination between infection and some other processes in bone, such as bone repair at the sites of previous orthopaedic procedures and in fractures (Waldvogel and Vasey 1980). The uses of radioisotope scanning techniques in bone disease, including infection, have recently been reviewed by Kirchner and Simon (1981).

Pathology of osteomyelitis

Staphylococcal osteomyelitis has been used in the past as an example of haematogenous osteomyelitis, and the same course will be followed here. Acute haematogenous osteomyelitis most often involves rapidly growing long bones in children, and the organisms settle in the metaphyseal region where there is a rich vascular network of capillaries on the metaphyseal side of the growth plate. Vessels pass into the epiphysis in infants, and this has been suggested as a reason why epiphyseal involvement may occur under the age of 1 year (Trueta 1959). The epiphyseal end of the bone may be involved if the growth plate has closed and there is continuity between the bone of the epiphyseal and metaphyseal regions, as occurs in the adult.

The colonies of organisms become established in the intertrabecular myeloid tissues, where suppurative inflammation develops (Fig. 10.3). Changes in pH, local oedema and the activity of leucocytes may all contribute to the necrosis, but vascular obstruction is probably one of the most important factors. The bone trabeculae die and become fragmented when they lose their blood supply (Fig. 10.4). Suppuration spreads to neighbouring bone through the Haversian and Volkmann canals, and large segments of osseous tissue undergo ischaemic necrosis because of inflammatory thrombosis of the arteries and veins passing down these canals. Large blocks of cortical bone become necrotic (Fig. 10.5) and form 'sequestra' which may separate entirely from the surrounding bone and come to lie freely in an abscess cavity (Fig. 10.6). Pus reaching the surface of the bone collects under the periosteum, where it further impairs the blood supply (Collins 1966). Osteoblastic activity at the margin of the lesion gives rise to appositional new bone formation on surviving trabeculae, but this thickened bone may in turn undergo necrosis as the infective process expands outwards. Living tissues in the wall of the suppurative focus, and especially

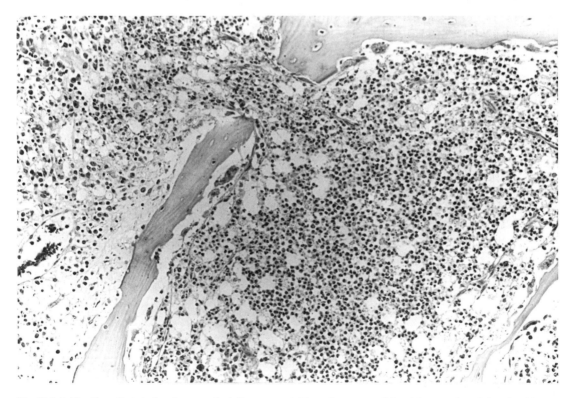

Fig. 10.3. Infiltration of intertrabecular space by inflammatory infiltrate in osteomyelitis, with resorption of the related bone. (H&E × 160)

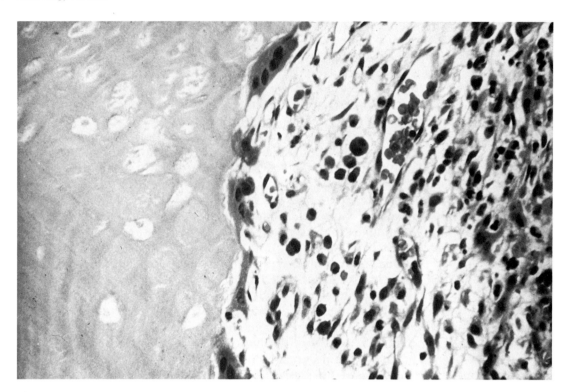

Fig. 10.4. Chronic osteomyelitis, showing necrotic bone (*left*), which is being resorbed by osteoclasts, and granulation tissue containing plasma cells (*right*). (H&E × 600)

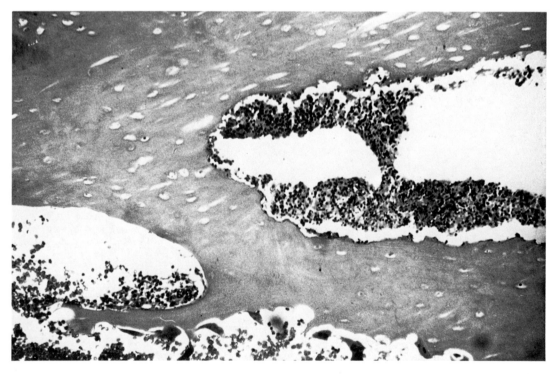

Fig. 10.5. Extensive necrosis of cortical bone in osteomyelitis, showing crenated margin caused by resorption and inflammatory infiltrate in the adjacent marrow space. (H&E × 160)

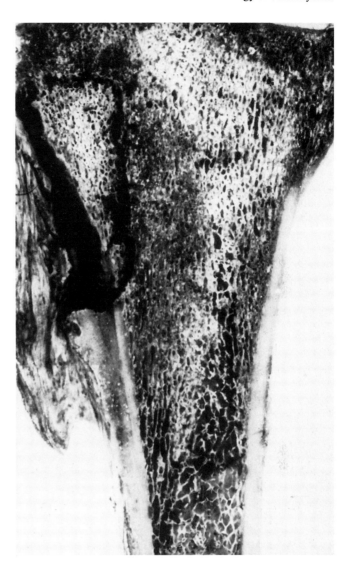

Fig. 10.6. Upper tibia in chronic osteomyelitis, showing complete separation of necrotic bone to form a 'sequestrum' (*top left*)

the elevated periosteal membrane, produce new bone, so that the area of osteomyelitis becomes enclosed in a shell of bone, the 'involucrum'. Where there is relatively slow evolution of the destructive process, osteoblastic activity on the surface of old trabeculae may cause these to become greatly thickened, and abnormally dense sequestra may be formed. Large amounts of reparative new bone in the medullary region, in conjunction with cortical thickening, can give rise to problems in radiological interpretation and be mistaken for a bone tumour. Sclerosis in areas of osteomyelitis may also be misleading from the histological point of view. The problem of osteomyelitis simulating a primary bone tumour has been reviewed recently by Lindenbaum and Alexander (1984), the cases being those with subacute osteomyelitis. A form of diffuse sclerosing osteomyelitis occurs in the mandible and has been reviewed by Jacobsson (1979). Similar changes are seen on occasion at other sites.

Complications of osteomyelitis

The development of a septicaemia in patients with osteomyelitis was a serious and often fatal complication in the pre-antibiotic era. Suppurative arthritis was also a major problem and even now may cause severe derangement of joints (Fig. 10.7). Osteomyelitis in the spine may spread from one vertebra into the adjacent intervertebral disc and vertebra causing considerable disruption with collapse and deformity. Destruction of the cortex of a long bone by the inflammatory process may be followed by pathological fracture. Chronic sinus formation with poor healing in the wall of the sinus and reactive hyperplasia of the squamous epithelium of the skin around the opening of the sinus may eventually lead to development of squamous carcinoma after 20–30 years (Fig. 10.8). Amyloidosis was formerly considered a significant complication of chronic osteomyelitis, though it is rarely seen nowadays (Waldvogel and Vasey 1980).

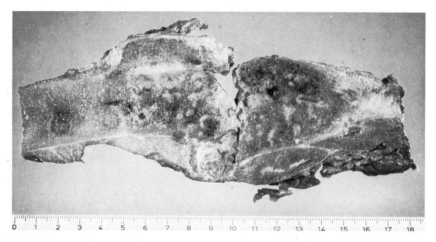

Fig. 10.7. Suppurative arthritis completely destroying the knee joint with extension from the lower femur (*left*) across the joint to involve the upper tibia (*right*)

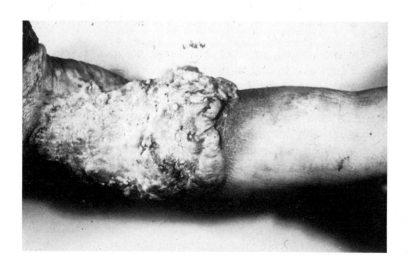

Fig. 10.8. Squamous carcinoma of the upper arm arising in relation to a sinus in osteomyelitis

Chronic bone abscess

A sharply delineated abscess cavity may sometimes develop in bone and is often known as a Brodie's abscess. The most common site for such a change is one of the metaphyses of the tibia or femur. There will frequently have been no prior symptoms. The abscess cavity may contain purulent or thicker slimy mucoid material; bacterial cultures often fail to grow an organism, though staphylococci or other bacteria may sometimes be demonstrable. The cavity is lined by granulation tissue or more mature collagenous tissue, outside which is sclerotic reactive bone.

Tuberculosis

Although tuberculosis of the skeleton may be caused by either human or bovine strains, most cases are now examples of the human type with pulmonary infection. Haematogenous spread of the organisms to bone occurs in both children and adults. Tuberculous osteomyelitis occurs in two main sites, the spine and the shafts of long bones. The third type of skeletal involvement, namely tuberculous arthritis, will not be considered here, except to state that involvement of the adjacent bone ends with osteomyelitis may occur in advanced cases.

Spinal disease accounts for about 25%–40% of all cases of skeletal tuberculosis (Jaffe 1972). The lower half of the spine is most frequently involved with a more or less equal incidence from the T-8 to L-4 vertebrae, according to Schmorl and Junghans (1971), though Collins (1966) considered the lower thoracic region to be the most frequently involved. Certainly the lumbosacral region, upper thoracic and cervical spine are less often affected. Although a single vertebra may be diseased, involvement of several adjacent bones is common. Rarely, isolated lesions may occur in widely separated vertebrae (Collins 1966). It should be borne in mind, however, that evaluations of the distribution of lesions are based on clinical data and that morbid anatomical studies may show small foci of tuberculosis at other levels not detected by radiology (Schmorl and Junghans 1971).

The early focus of tuberculosis is usually located near the superior or inferior end plate of the vertebral body, or anteriorly. It is less often situated posteriorly. Tuberculosis of the vertebral arches is rare. Caseating tuberculoid granulomas replace the fatty and haematopoietic tissues, and there is necrosis of bone trabeculae (Fig. 10.9). Osteolysis is accelerated by the spreading caseation, and sequestra are seldom formed. There is often little in the way of bone regeneration until resolution has commenced, so that a sclerotic margin may not be seen on radiological examination until the commencement of healing (Collins 1966). A personal review of a series of cases of spinal tuberculosis reveals, however, that other areas of bone may show only small granulomas (Fig. 10.10), often without significant caseation, intermingled with the bone marrow cells, and that very careful examination of sections may be needed for the detection of such lesions.

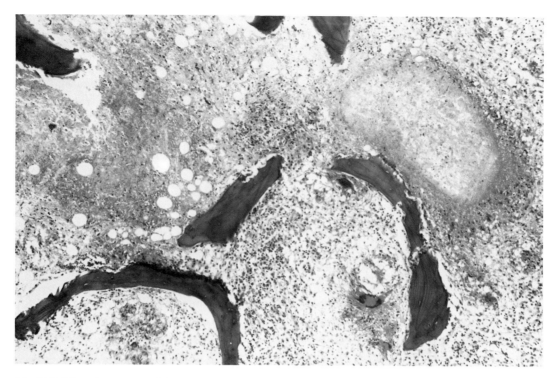

Fig. 10.9. Tuberculous osteomyelitis, showing caseating granulomas in the intertrabecular space and necrosis of bone trabeculae, which are undergoing resorption. (H&E × 80)

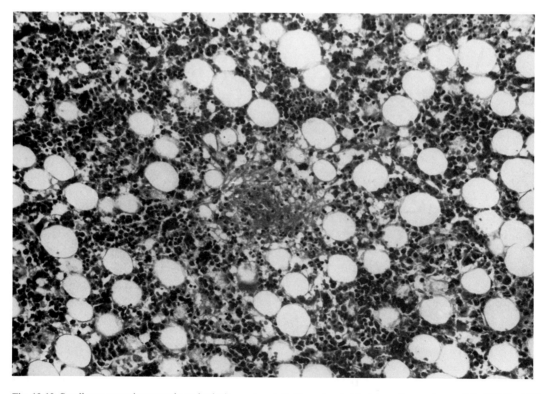

Fig. 10.10. Small non-caseating granuloma in the haematopoietic tissue (*centre*) in tuberculous osteomyelitis. (H&E × 160)

The presence of a paravertebral soft tissue shadow on the radiograph and narrowing of the intervertebral disc space are held to be useful features and there may be collapse and wedge-shaped deformity of vertebral bodies where there is advanced disease. No radiological feature is specific, however, and there may be complete absence of any radiological changes, as with other forms of osteomyelitis (see p. 240). It is the destruction of the trabeculae of the vertebral body which gives rise to collapse, and where two or more vertebral bodies with their intervening discs are affected an angular kyphosis or gibbus deformity may result (Figs. 10.11, 10.12). Occasionally, tuberculosis may be confined to the anterior part of the vertebra beneath the anterior longitudinal ligament. A tuberculous abscess forms in the absence of vertebral collapse under these circumstances. Cold abscesses may appear on the back, lateral abdominal wall, at the thigh, in the buttock or lower down the leg. Retropharyngeal abscesses occur in association with cervical spine involvement. Posterior extension of the tuberculous process may affect the spinal nerve roots within the intervertebral foramina. The healed stage of vertebral tuberculosis may present problems in its differentiation from congenital block vertebra or trauma with collapse and bony ankylosis of the spine.

Tuberculosis of long bones is rare and usually occurs in the metaphyseal region, like other osteomyelitis (Hayes 1961) (see p. 240). Such chronic tuberculosis may spread into the epiphysis, and in children involvement of the growth plate can interfere with bone development.

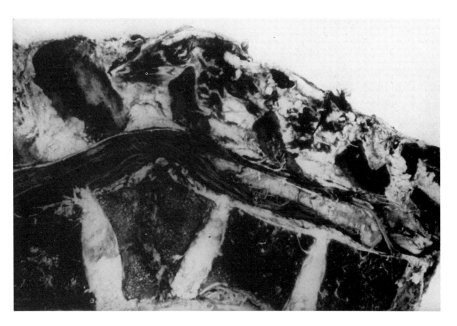

Fig. 10.11. Mid-line sagittal slice of lumbar spine, showing collapse of a tuberculous vertebral body, giving rise to an angular deformity

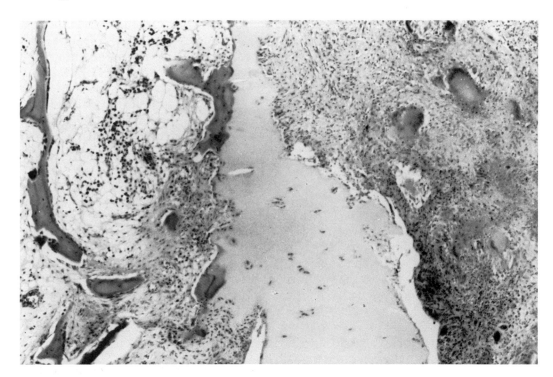

Fig. 10.12. Extension of tuberculous osteomyelitis from one vertebral body, in which the subchondral bone has been completely lost (*right*), across the intervertebral disc to involve the adjacent bone (*left*). (H&E × 80)

Other organisms

A large number of organisms may infect bone. It is not proposed to give detailed information about these in this chapter; however, descriptions of most are available in Jaffe (1972). The following sections will deal briefly with some of the other bacterial infections and the involvement of bone by viruses, fungi, treponemes and parasites.

Brucellosis

Brucellosis is caused by *Brucella melitensis, B. abortus* or *B. suis*, and the exact form of disease varies with the organism. The highest incidence of skeletal involvement occurs with *B. melitensis* infection. The bones most affected are the vertebrae (Lowbeer 1948). Like tuberculosis, the lumbar and dorsolumbar regions are involved, mainly in the anterior parts of the vertebral bodies. There is destruction of the intervertebral discs, and osteophyte-like overgrowth of reactive new bone occurs. Histological examination reveals the presence of epithelioid granulomas (Spink 1956), as seen in brucellosis elsewhere, although lesions in the spine may resemble low-grade suppurative osteomyelitis with limited necrosis, plentiful fibrosis and new bone formation (Lowbeer 1948). *B. melitensis* infection also affects large synovial joints (Makin et al. 1957).

Leprosy

Leprosy is a chronic infectious disease caused by *Mycobacterium leprae*, which affects bones in one of two ways, corresponding to the two basic types of lesion seen elsewhere. *Lepromatous leprosy* shows the presence of histiocytes (lepra cells), which are laden with large numbers of organisms. Such lepromatous lesions in bone cause cyst-like lesions and focal destruction of bone. Haematogenous osteomyelitis is very slowly progressive, and the foci of bone destruction usually occur in the ends of bones. Bone involvement usually occurs by direct spread from overlying dermal or mucosal lesions, so that the bones of the hands and the skull are those most often affected. In leprous periostitis there is normally little periosteal new bone formation unless secondary infection supervenes, when there may be abundant new bone.

The second histological appearance of leprosy is that of *tuberculoid leprosy*, in which epithelioid granulomas are formed. It is this type which involves peripheral nerves, thus causing sensory loss. The bone changes associated with this neurotrophic leprosy are much more severe than those caused by actual leprous osteomyelitis. There is marked atrophy of bones, which may eventually disappear completely. The changes first occur in the most distal parts of the limbs, in the phalanges, and advance slowly in a proximal direction. There is progressive resorption of bones from their outer surfaces. If fractures occur, healing and callus formation are poorly developed. The changes are made more severe by the fact that the leper is more prone to injury of anaesthetic limbs and by the effects of secondary infection with deep ulceration, thrombosis of vessels and gangrene. Reactive periostitis, osteitis, bone necrosis and sequestration may all contribute to the final result (Harris and Brand 1966).

Treponemal infections

Syphilis

The skeletal changes of syphilis may be divided into those occurring in the congenital and acquired forms of the disease. A detailed account of both is available in Jaffe (1972). Briefly, the lesions of *congenital syphilis* do not appear before the fifth month of intrauterine life, after which time there is an osteochondritis at sites of endochondral ossification. The growth plates of the long tubular bones and costochondral junctions may be the only areas affected, although in severe cases flat bones, short tubular bones and the vertebrae are also involved. Syphilitic neonates show widening of the zone of provisional calcification, in which there are long columns of calcified cartilage lacking new bone formation because of decreased osteoblastic activity. Vascular granulation tissue containing lymphocytes, plasma cells and spirochaetes is present between the calcified cartilage columns. This vascular tissue may itself invade the epiphyseal cartilage, and where a large amount of such granulation is present there is effectively a loss of continuity between epiphysis and metaphysis, so that epiphyseal separation may occur. The periostium is a second site of active bone formation in the developing fetus, and a periostitis is often seen. There is subperiosteal granulation tissue containing spirochaetes, and subperiosteal new bone growth is brought about by osteoblastic activity in the elevated periosteum (Collins 1966). According to Jaffe (1972), this change is seen in surviving neonates with congenital syphilis rather than fetuses and its combination with osteochondritis is exceptional. He also describes non-specific reactive and late reparative forms of periostitis, the former being a callus-like overgrowth in response to a partially detached epiphysis or cortical destruction, while the latter is a late stage in the healing of osteochondritis.

The bone changes of *acquired syphilis* occur during the tertiary stage of the disease. There may be reactive osteosclerosis in relation to the dense, often perivascular, lymphocytic infiltrate in the periosteum (Fig. 10.13). This thickened spongy new bone may eventually be condensed into compact, cortical bone with resorption of the original but encased bone cortex. Non-gummatous syphilitic osteomyelitis is found near to gummatous osteomyelitis, but only very rarely does this process occur more widely on its own. In gummatous periostitis and osteomyelitis there is bone destruction with necrosis. This necrotising osteomyelitis may penetrate cortical bone to produce holes, such

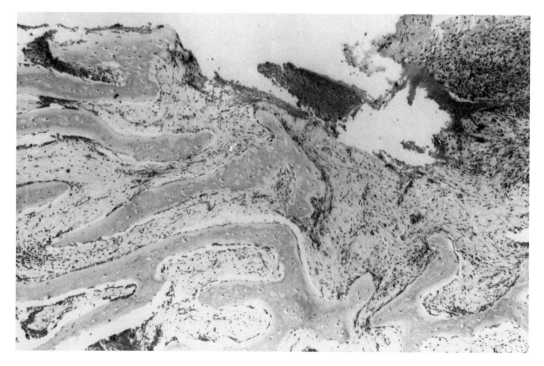

Fig. 10.13. Syphilitic periostitis, with a lymphocyte infiltrate in soft tissue (*top right*) and reactive new bone formation in cellular fibrous tissue. (H&E × 80)

as perforations in the skull and palate, or the collapse of vertebrae with development of kyphosis. Both gummatous and non-gummatous processes contribute to the changes seen late in congenital syphilis, such as the sabre tibia and the saddle nose.

Yaws

Yaws is due to infection with *Treponema pertenue* and occurs in the tropics. The primary (extragenital) lesion is followed by secondary involvement with widespread skin eruptions. Skin and bone involvement are seen in the tertiary phase. Osteochondritis does not occur, but the changes otherwise closely resemble those of syphilis and indeed are histologically indistinguishable. Diffuse sclerosis of the anterior part of the tibia gives rise to the sabre tibia appearance, while necrosis of the palate, nose and nasopharynx is known as 'gangosa'.

Fungi and actinomycosis

Systemic mycoses can no longer be regarded as exotic. The considerable mobility of people brought about by air travel and the widespread use of corticosteroid and cytotoxic drugs following transplant surgery and in malignant disease have all meant that fungal infections are now not unfamiliar problems to the pathologist. While tuberculosis is the most likely organism in immunosuppressed patients, fungal infections of bone may mimic bacterial osteomyelitis or tuberculosis both radiologically and histologically.

Actinomycosis

Actinomycosis is a low-grade, slowly progressive infection of man and cattle caused by *Actinomyces israelii*, a common saprophyte of the mouth and tonsils. It is now usually classified among the bacteria. Bone involvement in man is secondary to infection of adjacent tissue, such as osteomyelitis of the jaw in association with oral infection from a tooth socket. Other sites of infection are the lung, appendix and large intestine, while bone involvement may occur in the vertebral column or ribs (Beitzke 1934). Spinal involvement presents clinical problems in its differentiation from tuberculosis (Simpson and McIntosh 1927). Histological examination of affected bone shows colonies of organisms, often in matted clumps, necrotic tissue with polymorphonuclear leucocytes and histiocytes (Fig. 10.14), and fibrosis of surrounding bone marrow spaces. Erosion of bone with sinus formation occurs and there is some reactive new bone formation.

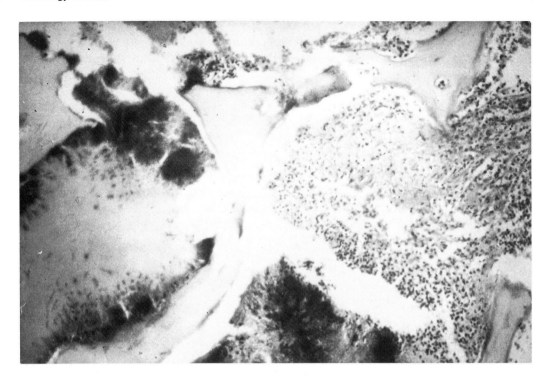

Fig. 10.14. Actinomycosis of bone. The necrotic bone trabeculae are poorly defined and there are matted clumps of organisms (*left* and *bottom*). (H&E × 120)

Blastomycosis

Blastomycosis is caused by a spherical yeast-like budding fungus, *Blastomyces dermatitidis*, and has its highest incidence in parts of the USA. The inflammatory reaction is granulomatous and/or suppurative and affects the skin and internal organs such as the lungs. Osseous involvement occurs as a result of direct spread from a soft tissue focus or by the haematogenous route. The vertebrae, ribs, tibia, ankle and wrist are the most common sites of infection. Radiological examination shows areas of radiolucency with sclerotic margins, and there may be widespread destruction of bone.

Coccidioidomycosis

Coccidioidomycosis is endemic in the arid south-western part of the USA. Pulmonary infection results from the inhalation of dust containing chlamydospores of *Coccidioides immitis*, which produce spherical endospore-filled encapsulated organisms in human tissues. The histological response is of tuberculoid granuloma formation, sometimes with caseation, which may be mistaken for tuberculosis if the fungi are not apparent in sections. Radiological examination of bones shows osteolytic lesions with reactive osteosclerosis, and the skeletal involvement is often widespread. In some cases, lesions may remain inactive for many years with only a slow reactive osteosclerosis present (Birsner and Smart 1956).

Cryptococcosis

Cryptococcosis is caused by a yeast-like organism, *Cryptococcus neoformans*, which has a predilection for the central nervous system but may also affect the skin, lungs and other sites including bones and joints. Collins (1950) found 17 examples of bone involvement in a series of 200 cases of cryptococcosis. The osseous lesions are osteolytic on radiological examination, with a variable amount of reactive new bone formation. Histological examination shows inflammatory tissue containing lymphocytes, histiocytes and giant cells together with the organisms.

Maduromycosis

Maduromycosis has a high incidence in southern India and most often affects the foot (Madura foot). Similar mycetomas occur in other parts of the world, however, and other anatomical sites, like the hand, are sometimes affected. The disease is typically one of bare-footed peoples since the infective organisms are present in the soil. The affected periphery is painful and enlarged and has numerous sinuses with raised margins. There is slowly progressive destruction of soft and hard tissues, so that the foot is grossly deformed with extensive loss of bone. Mycetomas typically occur on the extremities and are caused by a wide variety of organisms which are bacteria (*Nocardia, Streptomyces* and *Actinomyces* species) and fungi (*Madurella, Allescheria, Cephalosporium, Phialophora, Pyrenochaeta, Leptosphaeria* and *Neotestudina*). All these organisms are widely distributed in nature (Bindford and Dooley 1976). The histological hallmark of the mycetoma is the presence of one or more granules containing organisms.

Parasitic disease

Two parasitic infestations have been described in human bone, namely *echinococcosis* and *cysticercosis*, the latter being excessively rare (Boemke 1939). Involvement of bones with *hydatid disease* is unusual, affecting around 2% of cases. The most common site is the lower vertebrae, where the presentation is sometimes called 'hydatid Pott's disease', which can cause spinal cord compression and paraplegia (Sparks et al. 1976). The pelvis, humerus, tibia, fibula, femur and skull are other bones which may be affected. The single fluid-containing hydatid cyst, with germinal layer, outer chitinous layer, brood capsules, daughter cysts and scolices, which is found in the liver and other organs is not seen in bone. Instead, cancellous bone is filled with small thin-walled cysts containing gelatinous material in which brood capsules are unusual. The cysts spread through paths of least resistance giving rise to pressure atrophy of bone. A radiolucent area is seen on radiological examination, but a single large cystic lesion is not developed. If the cysts break out through the thinned bone cortex, the extraosseous component develops into the large cyst seen in classic soft tissue hydatid disease (Jaffe 1972).

Viral infections

Bone involvement with viral diseases is confined to smallpox and vaccinia, and examples of these are excessively rare. In smallpox, foci of necrosis in the bone marrow and stunted growth plates of affected bones have been noted. Osteomyelitis following vaccination against smallpox is very rare, and the development of vaccinia osteomyelitis cannot be assumed until virus has been isolated from the affected bone. A single such case is described by Cochran et al. (1963).

References

Adeyokunna AA, Hendrickse RG (1980) Salmonella osteomyelitis in childhood. A report of 63 cases seen in Nigeria of whom 57 had sickle cell anaemia. Arch Dis Child 55:175–184

Artz TD, Macys J, Salvati EA, Jacobs B, Wilson PD (1975) Hematogenous infection of total hip replacements. A report of four cases. J Bone Joint Surg [Am]57:1024 (abstr)

Beitzke H (1934) Aktinomykose der Knochen. In: Handbuch der speziellen Pathologischen Anatomie und Histologie, vol IX, part 2. Springer, Berlin (Cited by Collins 1966)

Bindford CH, Dooley JR (1976) Diseases caused by fungi and actinomycetes: deep mycoses. In: Binford CH, Connor DR (eds) Pathology of tropical and extraordinary diseases. An atlas, vol 2. Armed Forces Institute of Pathology, Washington DC, pp 551–560

Birsner JW, Smart J (1956) Osseous coccidioidomycosis. Am J Roentgenol 76:1052–1060

Boemke F (1939) Parasiten des Knochensystems. In: Handbuch der speziellen Pathologischen Anatomie und Histologie, vol IX, part 4. Springer, Berlin (Cited by Collins 1966)

Bornstein DL, Weinberg AN, Swartz MN, Kunz LJ (1964) Anaerobic infections. Review of current experience. Medicine (Baltimore) 43:207–232

Charnley J (1972) Post-operative infection after total hip replacement, with special reference to air contamination in the operating room. Clin Orthop 87:167–187

Charnley J, Eftekhar N (1969) Post-operative infection in total prosthetic replacement arthroplasty of the hip joint with special reference to the bacterial content of the air of the operating room. Br J Surg 56:641–649

Chow AW, Guze LB (1974) Bacteriodaceae bacteraemia: clinical experience with 112 patients. Medicine (Baltimore) 53:93–126

Cochran W, Connolly JH, Thompson ID (1963) Bone involvement after vaccination against smallpox. Br Med J II:285–287

Collins VP (1950) Bone involvement in cryptococcosis (torulosis). Am J Roentgenol 63:102–112

Collins DH (1966) Pathology of bone. Butterworths, London

Cruess RL, Bickel WS, von Kessler KL (1975) Infections in total hips secondary to a primary source elsewhere. Clin Orthop Res 106:99–101

Deysine M, Rosario E, Isenberg HD (1976) Acute hematogenous osteomyelitis; an experimental model. Surgery 79:97–99

Edwards MS, Baker CJ, Wagner ML, Taher LH, Barrett FF (1978) An etiologic shift in infantile osteomyelitis; the emergence of the group B streptococcus. J Pediatr 93:578–583

Felner JM, Dowell VR (1971) Bacteroides bacteraemia. Am J Med 50:787–796

Fink CW, Dick VQ, Howard J, Nelson JD (1977) Infection of bone and joints in children. Arthritis Rheum 20 (2):578–583

Fox L, Sprunt K (1978) Neonatal osteomyelitis. Pediatrics 62:535–542

Freeman MAR, Challis JH, Zelezonski J, Jarvis ID (1977) Sepsis rates in hip replacement surgery with special reference to the use of ultra clean air. Arch Orthop Unfallchir 90:1–14

Garcia A, Grantham SA (1960) Hematogenous pyogenic vertebral osteomyelitis. J Bone Joint Surg [Am] 42:429–436

Golding JSR, MacIver JE, Went LH (1959) The bone changes in sickle cell anaemia and its genetic variants. J Bone Joint Surg [Br] 41:711–718

Hall AJ (1974) Late infection about a total knee prosthesis. J Bone Joint Surg [Br] 56:144–147

Harris NH (1960) Some problems in the diagnosis and treatment of acute osteomyelitis. J Bone Joint Surg [Br] 42:535–541

Harris JR, Brand PW (1966) Patterns of disintegration of the tarsus in the anaesthetic foot. J Bone Joint Surg [Br] 48:4–16

Hayes JT (1961) Cystic tuberculosis of the proximal tibial metaphysis—with associated involvement of the epiphysis and epiphyseal plate. J Bone Joint Surg [Am] 43:560–567

Hunter G, Dandy D (1977) The natural history of the patient with an infected total hip replacement. J Bone Joint Surg [Br] 59:293–297

Jacobsson S (1979) Diffuse sclerosing osteomyelitis of the mandible. Acta Otolaryngol [Suppl] (Stockh) 360:61–63

Jaffe HL (1972) Metabolic, degenerative and inflammatory diseases of bones and joints. Lea and Febiger, Philadelphia

Kirchner PT, Simon MA (1981) Radioisotopic evaluation of skeletal disease. J Bone Joint Surg [Am] 63:673–681

Letts RM, Afifi A, Sutherland JB (1975) Technetium bone scanning as an aid in the diagnosis of atypical acute osteomyelitis in children. Surg Gynecol Obstet 140:899–902

Lim MO, Gresham EL, Franken EA, Leake RD (1977) Osteomyelitis as a complication of umbilical artery catheterisation. Am J Dis Child 131:142–144

Lindenbaum S, Alexander H (1984) Infections simulating bone tumours. Clin Orthop 184:193–203

Lowbeer L (1948) Brucellotic osteomyelitis of the spinal column in man. Am J Pathol 24:723–724

Makin M, Alkalaj I, Rozansky R (1957) Mono-articular brucellar arthritis. J Bone Joint Surg [Am] 39:1183–1186

Mallory TH (1973) Sepsis in total hip replacement following pneumonococcal pneumonia. J Bone Joint Surg [Am] 55:1753–1754

McHenry MC, Wellman WE, Martin WJ (1961) Bacteraemia due to bacteroides. Arch Intern Med 107:572–577

Ogden JA, Light TR (1979) Pediatric osteomyelitis: III anaerobic micro-organisms. Clin Orthop 145:230–237

Ortiz-Neu C, Marr JS, Cherubin CE, Neu HC (1978) Bone and joint infections due to *Salmonella*. J Infect Dis 138:820–828

Raff MJ, Melo JC (1978) Anaerobic osteomyelitis. Medicine (Baltimore) 57:83–103

Rinsky L, Goris ML, Schurman DJ, Nagel DA (1977) ^{99}Technitium bone scanning in experimental osteomyelitis. Clin Orthop 128:361–366

Roca RP, Yoshikawa TT (1979) Primary skeletal infections in heroin users. Clin Orthop 144:238–248

Schmorl G, Junghans H (1971) The human spine in health and disease. Grune and Stratton, New York

Simpson WM, McIntosh CA (1927) Actinomycosis of the vertebrae (actinomycotic Pott's disease). Arch Surg 14:1166–1186

Sparks AK, Connor DH, Neafie RC (1976) Echinococcosis. In: Binford CH, Connor DR (eds) Pathology of tropical extraordinary diseases. An Atlas, vol 2. Armed Forces Institute of Pathology, Washington DC, pp 530–533

Spink WW (1956) The nature of brucellosis. University of Minnesota Press, Minneapolis

Stone DB, Bonfiglio M (1963) Pyogenic vertebral osteomyelitis. Arch Intern Med 112:491–500

Treves S, Khettoy J, Broker FH, Wilkinson RH, Watts H (1976) Osteomyelitis: early scintigraphic detection in children. Pediatrics 57:173–186

Trueta J (1959) The three types of acute haematogenous osteomyelitis: a clinical and vascular study. J Bone Joint Surg [Br] 41:671–680

Waldvogel FA, Vasey H (1980) Osteomyelitis: the past decade. N Engl J Med 303:360–370

Waldvogel FA, Medoff G, Schwartz MN (1970) Osteomyelitis: a review of clinical features, therapeutic considerations and unusual aspects. N Engl J Med 282:198–206, 260–266, 316–322

Chapter 11

Bone Tumours and Tumour-like Conditions

Introduction

It is not proposed to give a detailed description of various bone tumours and tumour-like conditions in this chapter. There are already several excellent books which deal specifically with the subject (Jaffe 1958; Spjut et al. 1971; Lichtenstein 1972; Schajowicz et al. 1972; Dahlin 1978; Huvos 1979; Mirra 1980; Schajowicz 1981). The following account will be concerned with general aspects of the diagnosis of bone tumours, giving the briefest of descriptions of particular tumours and a discussion of the differential diagnosis of particular types of lesion. Current trends in diagnosis and treatment are summarised by Schajowicz (1983).

Classification of bone tumours

The histological features of bone tumours are a reflection of the fact that skeletal connective tissue cells are capable of varied differentiation. Tumours may produce cartilage, fibrous tissue or bone, and there may be variable numbers of osteoclastic giant cells present. Interpretation of histological appearances is complicated by the way that tumour tissue may undergo changes akin to those occurring in normal skeletal tissue, for example calcification and ossification in cartilaginous tumours. It is also necessary to recognise potentially misleading reactive tissue as distinct from the tumour, for example areas of reactive new bone within a tumour.

The classification of bone tumours is based on the differentiation shown by the cells present and the type of matrix produced. Although there are some differences between authors, the basic categories are those outlined in Table 11.1, from which tumour-like conditions have been omitted. Particular areas

Table 11.1. Classification of bone tumours

Origin or differentiation	Benign	Malignant
Cartilage	Osteochondroma Chondroma Chondroblastoma Chondromyxoid fibroma Juxtacortical chondroma	Chondrosarcoma: primary/secondary (Mesenchymal chondrosarcoma) (Dedifferentiated chondrosarcoma) (Juxtacortical chondrosarcoma)
Bone	Osteoid osteoma Osteoblastoma	Osteosarcoma (Periosteal osteosarcoma) (Parosteal osteosarcoma)
Bone marrow		Multiple myeloma Plasmacytoma Malignant lymphoma
Fibrous tissue	Desmoplastic fibroma Fibroma Periosteal desmoid fibromyxoma	Fibrosarcoma
Unknown origin	Giant cell tumour (Fibrous) histiocytoma	Malignant giant cell tumour Ewing's tumour Adamantinoma Malignant fibrous histiocytoma
Vascular	Haemangioma Glomus tumour Skeletal angiomatosis	Angiosarcoma Haemangioendothelioma Malignant haemangiopericytoma
Fat	Lipoma	Liposarcoma
Smooth muscle		Leiomysarcoma
Nerve	Neurilemmoma Neurofibromatosis	
Notochord		Chordoma

of difficulty arise in relation to giant cell lesions, some fibrous lesions, small round cell tumours and bone-forming osteoblastic lesions. As with other fields of tumour pathology, the histologist will sometimes have to admit his ignorance and give the opinion, 'Primary bone tumour, unspecified'.

General approach to bone tumour pathology

The need for close cooperation between pathologist, radiologist and orthopaedic surgeon in the diagnosis and treatment of bone tumours has become a well-known cliche (Spjut et al. 1971), which is nevertheless well worth repeating. There is no need for the pathologist to make a difficult area of his work more difficult by trying to make a diagnosis on inadequate biopsy material with inadequate clinical information and no idea of what the lesion looks like on a radiograph. He should insist on receiving all the available clinical information and seeing the radiographs for himself before offering a diagnostic opinion. The council of perfection is the discussion of each individual case by surgeon, radiologist and pathologist, planning together such matters as the likely best site for biopsy.

Clinical features

Bone tumours may cause local pain, swelling and limitation of movement, all of which are non-specific. Pain occurring with an osteoid osteoma is characteristically worse at night and relieved by salicylates (see p. 274). Trauma to the affected part is important only in bringing attention to a tumour and is not likely to be directly responsible for its development. Patients with Ewing's tumour sometimes have a fever, localised increase in temperature near the lesion, leucocytosis and secondary anaemia, so that osteomyelitis enters the differential diagnosis.

It is essential to have accurate details of the age of the patient, the bone involved and the location in the bone (epiphysis, metaphysis, diaphysis, cortical, central, parosteal etc.), since certain tumours occur in particular age groups and most commonly at certain sites (Tables 11.2–11.4). Laboratory investigations are of value in certain circumstances. Raised alkaline phosphatase levels in the blood may be present with primary bone-forming tumours but may equally be found with metastatic disease, Paget's disease of bone and non-osseous pathology. Metastatic prostatic carcinoma may cause elevated acid phosphatase levels. Hypercalcaemia, hyperuricaemia and an elevated

Table 11.2. Usual age of presentation of bone tumours and tumour-like lesions

Tumour or tumour-like lesion	1	2	3	4	5	6	7	8
Non-ossifying fibroma/ metaphyseal fibrous defect	+	+ +	+					
Osteochondroma	+	+ +	+ +	+				
Aneurysmal bone cyst	+	+ +	+ +					
Chondromyxoid fibroma	+ +	+ +	+ +	+	+	±		
Ewing's tumour	+ +	+ + +	+ +	+				
Osteoblastoma	±	+ +	+ +	+				
Osteoid osteoma	+	+ +	+					
Simple cyst	+	+	±					
Adamantinoma		+	+ +	±				
Chondroblastoma	±	+ +	+	+	+			
Chondroma	+	+ +	+ +	+ +	+ +	+		
Fibrosarcoma		+	+	+	+	+		
Giant cell tumour		+	+ + +	+ +	+			
Haemangioma/ haemangiosarcoma		+	+ +	+ +	+ +	+		
Malignant lymphoma		+	+	+	+	+ +	+ +	+
Osteosarcoma	±	+ + +	+ +	±	±	+	+	
Carcinoma, metastatic				+	+ +	+ +	+ +	+
Chondrosarcoma			±	+	+	+ +	+ +	+
Chordoma				+	+	+ +	+	
Myeloma				+	+ +	+ +	+	

The scoring is meant to give a rough guide to the age distribution, showing the proportion of cases of a particular tumour by decade. There is no attempt to equate the scoring for one tumour with that of another (i.e. the chart should only be read across the rows).

blood urea level may be present in myelomatosis, in which alterations in serum globulin, Bence Jones proteinuria and abnormalities in the serum and urine electrophoretic strip are familiar features.

Table 11.3. Type of bone affected by different tumours and tumour-like conditions in broad categories

Long bones	Adamantinoma
	Chondroblastoma
	Chondromyxoid fibroma
	Chondroma
	Osteochondroma
	Chondrosarcoma
	Ewing's tumour
	Non-ossifying fibroma/metaphyseal fibrous defect
	Fibrous dysplasia
	Fibrosarcoma/malignant fibrous histiocytoma
	Haemangioma
	Liposarcoma
	Osteoid osteoma
	Osteoblastoma
	Osteosarcoma
	Simple cyst
	Aneurysmal bone cyst
	Eosinophilic granuloma
	Metastatic carcinoma
	Synovial chondromatosis
	Pigmented villonodular synovitis/nodular synovitis
Limb girdle	Chondroblastoma
	Chondromyxoid fibroma
	Chondrosarcoma
	Osteoid osteoma
	Osteosarcoma
	Multiple myeloma
	Aneurysmal bone cyst
	Metastatic carcinoma
Rib/sternum	Chondroblastoma
	Chondromyxoid fibroma
	Chondrosarcoma
	Fibrous dysplasia
	Multiple myeloma/plasmacytoma
	Metastatic carcinoma
	Eosinophilic granuloma
Spine	Chondroma
	Haemangioma
	Osteoblastoma
	Multiple myeloma
	Aneurysmal bone cyst
	Metastatic carcinoma
Skull	Haemangioma
	Multiple myeloma
	Aneurysmal bone cyst
	Fibrous dysplasia
	Metastatic carcinoma
	Eosinophilic granuloma
Hand/foot	Chondroma
	(Chondroblastoma)
	(Chondromyxoid fibroma)
	(Osteoid osteoma/osteoblastoma)
	Pigmented nodular synovitis/nodular synovitis

Table 11.4. Position in long bone of bone tumours and other conditions

Epiphyseal	Chondroblastoma
	Giant cell tumour
Metaphyseal	Adamantinoma
	Aneurysmal bone cyst
	Chondromyxoid fibroma
	Chondrosarcoma
	Ewing's tumour
	Fibrosarcoma
	Non-ossifying fibroma/metaphyseal fibrous defect
	Haemangioma
	Osteochondroma
	Osteoblastoma
	Osteoid osteoma
	Osteosarcoma
	Osteomyelitis
	Malignant lymphoma
	Multiple myeloma
	Adamantinoma
	Ewing's tumour
	Haemangioma
Diaphyseal	Osteoblastoma
	Osteoid osteoma
	Multiple myeloma
	Aneurysmal bone cyst

Radiological features

Examination of the radiographs by the pathologist will provide important information, even to those not used to dealing with bone tumours. They will often give a clear idea of the exact site and size of the lesion, the latter being particularly useful in assessing the adequacy of the biopsy submitted for diagnosis. Basic considerations in the interpretation of the radiographic features of bone tumours rest with an understanding of the pathological processes which may be occurring in the bone. The tumour may be locally destructive. There may be resorption of surrounding bone or reactive new bone formation. The end result seen in the radiograph depends on the relative proportions of these features (Milch and Changus 1956). The particular radiological pattern at the margins of lesions may be helpful (e.g. moth-eaten appearance in myeloma, onion-skin appearance in Ewing's tumour), as may the type of periosteal new bone growth in assessing the nature of the tumour growth and its extension. Attention should be paid to the tumour itself with respect to radiolucency, evidence of calcification or ossification and its overall shape (e.g. cystic, lobular, oval in the long-axis of the bone etc.). It does not seem appropriate to attempt detailed descriptions. The radiological features of individual tumours are well illustrated elsewhere (Jaffe 1958; Spjut et al. 1971; Murray and Jacobson 1971; Lichtenstein 1972; Eidekin and Hodes 1973; Netherlands Committee on Bone Tumours 1973; Dahlin 1978). Arteriography has been found useful in the demonstration of tumours in bones and related soft tissues (Strickland 1959). Computerised axial tomography (CAT scanning) is beginning to be used more widely.

Radioisotopic scanning is on occasions a useful adjunct to the diagnosis and localisation of bone tumours. A recent review of the subject has been provided by Kirchner and Simon (1981). ^{99m}Tc-labelled phosphorous complexes (condensed phosphates or phosphonates) are rapidly distributed throughout the extracellular fluid and taken up by skeletal tissue after intravenous injection. The normal skeletal distribution is to trabecular rather than cortical bone, and accumulation is especially high in the metaphyseal and periarticular regions of adults and the growth plate and epiphyseal regions of children and adolescents. Since most cases of regional bone disease show some related reactive bone formation, increased uptake (a 'hot spot') is usually found where there is pathology. Necrosis, aggressive metastatic tumours, fulminant osteomyelitis and multiple myeloma are situations where there may be no significant bone reaction and they may even show as absence of uptake ('cold spot') at some stage in their development, although a more characteristic 'hot lesion' develops later. ^{99m}Tc-labelled sulphur colloid is taken up by the cells of the mononuclear phagocyte system (reticuloendothelial system) and can be used to demonstrate the normal bone marrow distribution in the axial skeleton and proximal long bones of adults, with uptake by the limb bones seen additionally in children.

The most frequent indication for scintigraphic scanning of the skeleton is in the search for metastatic tumour, over 95% of which is detected by this method (Fig. 11.1). Radiological bone surveys are no longer justifiable in the

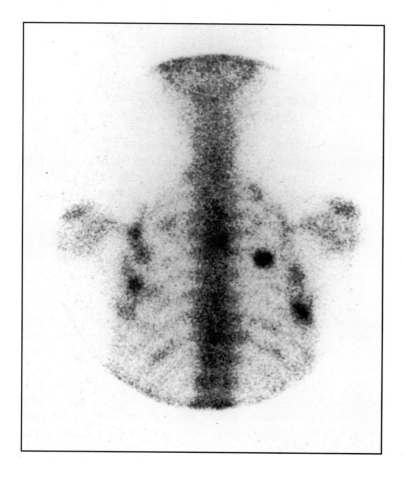

Fig. 11.1. Radioisotope scan showing deposits of secondary carcinoma of the breast in the ribs. Gamma camera, ^{99m}Tc-methylene-diphosphonate (^{99m}Tc-MDP)

search for metastatic tumour, being less sensitive, more costly and causing unnecessary radiation exposure. Most skeletal secondary deposits show increased isotope uptake and are therefore not distinguishable from other benign, inflammatory or traumatic bone disease. Demonstration of 'hot spots' in bone in patients likely to have metastatic disease is nevertheless useful in assessing the extent of the involvement. Primary malignant tumours of bone uniformly display increased focal accumulation of technetium phosphate tracer (Fig. 11.2). Most benign tumours also take up tracer, although simple bone cysts, non-ossifying fibromas and osteochondromas in adults, are occasional exceptions. Technetium scanning is effective in localising multiple foci of skeletal involvement in enchondromatosis, multifocal fibrous dysplasia, multiple osteochondromata and histiocytosis X, as well as in the detection of skeletal metastases of Ewing's tumour and osteosarcoma. When ^{99m}Tc-labelled sulphur colloid is used, extension of the bone marrow to a pattern more like that of the child may be seen in the presence of replacement of

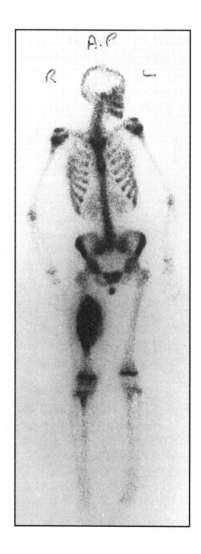

Fig. 11.2. Whole body radioisotope scan (^{99m}Tc-MDP) showing primary bone tumour in the shaft of the right femur. Same case as Fig. 11.21

haematopoietic tissue by malignant disease, some infective inflammatory processes and fibrosis. With this type of tracer, cold spots in the bone marrow are a reflection of primary or secondary tumour in bone and bone marrow necrosis.

Histopathological diagnosis

Establishment of a histological diagnosis is imperative in the case of any bone lesion suspected of being neoplastic, even where the clinical and radiological evidence is overwhelmingly in favour of a particular tumour. The exact method of biopsy must vary according to the individual surgeon and pathologist working together, and with respect to the surgical possibilities at a particular site. Needle biopsies have been successfully used by Schajowicz (Schajowicz 1955; Schajowicz and Derqui 1968), among others. They are particularly useful with vertebral lesions, where extensive surgery to obtain a biopsy can be avoided. It is sometimes necessary to resort secondarily to open biopsy when the lesion has been missed, is necrotic, or crushed (Spjut et al. 1971). Needle biopsies are not appropriate to low-grade chondrosarcomas, where a large sample is required in order to detect malignancy.

Fresh-frozen sections of an open biopsy are advocated by Dahlin (1978) on the basis that they provide instant appraisal of the adequacy of the biopsy specimen and a rapid diagnosis, so that the surgeon can institute bacteriological studies if the lesion proves to be inflammatory and immediate ablative therapy of a tumour if appropriate. Permanent fixed haematoxylin/eosin-stained sections can usually be prepared within 24 h if the soft portions of the lesion are selected and rapidly processed. Ideally, the pathologist should have seen and discussed the relevant radiographs with the surgeon and radiologist in advance of receiving the biopsy.

A wide variety of different techniques can be applied to the further investigation of the tumour if the biopsy is received fresh from the operating theatre. The cytology of bone tumours in imprint preparations can be studied (Sanerkin 1980), and frozen sections and imprints used for enzyme histochemistry (e.g. the demonstration of alkaline phosphatase). Such freshly obtained material fixed for electron microscopy from the outset will give better ultrastructural detail than formalin-fixed tissue. Fixation in 80% ethyl alcohol is preferable when the demonstration of glycogen in small round cell tumours is to be performed, though the present author has found success with routinely fixed tissue, so long as sections are 'floated out' on alcohol before staining. Immunohistochemical staining with the peroxidase-antiperoxidase technique may occasionally be useful and is easily performed on formalin-fixed soft tissue, although the author has not obtained consistent results when the tissue has undergone decalcification. All these methods are applicable as aids to the diagnosis of bone tumours. The ideal is to be able to give a correct diagnosis on the haematoxylin/eosin sections with the shortest possible delay.

An area of bone tumour pathology sometimes neglected is the method of handling the resected bone or amputation specimen after a definitive operation has been performed. It is not sufficient merely to confirm the biopsy diagnosis by taking further small samples from the tumour. The tumour should be thoroughly assessed with respect to surgical limits of excision, proximal limit of extension in the bone, possible vascular and lymph node involvement and extension into soft tissues, in just the same way that an excised tumour in an organ would be examined. Hard tissues may be sawn by hand using a meat/ hacksaw, with recourse to an electric hand saw or band saw if necessary and available. We use a combination of all three types and in addition have a water-cooled circular cutting device in which carborundum- or diamond-impregnated wheels may be used. Radiographic examination of the specimen is useful, and comparison of slab radiographs with the clinical radiograph is often rewarding.

Hard tissue may be decalcified in formic acid or ethylenediaminetetraacetic acid (EDTA), though the author's preference is for the former. Rapid decalcification methods based on hydrochloric or nitric acids are available, but have not proved especially advantageous in the author's laboratory. The use of undecalcified methylmethacrylate sectioning methods enables early assessment of hard parts of the tumour and limits of excision.

Particular types of bone tumour

A description of the histopathology of all the various bone tumours and tumour-like conditions will not be attempted here. Particular lesions are described below under broad categories:

1. Cartilaginous tumours
2. Bone-forming tumours
3. Giant cell tumour
4. Malignant fibrous tumours
5. Round cell tumours

The descriptions of these tumours are in no way meant to be comprehensive, but may be of assistance. A guide to the differential diagnosis of bone tumours and tumour-like conditions according to the histological features present is given in Table 11.5. It is hoped that this table and the others in this chapter may provide a way of sifting out the possibilities for the pathologist faced with a particular lesion.

Cartilaginous tumours

Osteochondroma (cartilage-capped exostosis)

An osteochondroma is a cartilage-capped protrusion usually occurring in the metaphyseal region of a long bone in the limb of a child or young adult. The question of the origin of these lesions has been discussed by Milgram (1983),

Table 11.5. A guide to the differential diagnosis of bone tumours and tumour-like conditions according to presence of histological features

Spindle-celled/fibrous	*Giant cells*	*Osteoid*
Non-ossifying fibroma/ metaphyseal fibrous defect	Chondromyxoid fibroma	Osteoblastoma
Fibrous dysplasia	Fibrous histiocytoma	Osteoid osteoma
Fibrous histiocytoma	Fibrosarcoma	Osteosarcoma
Fibrosarcoma	Non-ossifying fibroma/ metaphyseal fibrous defect	(Parosteal osteosarcoma)
Chondrosarcoma	Simple cyst	Osteochondroma
(Mesenchymal chondrosarcoma)	Osteosarcoma	Chondrosarcoma
Osteosarcoma	(Parosteal osteosarcoma)	Giant cell tumour
(Parosteal osteosarcoma)	(Telangiectatic osteosarcoma)	Haemangioma
Adamantinoma	Aneurysmal bone cyst	Aneurysmal bone cyst
Aneurysmal bone cyst	Giant cell tumour	Simple cyst
Simple cyst	Osteoblastoma	Heterotopic ossification
Metastatic carcinoma	Osteoid osteoma	Fibrous dysplasia
Chondromyxoid fibroma	Chondroblastoma	
Heterotopic ossification	Chondrosarcoma	*Small round cell*
Nodular tenosynovitis	Hyperparathyroidism	Ewing's tumour
Smooth muscle tumours		Malignant lymphoma
Neurogenic tumours	*Chondroid*	(multiple myeloma)
Fibroma desmoplastic	Chondroblastoma	Chondrosarcoma
	Chondroma	(Mesenchymal chondrosarcoma)
Myxoid	Osteochondroma	Osteosarcoma
Chondroma	Chondromyxoid fibroma	Liposarcoma
Chondromyxoid fibroma	Chondrosarcoma	
Chondrosarcoma	Osteosarcoma	
Chordoma	(Parosteal osteosarcoma)	
Liposarcoma	Chondroma	
Nerve sheath tumour		

with particular reference to the relationship with the growth plate. It is one of the commonest benign bone lesions and may present with pain and/or swelling. The lower femur and upper tibia are particularly affected, though other sites include the upper humerus and upper femur, and almost any bone has occasionally been involved (Spjut et al. 1971; Dahlin 1978). Radiological examination shows a bony sessile or pedunculated projection on the outside of the bone, frequently pointing away from the epiphysis and showing continuity of its cortical and medullary bone with that of the bone of origin (Fig. 11.3). There may be irregular calcification in the cartilage cap. Macroscopic examination confirms the features seen on the radiograph. The cartilage cap may be thin and smooth or knobbly and lobulated, depending partly on the age of the patient. If the cartilage cap is thin and regular, the tumour is always benign, and exostoses in which growth has ceased may show minimal distal cartilage. Excessive thickening and irregularity of the cartilage cap should arouse the suspicion of chondrosarcomatous change when seen in an adult. Malignant change is rare and occurs more frequently in cases with multiple exostoses (see p. 270). Cartilaginous exostoses have been described in small children following radiotherapy for neuroblastoma, Wilms' tumour and eosinophilic granuloma, occurring within or near the field of radiation therapy (Murphy and Blount 1962; Cole and Darte 1963).

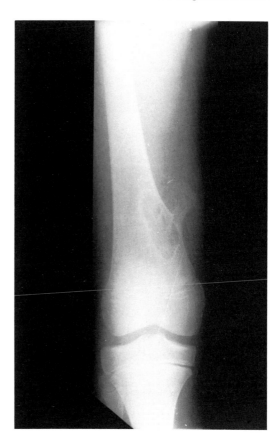

Fig. 11.3. Osteochondroma (cartilage-capped exostosis) at the lower end of the femur. There is a pedunculated mass arising on the outside of the bone at the metaphysis and this point upwards, that is away from the epiphysis. In this particular example, there is also a metaphyseal fibrous defect within the bone

Chondroma

Chondromas are benign tumours made up of mature hyaline cartilage which usually occur centrally in the affected bone and are then often called 'enchondromas'. The origins of these lesions have recently been discussed by Milgram (1983). Periosteal lesions also occur, and in sites such as the ribs, scapula or pelvis the exact site of origin is not always easy to define. Chondromas may present at any age but most frequently between the ages of 10 and 40 years. The short tubular bones of the hands and feet are most commonly affected (Fig. 11.4), and a chondroma is likely to be asymptomatic and found fortuitously on radiological examination. Radiologically, there is a centrally placed area of radiolucency, most often in the diaphyseal region and showing mottled calcification or ossification within the tumour mass. Naked-eye examination shows a lobular bluish-grey semi-transparent lesion resembling cartilage with variable presence of calcified and ossified foci. Large lesions should arouse the suspicion of chondrosarcoma, and multiple sections of such tumours should be examined to exclude this possibility. Histologically, the tumour comprises small chondrocytes with regular nuclei in a hyaline chondroid matrix. Areas may show marked cellularity and there may be arrangement of cells into large clusters. Chondrocytes with large nuclei and multinucleate forms suggest the possibility of malignancy. There may be focal calcification, endochondral ossification or myxoid change.

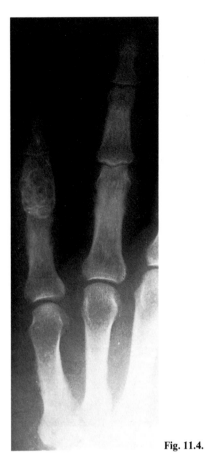

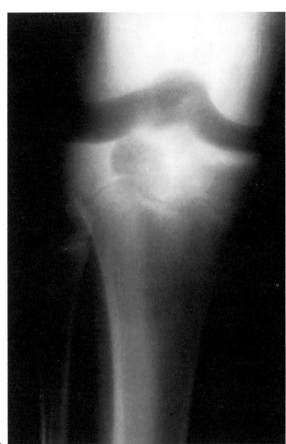

Fig. 11.4.

Fig. 11.5.

Fig. 11.4. Enchondroma in middle phalanx of little finger

Fig. 11.5. Chondroblastoma in the upper epiphysis of the tibia

Chondroblastoma

Chondroblastoma is a rare tumour usually occurring in the epiphyseal part of a long bone, mostly the femur, tibia or humerus. The majority of patients are aged between 10 and 20 years. Localised pain of some duration is an almost constant clinical feature, and there may be local tenderness. Radiologically, there is a radiolucent area of bone destruction in the epiphysis, surrounded by a narrow margin of sclerosis (Fig. 11.5). Mottled areas of calcification are seen within the tumour in some cases (McLeod and Beabout 1973). Macroscopically, the tumour, which is not usually large, has a greyish-blue or grey-brown surface and may be gritty or undergo cystic change. Microscopy shows it to be composed of chondroblasts, which are polygonal, round or spindle-shaped cells with oval nuclei (Fig. 11.6). There is some chondroid matrix between the cells, and the presence of benign multinucleate giant cells may suggest the erroneous diagnosis of giant cell tumour. Lace-like focal calcification of the chondroid matrix is a helpful diagnostic feature (Spjut et al. 1971; Fig. 11.7).

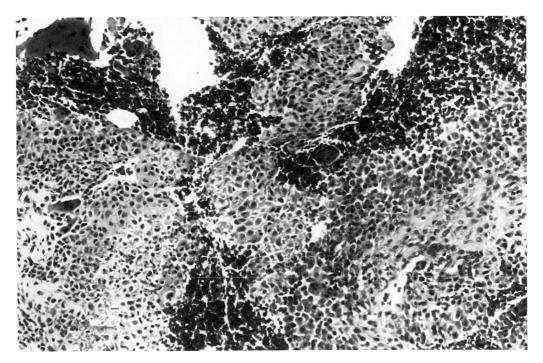

Fig. 11.6. Large collections of polygonal and oval chondroblasts in a chondroblastoma
Note: Occasional giant cells in this example. (H&E × 160)

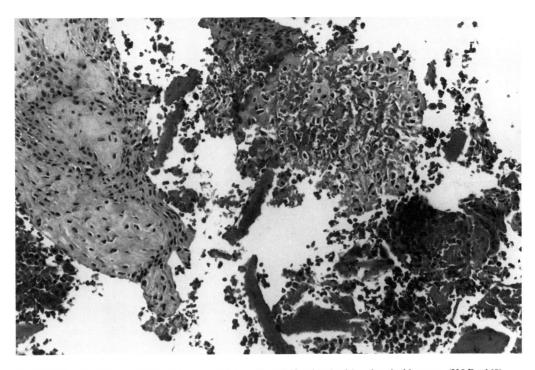

Fig. 11.7. Chondroid tissue (*left*) and tumour with lace-like calcification (*right*)—chondroblastoma. (H&E × 160)

Chondromyxoid fibroma

Chondromyxoid fibroma is a rare localised tumour characterised by lobulated areas of spindle-shaped and stellate cells with myxoid or chondroid matrix. It was first described by Jaffe and Lichtenstein (1948) and affects males more often than females (Dahlin 1978). Although it may occur at any age in adults, presentation in the second and third decades is usual. The metaphyseal region of a long bone, especially in the lower limb is a common site (Spjut et al. 1971; Dahlin 1978). Like chondroblastoma, local pain of some duration is a common presenting symptom, and there may be local tenderness. Radiological examination shows an eccentric well-circumscribed area of rarefaction, sometimes causing expansion of the outline of the bone. There may be a surrounding thin line of sclerosis and the appearances are those of a benign lesion (Turcotte et al. 1962). Macroscopically, it is a well-circumscribed lobulated solid grey-white mass often representing hyaline cartilage, though there may be myxoid, cystic or haemorrhagic areas present. The histological features of the tumour are well summarised by its name, since there may be myxomatous and fibrous areas together with distinctly chondroid features. The cells present have variably shaped nuclei, which are round, oval or spindle shaped. Foci of cells may bear a strong resemblance to chondroblasts as seen in chondroblastoma. Large cells with nuclei of irregular size and shape and occasional multinucleate chondroid cells may be present, but in the presence of the other features do not detract from the diagnosis and should not be mistaken for chondrosarcoma. The characteristic lobulated pattern may be difficult to distinguish in a small curetted biopsy, but the increased concentration of nuclei towards the clearly demarcated edge of lobules is a helpful feature, though it should be borne in mind that a similar increased cellularity is seen in some chondrosarcomas. The lobular areas are separated by cellular tissue containing abundant spindle-shaped cells and variable numbers of macrophages and benign giant cells.

Chondrosarcoma

Chondrosarcoma is a malignant cartilage-forming tumour of bone, which is usually primary, that is arising *de novo*, but may be secondary, namely arising in a previously benign cartilaginous tumour such as an osteochondroma. It is difficult to prove that a pre-existing osteochondroma was a precursor to a solitary chondrosarcoma. Malignant transformation in hereditary multiple exostoses and enchondromatosis is, however, well recognised (Spjut et al. 1971). A recent study suggests the incidence of malignant change may be fairly low (Voutsinas and Wynn-Davies 1983).

Chondrosarcoma is a tumour of adults, most frequently occurring in the age range 30–60 years and affecting men more often than women. The pelvic bones are the most common site of involvement, though others include the scapula, ribs, humerus and femur. Other bones may sometimes be affected, but involvement of the small bones of the hand and foot is exceptional (Jakobson and Spjut 1960; Dahlin 1978). Local pain and/or swelling are the presenting symptoms and evolution is usually slow. Tumours of the pelvis may reach a large size before becoming clinically apparent. Radiological examination shows a lobulated mass projecting from a long or flat bone with mottled radio-

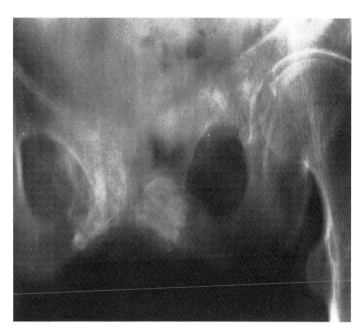

Fig. 11.8. Chondrosarcoma arising in the region of the symphysis pubis

densities caused by calcification or ossification within the substance of the lesion (Fig. 11.8). Central chondrosarcomas are more difficult to recognise. They produce a radiolucent area with a local fusiform swelling with or without cortical destruction. Speckled calcification may be helpful in suggesting the diagnosis. Tumours of the innominate bone, especially near the acetabulum, may be especially difficult to recognise.

Macroscopic examination shows a bluish-grey lobular cut surface. There may be cystic, necrotic or calcified foci. Central tumours may have a well-defined border but often cause destruction of the adjacent cortex. Tumours arising externally form sessile or pedunculated masses, which may reach large size in the pelvis. Chondrosarcomas of the rib most commonly affect the costochondral junction. Most pathologists will have no difficulty with the histological diagnosis of the highly malignant poorly differentiated chondrosarcoma. The cartilage cells have large pleomorphic nuclei (Fig. 11.9). There are multinucleate tumour cells and mitoses, some of which may be abnormal. The problem arises in deciding between a low-grade chondrosarcoma and a benign cartilage tumour. The presence of many cells with plump nuclei, more than the occasional binucleate cell and giant cells with large single or multiple nuclei are helpful features (Lichtenstein and Jaffe 1943). Observation of the general rules of examining bone tumours described at the beginning of this chapter—adequate clinical details, inspection of the radiograph and examination of multiple blocks from the tumour—are especially important in this difficult area of bone tumour pathology.

Certain histological patterns are recognisable amongst the malignant cartilage-forming tumours and it seems worthwhile to mention these here. More detailed accounts are available elsewhere.

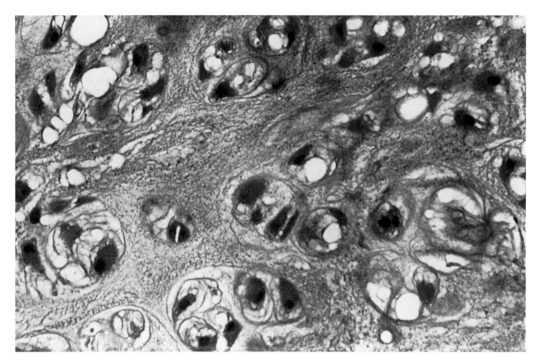

Fig. 11.9. Chondrosarcoma. Nuclear and cellular pleomorphism and occasional binucleate tumour cells. (H&E × 400)

Mesenchymal chondrosarcoma

This tumour was first described by Lichtenstein and Bernstein (1959). It is characterised by a biphasic histological pattern in which there are sheets and clusters of small undifferentiated round cells, also sometimes spindle-shaped, between islands of chondroid tumour, which itself varies in the extent to which it shows malignant features (Fig. 11.10). The age range of patients affected is a little lower than that for conventional chondrosarcoma, and males are more frequently affected than females. Radiological examination shows a lytic destructive lesion with mottled calcification, and the appearances do not differ significantly from those of conventional chondrosarcoma. Confusion with Ewing's sarcoma is possible if only a small biopsy is available and the chondroid element is not recognised. Further details and references are available in Dahlin (1978).

Dedifferentiated chondrosarcoma

The concept of dedifferentiation in chondrosarcoma has been introduced over recent years. A small number of chondrosarcomas show the presence of areas of spindle-celled fibrosarcomatous tissue. Some may show osteoid production by tumour cells, when the question of osteosarcoma arises. It is difficult to generalise on clinical features such as the site of such tumours, since relatively few cases have been described, but the age and localisation appear to be similar to those for conventional chondrosarcoma. Histological examination shows a transition between chondrosarcomatous and poorly differentiated

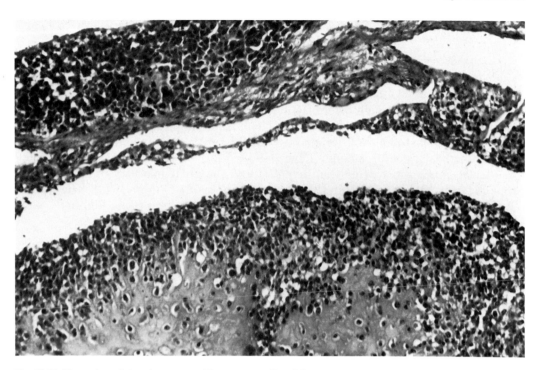

Fig. 11.10. Mesenchymal chondrosarcoma. Numerous small undifferentiated round cells and tumour showing chondroid differentiation (*bottom*) (H&E × 160)

fibrosarcomatous tissue. Dedifferentiated chondrosarcoma has a much poorer prognosis than ordinary chondrosarcoma. Further information on these tumours is available in publications by Dahlin and Beabout (1971), Mirra and Marcove (1974) and Dahlin (1978).

Clear cell chondrosarcoma

A small number of tumours, which have been designated clear cell chondrosarcoma, may be mistaken for chondroblastoma or osteoblastoma (Unni et al. 1976a; Dahlin 1978; Le Charpentier et al. 1979). Practically all the cases have involved the ends of long bones, most often the femoral head and neck. Both Unni et al. (1976a) and Le Charpentier et al. (1979) felt that clear cell chondrosarcoma was epiphyseal in location, in contrast to the metaphyseal site of ordinary chondrosarcoma of long bones. The tumour has a benign radiological appearance and is lytic, sometimes with focal calcification. There is a sclerotic margin and expansion of the bone. Macroscopically, the lesion is solid or cystic, but lacks a recognisable glistening cartilaginous appearance. Histologically, there are lobular areas of conventional chondrosarcoma, but a large amount of the tumour comprises sheets of cells with small nearly uniform nuclei and abundant clear cytoplasm. Foci of osteoid are present, though these are bordered by non-neoplastic osteoblasts. Multinucleate osteoclast-like cells are present throughout these tumours. Some show fine lace-like calcification between the tumour cells. The resemblance to chondroblastoma, osteoblastoma and even aneurysmal bone cyst may lead to confusion, but the recognition of clear cell areas and chondrosarcomatous areas excludes the last two diagnoses (Unni et al. 1976a).

Bone-forming tumours

Osteoid osteoma

Osteoid osteoma is a benign osteoblastic tumour which is clearly demarcated and surrounded by new bone formation. There is a marked histological similarity to osteoblastoma, and lesions less than 1 cm in diameter have come to be defined as 'osteoid osteoma' (Byers 1968; McLeod et al. 1976). Males are affected much more often than females, and the great majority of cases occur between the ages of 5 and 24 years (Byers 1968; Dahlin 1978). The diaphyses or metaphyses of the long bones in the lower limb (tibia, femur) are common localisations (Fig. 11.11). Osteoid osteoma generally causes progressively more severe pain, and relief from this is obtained by the use of salicylates. Development of a limp and muscle atrophy in the affected limb are common. A friable red-grey discrete 'nidus' of tumour surrounded by sclerotic new bone is seen on macroscopic examination and this gives the radiologically classic appearance of a central radiolucent or dense area with a dense periphery. Location of the nidus of an osteoid osteoma in a pathological specimen may be difficult, especially where the surgeon has removed the affected area of bone piecemeal rather than as a single block of bone. Radiological examination of the specimen may help in detecting the nidus. Histologically, the nidus is composed of cellular, highly vascular tissue containing islands of osteoid trabeculae which are totally random in arrangement. These trabeculae undergo calcification to a variable degree, and the osteoblasts lining the trabecular surfaces are always uniform and benign in appearance (Fig. 11.12). Variable numbers of benign giant cells are present. There is no cartilage formation. Well-organised newly formed trabeculae make up the surrounding sclerotic bone (Spjut et al. 1971; Schajowicz et al. 1972; Dahlin 1978).

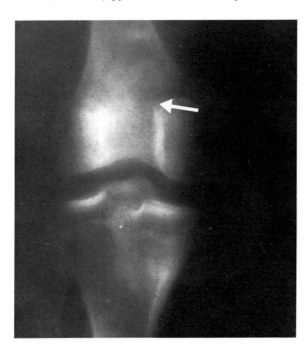

Fig. 11.11. Osteoid osteoma. Localised sclerotic area in the upper metaphysis of the tibia (*arrow*)

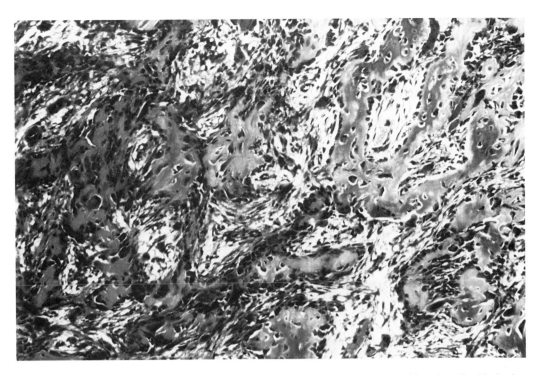

Fig. 11.12. Nidus of an osteoid osteoma, showing randomly arranged osteoid trabeculae with surfaces lined by benign osteoblasts. (H&E × 160)

Osteoblastoma

Osteoblastoma is related to osteoid osteoma and there are no specific histological criteria for their separation. Indeed, occasional lesions could quite reasonably be placed in one or the other category. The question of size enters into the definition of an osteoblastoma, and McLeod et al. (1976) considered lesions more than 1.5 cm in diameter to fall into this category. The chief differences from osteoid osteoma are the clinical presentation, site, radiological appearances and changes in the surrounding bone. Surrounding reactive new bone is not often present in relation to osteoblastomas. Teenagers and young adults are usually affected (age range usually 10–35 years), and, like osteoid osteoma, osteoblastoma is more common in males. There is a marked tendency for the tumour to occur in the vertebrae, and other sites include the ilium, ribs, hand and foot bones and long bones (Jaffe 1958; Spjut et al. 1971; Lichtenstein 1972; Dahlin 1978). Three-quarters of the lesions of long bones were diaphyseal in the series of McLeod et al. (1976). Although pain may be present, it is not such a marked feature as in osteoid osteoma. The radiological appearances are non-specific, the lesion being sometimes radiolucent, sometimes more dense, with a variable degree of demarcation and sclerosis at the margin. They may be mistaken for those of osteosarcoma, chondrosarcoma, aneurysmal bone cyst or osteoid osteoma (Pochachevsky et al. 1960). Macroscopically, the tumour has a vascular and haemorrhagic dark purple, red-grey or brown gritty cut surface. Areas may show more developed trabecular bone. A dense sclerotic reactive margin is not usually seen in the adjacent bone, though there may be a thin shell of new bone around the tumour. Histological examination shows a cellular connective tissue stroma containing osteoid and primitive bone trabeculae formed by benign osteoblasts. Areas of the intertrabecular tissue often contain numerous thin-walled capillary type vessels. There are strong similarities to osteoid osteoma. More cellular osteoblastic areas with mitoses may be seen and numerous giant cells are sometimes present. Occasionally the problem arises as to whether the osteoblasts are malignant; differentiation from an osteosarcoma may then be difficult.

The concept of 'malignant or aggressive osteoblastoma' (Schajowicz and Lemos 1976; Revell and Scholtz 1979) has been introduced in recent years to describe tumours which are locally aggressive and tend to recur locally. These lesions present characteristics of osteoblastoma but with areas having more cellular and aggressive features suggestive of a low-grade osteosarcoma. The author prefers the term 'aggressive osteoblastoma' to indicate that these lesions are likely to behave less well than most osteoblastomas. The question arises as to whether osteoblastoma may undergo malignant transformation (Dorfman 1973) to give the picture seen as 'malignant or aggressive osteoblastoma', or whether these lesions should be regarded as a low-grade osteosarcoma from the outset.

Osteosarcoma (general considerations)

An osteosarcoma is a malignant tumour showing evidence of osteoid or bone formation by the malignant tumour cells. Osteosarcomas are divisible into several different histological types mainly for descriptive purposes. Thus, for example, they may be described as osteoblastic, chondroblastic or fibroblastic, depending on whether osteoid, chondroid or fibromatoid elements predominate. Precise definition of a particular tumour may be impossible on occasions, especially since there are no stains specific for osteoid, which may itself be indistinguishable from collagen and cartilage matrix and difficult to find with certainty in a predominantly cartilaginous or fibrous tumour. Brief descriptions are given below of special types of osteosarcoma such as telangiectatic (see p. 280), periosteal (see p. 282), parosteal (see p. 282), osteosarcoma in Paget's disease of bone (see p. 285) and post-radiation tumours (see p. 286).

Most cases of osteosarcoma occur between the ages of 10 and 20 years, and boys are affected more often than girls. Osteosarcoma may occur in any bone, but the metaphyseal ends of long bones (lower femur, upper tibia, upper femur, upper humerus) are the most frequently involved. The sites of involvement in five series are summarised by Revell (1981), and one large series is that of Dahlin and Unni (1977). Pain and local swelling, which are both non-specific yet important symptoms, are the most common modes of presentation. A long history is uncommon.

The radiological appearances are variable, but usually include evidence of bone destruction (Fig. 11.13; see also Fig. 9.8, p. 213), new bone formation in relation to cortical destruction and subperiosteal new bone formation. The degree to which radiodensity is seen within the tumour mass will naturally depend upon the amount of ossifying or calcifying osteoid present. The radiological appearances are often thought to be specific, but a large minority of cases have none of the characteristic features such as 'Codman's triangle', about which all medical students learn. Skeletal surveys, computerised

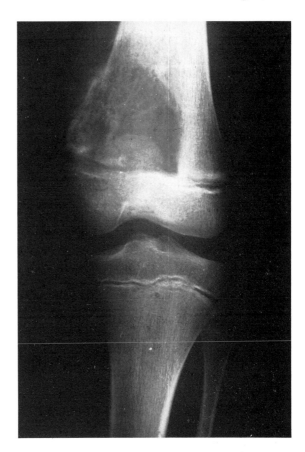

Fig. 11.13. Osteosarcoma, lower metaphysis of the femur in a 9-year-old showing osteolytic destructive lesion extending outside the bone. There is a pathological fracture through the tumour. Histological examination revealed a telangiectatic osteosarcoma (see Fig. 11.20)

tomography and radioisotope scanning may all be valuable in assessing a case clinically for extent of disease. Multifocal osteosarcoma has been described and discussed (Lowbeer 1968; Amstutz 1969; Dahlin 1978).

The typical osteosarcoma arises centrally in the metaphysis and has usually penetrated the cortex and invaded soft tissue by the time of presentation. The macroscopic appearances vary according to the amount of cartilaginous, fibrous or bony tissue in the tumour. There are often softer areas towards the periphery which can be processed rapidly. Areas of cyst formation, haemorrhage and necrosis may be present, and some tumours may have a dark-red cystic and sponge-like appearance. In assessing a surgical specimen for completeness of surgical excision it is important to be aware that tumour may extend much further within the medullary region than is apparent on the clinical radiograph, and that separate 'skip' metastasis may be present in the bone adjacent to the main mass (Lewis and Lotz 1974; Enneking and Kagan 1975a,b). Haematogenous metastasis to the lungs and other bones is the usual form of spread.

The histological appearances are extremely variable and depend on the amount of tumour bone produced, the pleomorphism of the tumour cells and the extent to which myxoid, chondroid or fibrous elements are present (Spjut et al. 1971; Schajowicz et al. 1972; Dahlin 1978). Classically, a malignant proliferation of spindle-shaped and oval cells with variable numbers of mitoses and some multinucleate cells shows evidence of direct formation of osteoid or bone (Figs. 11.14, 11.15). Islands of osseous tissue are seen with pleomorphic malignant osteoblasts present along their surfaces. Recognition of small areas of tumour osteoid in a highly cellular osteosarcoma is sometimes aided by Van Gieson, MSB or similar stain for the demonstration of collagen (Fig. 11.16). Problems may still remain in the differentiation of fibrous tissue stroma and osteoid, but formation of a trabecular structure is helpful. Broadly speaking, the predominant differentiation of the tumour may be to bone (the commonest), cartilage or fibrous tissue. Some tumours may contain vascular areas with numerous thin-walled vessels, others may have a telangiectatic appearance throughout (see p. 280).

Histochemical studies have demonstrated the presence of alkaline phosphatase in tumour cells (Jeffree and Price 1965), and, if available, this method may help in identification of osteosarcoma in smears or frozen sections (Fig. 11.17; Sanerkin 1980; Sanerkin and Jeffree 1980). Liposarcoma (Pardo-Mirdan et al. 1981) and angiosarcoma may contain alkaline phosphatase in the tumour cells, but these two sarcomas are excessively rare in bone and should not present a problem of differentiation from osteosarcoma. Electron microscopic studies of osteosarcoma have been performed by a number of authors, including Kay (1971), Paschall and Paschall (1975), Williams et al. (1976) and Reddick et al. (1980). The electron microscopy of bone tumours has been reviewed by Roessner and Grundman (1982).

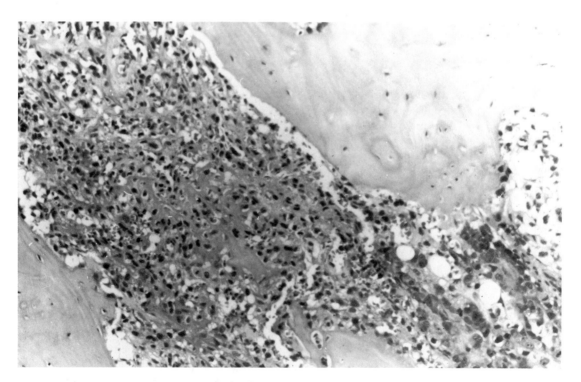

Fig. 11.14. Osteosarcoma invading bone, showing replacement of the intertrabecular tissue by spindle-shaped and oval tumour cells which are forming tumour osteoid. (H&E × 160)

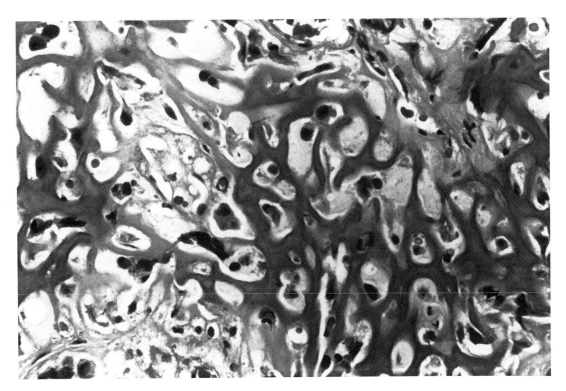

Fig. 11.15. Osteosarcoma. Formation of osteoid by pleomorphic osteoblastic tumour cells. (H&E × 600)

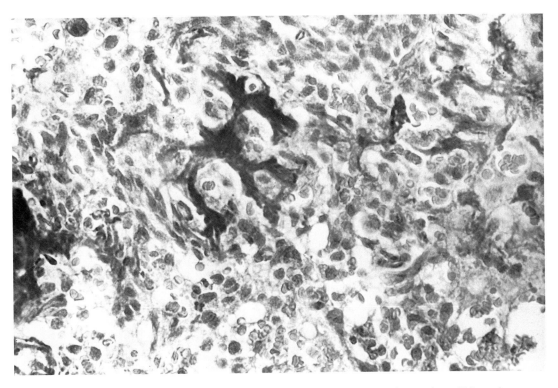

Fig. 11.16. Cellular osteosarcoma stained to demonstrate collagen to aid the detection of areas of osteoid formation. (van Gieson × 400)

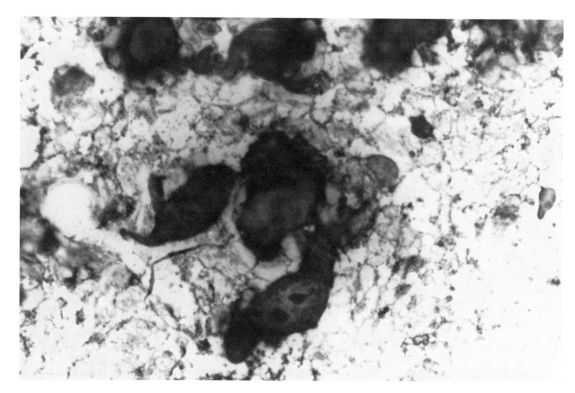

Fig. 11.17. Imprint preparation from an osteosarcoma stained for alkaline phosphatase, showing reaction product in individual tumour cells. (Gormori alkaline phosphatase × 1000)

Telangiectatic osteosarcoma

This tumour does not differ significantly in clinical presentation from conventional osteosarcoma. Radiological examination shows a destructive lesion which may appear lytic throughout. Macroscopically, there are cystic spaces filled with clotted blood and necrotic debris and there may be more spongy areas (Fig. 11.18). Histological examination shows cystic spaces lined by anaplastic spindle cells and variable numbers of giant cells (Matsuno et al. 1976). Confusion with aneurysmal bone cyst may occur on low-power examination (Fig. 11.19), and there may be little evidence of tumour osteoid production by the cells in the walls of the blood-filled cysts (Fig. 11.20).

Osteosarcoma on the outside of the bone

A small percentage of osteosarcomas arise not in the more usual central part of the affected bone but on the outside of the bone. These lesions have been separated into periosteal and parosteal (or juxtacortical) osteosarcomas, and it is important to distinguish clearly between these two types and conventional osteosarcoma occurring on the outside of the bone (Wold et al. 1984).

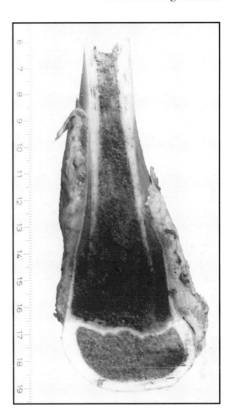

Fig. 11.18. Sagittal section of a telangiectatic osteocarcoma in the lower metaphysis of the femur. There is a spongy destructive lesion containing many blood-filled spaces and this extends beyond the outline of the original bone. Periosteal new bone formation is best seen anteriorly (*left*). (Same case as Fig. 11.15)

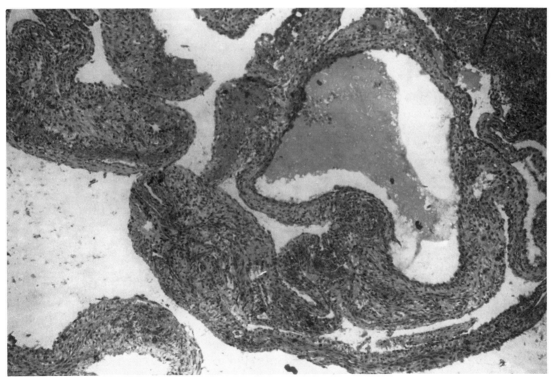

Fig. 11.19. Low-power view of telangiectatic osteosarcoma. There are numerous cystic spaces lined by spindle-celled tissue containing occasional giant cells. (H&E × 50)

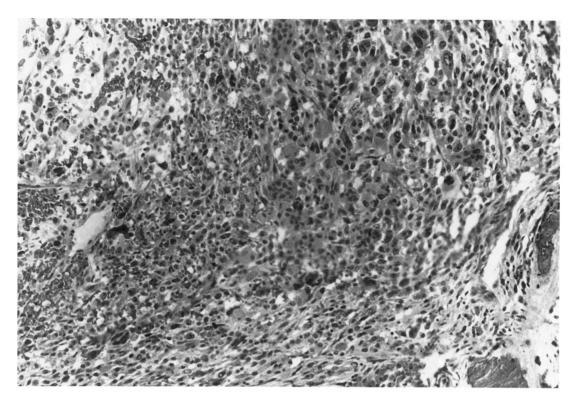

Fig. 11.20. Higher power view of telangiectatic osteosarcoma shown in Fig. 11.21. This is a highly cellular tumour showing cellular pleomorphism and occasional mitoses. Same case as that shown in Figs. 11.15 and 11.18. (The patient died 1 year after amputation with pulmonary metastases). (Methylmethacrylate, H&E × 160)

Periosteal osteosarcoma

Periosteal osteosarcoma is a rare type of bone tumour, also sometimes referred to as 'cortical osteosarcoma'. The tibia and femur are the sites most commonly affected. The tumours are large fusiform or cauliflower-like projections towards the mid-shaft of the bone in radiographs (Figs. 11.21, 11.22, 11.23) and show a predominance of chondroid differentiation so that chondrosarcoma is strongly suggested on histological examination (Fig. 11.24). However, the eosinophilic matrix towards the centre of the chondroid lobules resembles osteoid, and there are typical spicules of new bone present near the underlying cortex. For further details see Unni et al. (1976c).

Parosteal osteosarcoma

Parosteal (or juxtacortical) osteosarcoma is the other type of malignant bone-forming tumour found on the outside of the bone. It should be separated from periosteal because its behaviour is less malignant. This is borne out by the first description of the tumour as a separate entity by Geschickter and Copeland (1951), who designated it as 'parosteal osteoma' and thought it a benign lesion which underwent malignant change (Copeland and Geschickter 1959). It is a rare lesion affecting females more often than males and occurring in older patients than those with conventional osteosarcoma, in the second to fourth decades of life (Van der Heul and Von Ronnen 1967; Unni et al. 1976b).

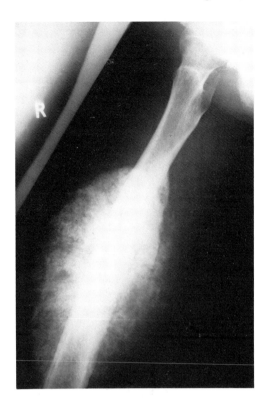

Fig. 11.21. Periosteal osteosarcoma. Large fusiform tumour arising in the midshaft of the femur of a teenager

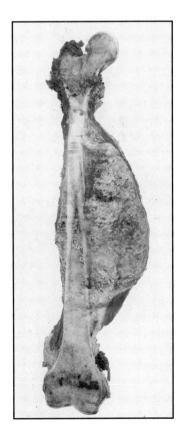

Fig. 11.22. Periosteal osteosarcoma, same case as Fig. 11.23. Specimen obtained at disarticulation through the hip joint, showing large fusiform tumour mainly on the medial aspect (*right*) but extending around the bone to the lateral side (*left*). A small amount of tumour is present in the medullary cavity in this advanced lesion

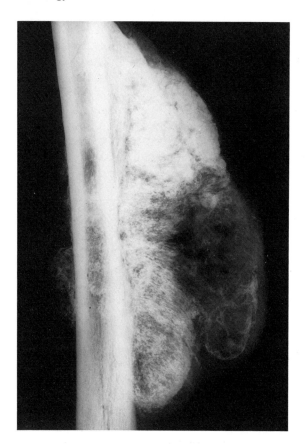

◁ **Fig. 11.23.** Radiograph of a slice of the specimen shown in Fig. 11.22

Fig. 11.24. Periosteal osteosarcoma. Malignant tumour showing predominantly chondrosarcoma-like appearance but with formation of osteoid. (H&E × 160)
▽

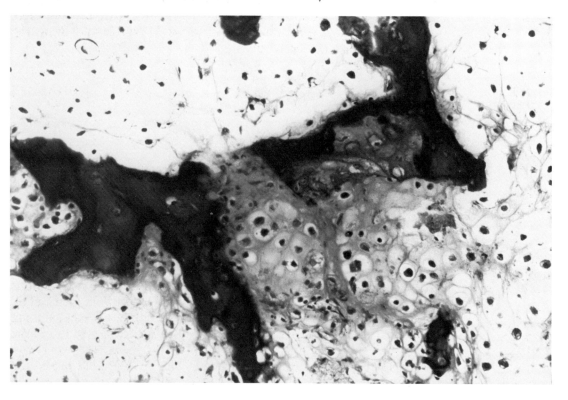

Swelling, often of some duration, is the most common presenting symptom and physical sign. This may or may not be painful. Some patients have pain alone. Sometimes there may be a history of a previous excision of a lesion regarded as an atypical osteochondroma. Dahlin (1978) regards this latter presentation as almost pathognomonic.

Radiological examination shows a dense lobulated mass arising on the outer aspect of the metaphyseal region of a long bone. Large tumours have a tendency to encircle the bone without becoming attached to it except at the site of origin (Stevens et al. 1957; Unni et al. 1976b). Ill-defined radiolucent areas in the tumour mass correspond to fibrous and cartilaginous elements. Medullary involvement does not usually occur. Differentiation from heterotopic ossification (myositis ossificans) is important and careful examination of different views and tomograms should reveal the difference between a lesion arising separately from the bone yet abutting it and one attached to the bone on a broad base. Macroscopically, parosteal osteosarcomas are predominantly hard osseous tumours, though there are soft fibrous and chondroid foci, especially towards the periphery. The above comments with respect to radiological differentiation from myositis ossificans apply equally well to the naked eye appearances. Histological examination shows a low-grade, bone-forming sarcoma with well-formed irregularly shaped bone trabeculae covered with a layer of osteoblasts or spindle cells. The more immature trabeculae show evidence of 'normalisation' (i.e. becoming more mature; Dahlin 1978). There may be chondrosarcomatous areas present and even a cartilage cap, suggesting osteochondroma as a differential diagnosis (Unni et al. 1976b). The tissue between the trabeculae of tumour bone comprises atypical spindle-shaped cells with variable members of mitoses in parosteal osteosarcoma, whereas in osteochondroma fat and bone marrow are present in the intertrabecular spaces. Confusion with myositis ossificans may arise because there may be intermingling of bone-forming tumour with muscle and fat at the periphery of a parosteal osteosarcoma.

Osteosarcoma in abnormal bone

Although osteosarcoma is usually a tumour of the younger age groups, it may also occur in older people. When it does so, associations with Paget's disease or previous radiotherapy are likely features.

Osteosarcoma in Paget's disease of bone

The development of osteosarcoma in bone affected with Paget's disease, sometimes called 'Paget's sarcoma', has been known for many years. About 1% of all patients with Paget's disease suffer the development of sarcomatous change (Porretta et al. 1957; McKenna et al. 1964; Dahlin 1978; Wick et al. 1981). Osteosarcomas predominate, though fibrosarcoma, chondrosarcoma and even giant cell tumour (Jacobs et al. 1979) also occur. In a Mayo Clinic series, 3% of all osteosarcomas were associated with Paget's disease (Wick et al. 1981). The age of presentation is over 60 years in most cases, and the site of involvement is different from osteosarcoma occurring in young people.

The distribution reflects the pattern of involvement by Paget's disease so that the pelvis, femur, humerus and skull are common sites. All the cases described by Wick and his colleagues had radiological evidence of polyostotic Paget's disease.

The histological pattern is not different from that of ordinary osteosarcoma. Occasional cases have fibrosarcomatous or malignant fibrous histiocytoma-like appearances. No parosteal or periosteal osteosarcomas were seen by Wick et al. (1981). Occasional cases of 'multicentric' Paget's sarcoma have been reported (Wick et al. 1981), but it is not possible to be sure whether these are the result of several tumours arising *de novo* or metastases to other bones from a single primary tumour (Dorfman 1973). An excellent source of further references to osteosarcoma in Paget's disease is the paper by Wick et al. (1981).

Post-radiation osteosarcoma

The development of sarcomas in bone that has been previously subjected to ionising radiation is well recognised (Sabanas et al. 1956; Steiner 1964; Sim et al. 1972). Absolute proof of a causal relationship is difficult to obtain, but if certain criteria are met then a diagnosis of post-radiation sarcoma can be made. The criteria suggested by Spjut et al. (1971) are:

1. There must be microscopic evidence of a benign primary lesion or radiological evidence of normal bone in the site of the subsequent sarcoma at the time of radiation.
2. There must have been radiation to the field in which the sarcoma later develops.
3. A relatively long symptom-free period (measured in years) after radiation must be established.
4. There must be microscopic evidence of a sarcoma.

Most tumours have been osteosarcomas or fibrosarcomas. The site of involvement obviously depends on the site of previous radiation therapy. Sarcomas of the pelvis following radiotherapy of uterine cervical carcinoma and of the ribs and humerus following treatment of breast carcinoma are good examples (Spjut et al. 1971; Dahlin 1978). Further information with respect to sites and reasons for previous radiotherapy are available in these two references.

Giant cell tumour

Giant cell tumour is a characteristic neoplasm occurring mostly in the age range 20–55 years with a predominance of cases in women in most series (Schajowicz 1961; Hutter et al. 1962; Goldenberg et al. 1970; Dahlin 1978). The presence of giant cells, often in considerable numbers in other bone tumours and lesions, leads to confusion in the literature and may also do so for the working pathologist. Non-osteogenic fibroma, chondroblastoma, chondromyxoid fibroma, giant cell reparative granuloma, aneurysmal bone cyst, hyperparathyroidism and even mesenchymal chondrosarcoma and osteosarcoma are among the lesions which may be mistaken for giant cell tumour (see Table 11.5).

Most giant cell tumours are localised in the epiphyseal region of long bones, frequently around the knee. A lesion *arising* in the metaphysis is almost certainly not a giant cell tumour. Almost any bone may be affected, and in Dahlin's series a significant number were present in the sacrum (Dahlin 1978). Care is needed in making the diagnosis at certain sites. For example, a giant cell lesion in the jaws is most probably reparative granuloma (Jaffe 1953), while a similar lesion in the small bones of the hand or foot is more likely to be due to hyperparathyroidism or bone involvement with localised nodular tenosynovitis (Murphy and Ackerman 1956). Clinical presentation of giant cell tumour is with pain and swelling, and physical examination shows a mass which may give crepitation on palpation. There are no specific radiological features, though epiphyseal location of a lytic lesion lacking a sclerotic margin is suggestive (Fig. 11.25). Eccentric position of the tumour was noted by Gee and Pugh (1958), but again is not specific (see Spjut et al. 1971; Dahlin 1978). Naked-eye examination shows a heterogeneous appearance with solid yellowish fibrous and osseous areas, grey-red vascular tissue, cysts and necrotic areas which sometimes contain blood. The bone is expanded and the overlying cortex thinned. There may be a pathological fracture. Light microscopy shows numerous plump oval or spindle-shaped cells interspersed with giant cells having up to 100 nuclei (Fig. 11.26). There may be moderate vascularity, haemorrhage, necrosis and foam cells present, and osteoid is not uncommon. The presence of secondary reparative changes, for example in response to pathological fracture, may complicate the histological picture. The presence of cartilage is extremely unusual and suggests the possibility of chondroblastoma

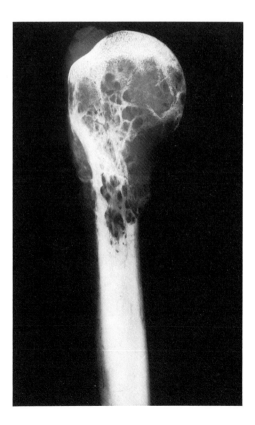

Fig. 11.25. Giant cell tumour. Upper humerus showing destructive lesion in the epiphysis and extending into the metaphysis. Radiograph of a slice from a pathological specimen obtained at the time of prosthetic replacement

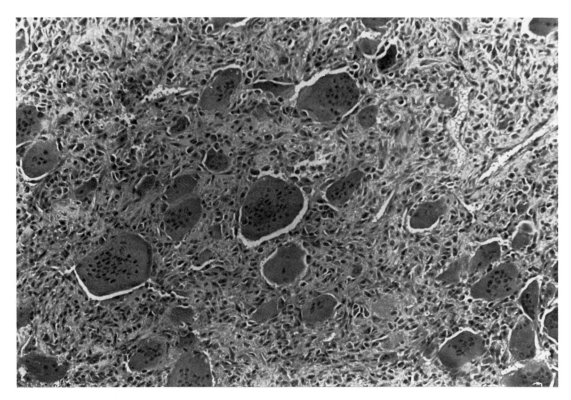

Fig. 11.26. Giant cell tumour of bone. Spindle-shaped cells with giant cells containing numerous nuclei. (H&E × 200)

or even osteosarcoma, depending on the arrangement and differentiation of the chondroid element. Systems of grading of giant cell tumour have been evolved by Jaffe et al. (1940) and Hutter et al. (1962). Unfortunately, some tumours with an apparently benign histological appearance may unexpectedly assume a malignant course, so that grading is regarded as of limited or no value (Spjut et al. 1971; Dahlin 1978). The presence of giant cell tumour in vessels at the margin of the lesion (Fig. 11.27) is not an indicator of potentially metastatic behaviour and is seen fairly frequently in tumours which subsequently have a benign course. The cases categorised by Dahlin (1978) as malignant giant cell tumour contained frankly sarcomatous tissue and presented no diagnostic problem.

Malignant fibrous tumours

Malignant fibrous lesions of bone have become a confusing area of tumour pathology over recent years. Fibrosarcoma, regarded as a relatively rare primary bone tumour, occurs predominantly in the long bones, particularly around the knee, though many other sites have been reported. The clinical and radiological appearances are non-specific and difficult to distinguish from osteosarcoma. Macroscopically, fibrosarcomas have a fairly homogeneous whitish-yellow surface in which there may, however, be areas of cystic change,

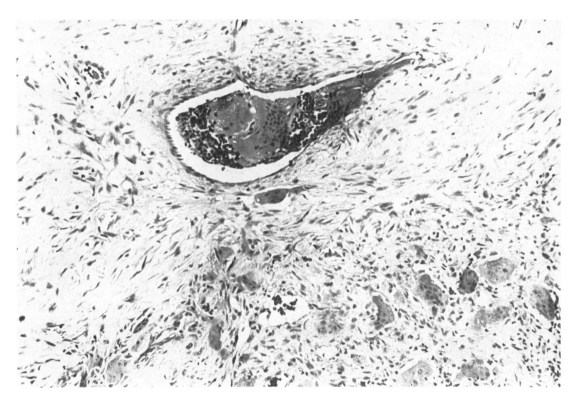

Fig. 11.27. Tumour in the lumen of a vessel at the edge of a giant cell tumour of bone. (H&E × 160)

necrosis and haemorrhage. Characteristically they have discretely delineated margins, destroy the cortex but are confined within the periosteum (Spjut et al. 1971). The histological appearances are the same as those of fibrosarcoma of soft tissue origin. Spjut et al. (1971) were in favour of the concept of primary fibrosarcoma of bone and cited other authors of the same opinion. Unfortunately, the existence of the tumour has been called into question (Geschickter 1932) on the basis that such lesions are either tumours of related soft tissues or are examples of fibroblastic osteosarcoma. More recently the concept of malignant fibrous histiocytoma of bone has been introduced (Spanier et al. 1975), and many malignant fibrous lesions of bone are now being placed in this category. Malignant fibrous histiocytomas are fibrogenic tumours containing spindle cells and arranged in a 'storiform' pattern (Fig. 11.28). Some of the cells have appearances similar to those of histiocytes with indented nuclei and abundant cytoplasm. Multinucleate malignant giant cells are an important feature. Too few cases have been accurately documented to give detailed overall clinical features, but malignant fibrous histiocytoma seems to occur at almost any age in the adult, with many different bones being affected. The radiological features are non-specific but indicate a malignant tumour. According to Dahlin (1978), osteosarcomas, dedifferentiated chondrosarcomas and fibrosarcomas may all have areas with a malignant fibrous histiocytoma pattern.

There is a trend at present to avoid the diagnosis of fibrosarcoma and to favour that of malignant fibrous histiocytoma. It seems unnecessary, and also illogical, to drop the designation fibrosarcoma completely. If, for example,

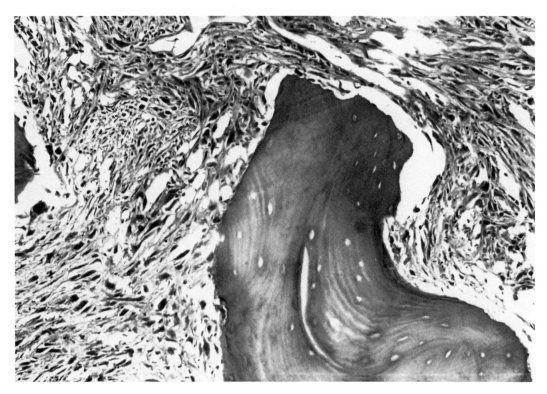

Fig. 11.28. High-power view of part of a malignant fibrous hystiocytoma of bone, showing pleomorphic spindle-celled tumour with occasional giant cells and necrotic original bone trabecula which shows evidence of being resorbed (*top*). (H&E × 160)

it is possible to have fibrosarcomatous (and for that matter malignant fibrous histiocytoma-like) areas in osteosarcomas, then why should there not exist pure fibrosarcomas of bone? What is essential is that the full range of possibilities should be considered in each case of a malignant fibrous tumour in bone. This differential diagnosis should include not only fibrosarcoma and malignant fibrous histiocytoma but also osteosarcoma, malignant giant cell tumour, malignant lymphoma, plasma cell tumours with a marked spindle cell element, leiomyosarcoma (Sanerkin 1979) and secondary carcinoma, especially those types like renal carcinoma which may show spindle cell differentiation.

Round cell tumours

Tumours of bone which are made up of small round cells present a particular problem of differential diagnosis. Nevertheless, it is important to attempt a differentiation since the treatment and prognosis of the various small round cell tumours vary considerably.

The main tumours concerned are Ewing's sarcoma, malignant lymphoma of bone, metastatic neuroblastoma and metastatic carcinoma, especially oat cell carcinoma. Small cell variants of osteosarcoma and even primary liposarcoma of bone also need to be considered on occasions. Obviously the age of the patient and site of the lesion give some help in narrowing down the list of possibilities in any individual case.

In children, careful attention to clinical details, especially the possibility of an adrenal mass, is required in the differentiation of Ewing's sarcoma and neuroblastoma. The determination of levels of catecholamine metabolites provides a useful discriminant (Gitlow et al. 1970), and this is worth recommending to clinicians. An analysis of the distinguishing features of Ewing's sarcoma and reticulum cell sarcoma (malignant lymphoma), including observer variation in detecting these features, has been performed by five separate bone pathologists (Ball et al. 1970). This article gives interesting insights into the confidence with which histological features may be recognised and to the accuracy and consistency of individual pathologists. It is proposed here to discuss only Ewing's sarcoma and malignant lymphoma and to provide further references which may be helpful in coming to grips with the overall problem. Ewing's sarcoma is one of the tumours sometimes mistakenly diagnosed when there is osteomyelitis (Lindenbaum and Alexander 1984).

Ewing's sarcoma

Ewing's sarcoma is an uncommon primary malignant tumour which may arise in almost any bone, although usual sites are the mid-shaft or the metaphysis of the femur, humerus or tibia, the ilium and ribs. Two-thirds of cases present before the age of 20 years (Dahlin et al. 1961; Spjut et al. 1971), and there is a male predominance among those afflicted. The radiological appearances are often non-specific, though a lytic lesion with surrounding multiple layers of subperiosteal reactive new bone giving an 'onion-skin' appearance is helpful. Equally likely, the lesion may be difficult to distinguish radiologically from osteosarcoma, eosinophilic granuloma, malignant lymphoma, metastatic malignant tumour or osteomyelitis.

Macroscopically, the centrally placed tumour is soft and grey-white, sometimes with haemorrhagic areas present. Light microscopy shows a neoplasm made up of small round cells in sheets, cords or nests, characteristically separated by fibrous septa (Fig. 11.29). A rosette pattern may be seen, caused by the collection of cells around small vascular spaces. The differentiation from other small round cell tumours of bone may be extremely difficult. The presence of glycogen granules in the cells of Ewing's sarcoma has been demonstrated by Schajowicz (1959) at the light microscopic level and confirmed ultrastructurally by Friedman and Gold (1968). Ball et al. (1977) provided an analysis of the light microscopic features often considered as helpful in the differentiation of Ewing's sarcoma and reticulum cell sarcoma (malignant lymphoma; Fig. 11.30). Pale nuclei, slight nuclear pleomorphism, lack of reticulin around individual tumour cells and the presence of intracellular glycogen showed an overall tendency to cluster, as did the opposites of these features (viz. dark nuclei, marked nuclear pleomorphism, reticulin around individual cells and lack of glycogen). Cases in the former group (Ewing's sarcoma) had a mean age of 16 years, while for those in the latter ('reticulum cell sarcoma') it was 48 years.

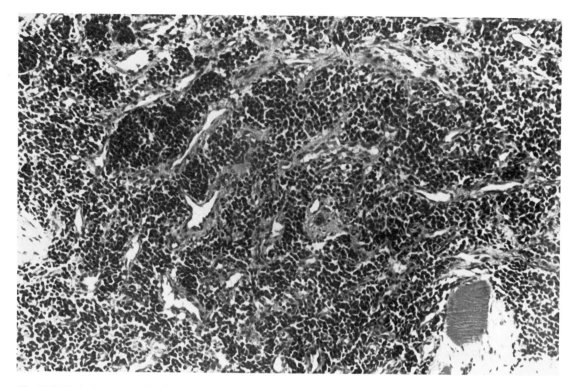

Fig. 11.29. Ewing's sarcoma. Small round cells separated in areas by fibrous septa and small vessels. (H&E × 160)

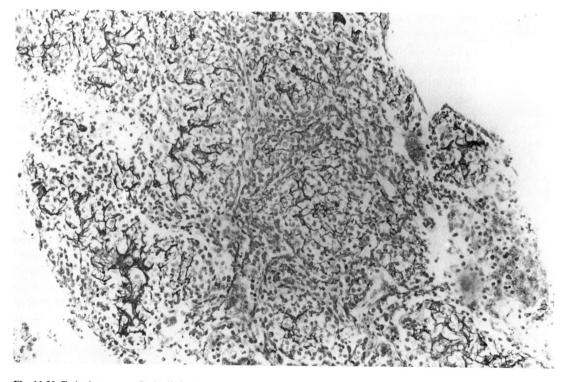

Fig. 11.30. Ewing's sarcoma. Reticulin is present mainly around small groups of cells rather than individual cells. (Reticulin × 160)

The ultrastructural features of Ewing's sarcoma are described by Llombart-Bosch et al. (1978), who discuss the differentiation from 'reticulum cell sarcoma' and other round cell sarcomas. They consider that the demonstration of glycogen in tumour cells is of limited value and quote references for its demonstration in the mononuclear cells present in giant cell tumours, chondrosarcoma and some forms of leukaemia and lymphoma. However, most childhood lymphomas are of a high-grade malignancy, for example, lymphoblastic Burkitt-type (B cell) or convoluted-cell (T cell) type. Cells of Burkitt-type lymphoblastic lymphoma are not PAS positive and those of convoluted-cell lymphoblastic lymphoma show the presence of diastase-resistant PAS-positive reaction in a single clumped pattern in the cytoplasm (Lennert 1978), so that the demonstration of glycogen in small round cells is still of value in the diagnosis of Ewing's sarcoma. A recent review of the ultrastructural features is that of Roessner and Grundmann (1982). A combined electron microscopic, immunohistochemical and cytochemical study by Navas-Palacios et al. (1983) also discusses the histogenesis of Ewing's tumour.

Primary malignant lymphoma

The classification of malignant lymphomas has been a subject of debate and some confusion over recent years. Lymphoid neoplasms of bone have in the past been called 'reticulum cell sarcoma' of bone, and this old term is now usually considered synonymous with the poorly differentiated types of lymphoma. It is difficult to relate the modern classifications of lymphomas to the older descriptions of primary lymphoreticular bone tumours. Histochemical and immunological methods of investigation must be applied to these in an attempt to see whether there are categories which coincide with those found in the lymphoid tissues in general.

Malignant lymphoma of bone (reticulum cell sarcoma) presents as a focally destructive lesion on radiological examination and macroscopically is a homogeneous grey or reddish-grey colour with necrotic areas. The histological appearances are varied, probably reflecting the fact that several different entities are being considered in the same category at present. Some tumours have pleomorphic round tumour cells with an admixture of lymphocytes, while in others the appearances are suggestive of histiocytic differentiation. The differentiation of Ewing's sarcoma from so-called reticulum cell sarcoma has already been discussed (see above).

References

Allan CJ, Soule EM (1971) Osteogenic sarcomata of the somatic soft tissues: clinico-pathologic study of 26 cases and review of the literature. Cancer 27:1121–1133

Amstutz HC (1969) Multiple osteogenic sarcomata—metastic or multicentric? Report of two cases and review of literature. Cancer 24:923–931

Ball J, Friedman L, Sissons HA (1977) Malignant round cell tumours of bone; an analytical histological study from the Cancer Research Campaign's Bone Tumour Panel. Br J Cancer 36:254–268

Byers PD (1968) Solitary benign osteoblastic lesions of bone: osteoid osteoma and benign osteoblastoma. Cancer 22:43–57

Cole ARC, Darte JMM (1963) Osteochondromata following irradiation in children. Pediatrics 32:285–288

Copeland MM, Geschickter CF (1959) The treatment of parosteal osteoma of bone. Gynecol Obstet 108:537–548

Dahlin DC (1978) Bone tumors. General aspects and data on 6221 cases, 3rd edn. Thomas, Springfield, Ill

Dahlin DC, Beabout JW (1971) Dedifferentiation of low-grade chondrosarcoma. Cancer 28:461–466

Dahlin DC, Unni KK (1977) Osteosarcoma of bone and its important recognizable varieties. Am J Surg Pathol 1:61–72

Dahlin DC, Coventry MB, Scanlon PW (1961) Ewing's sarcoma. A critical analysis of 165 cases. J Bone Joint Surg [Am] 43:185–192

Dahlin DC, Unni KK, Matsuno T (1977) Malignant (fibrous) histiocytoma of bone—fact or fancy? Cancer 39:1508–1516

Dorfman HD (1973) Malignant transformation of benign bone lesions. Proc Natl Cancer Conf 7:901–913

Eidekin J, Hodes PJ (1973) Roentgen diagnosis of diseases of bone, 2nd edn, vols 1 and 2. Williams and Wilkins, Baltimore

Enneking WF, Kagan A (1975a) 'Skip' metastases in osteosarcoma. Cancer 36:2192–2205

Enneking WF, Kagan A (1975b) The implications of 'skip' metastases in osteosarcoma. Clin Orthop 111:33–41

Friedman B, Gold H (1968) Ultrastructure of Ewing's sarcoma of bone. Cancer 22:307–322

Gee VR, Pugh DG (1958) Giant cell tumour of bone. Radiology 70:33–45

Geschickter CF (1932) So-called fibrosarcoma of bone. Bone involvement by sarcoma of the neighbouring soft parts. Arch Surg 24:231–291

Geschickter CF, Copeland MM (1951) Parosteal osteoma of bone: a new entity. Ann Surg 133:790–807

Gitlow SE, Bertani LM, Ransen A, Gribetz O, Dziedzig SW (1970) Diagnosis of neuroblastoma by qualitative and quantitative determination of catecholamine metabolites in urine. Cancer 25:1377–1383

Goldenberg RR, Campbell CJ, Bonfiglio M (1970) Giant-cell tumour of bone. An analysis of two hundred and eighteen cases. J Bone Joint Surg [Am] 52:619–664

Hutter RVP, Worcester JN, Francis KC, Forte FW, Stewart FW (1962) Benign and malignant giant cell tumours of bone. A clinicopathological analysis of the natural history of the disease. Cancer 15:653–690

Huvos AG (1979) Bone tumors. Diagnosis, treatment and prognosis. Saunders, Philadelphia

Jacobs TP, Michelsen J, Polay JS, D'Adamo AC, Canfield RE (1979) Giant cell tumour in Paget's disease of bone. Familial and geographic clustering. Cancer 44:742–747

Jaffe HL (1953) Giant cell reparative granuloma, traumatic bone cyst and fibrous (fibro-osseous) dysplasia of the jawbones. Oral Surg 6:159–175

Jaffe HL (1958) Tumors and tumorous conditions of the bones and joints. Lea and Febiger, Philadelphia

Jaffe HL, Lichtenstein L (1948) Distinctive benign tumour likely to be mistaken especially for chondrosarcoma. Arch Pathol 45:541–551

Jaffe HL, Lichtenstein L, Portis RB (1940) Giant cell tumor of bone. Its pathologic appearance, grading, supposed variants and treatment. Arch Pathol 30:993–1031

Jakobson E, Spjut HJ (1960) Chondrosarcoma of the bones of the hand. Report of 3 cases. Acta Radiol 54:426–432

Jeffree GM, Price CHG (1965) Bone tumours and their enzymes. A study of phosphatases, non-specific esterases and beta glucuronidase of osteogenic and cartilaginous tumours, fibroblastic and giant cell lesions. J Bone Joint Surg [Br] 47:120–136

Kay S (1971) Ultrastructure of an osteoid type of osteogenic sarcoma. Cancer 28:437–445

Kirchner PT, Simon MA (1981) Radioisotopic evaluation of skeletal disease. J Bone Joint Surg [Am] 63:673–681

Larssen S-E, Lorentzon R, Boquist L (1975) Giant cell tumour of bone: a demographic, clinical and histopathological study of all cases recorded in the Swedish Cancer Registry for the years 1958 through 1968. J Bone Joint Surg [Am] 57:167–173

Le Charpentier Y, Forest M, Postel M, Tomeno B, Abelanet R (1979) Clear cell chondrosarcoma. A report of five cases including ultrastructural study. Cancer 44:622–629

Lennert K (1978) Malignant lymphomas. Springer, Berlin Heidelberg New York

Lewis RJ, Lotz MJ (1974) Medullary extension of osteosarcoma; implications for rational therapy. Cancer 33:371–375

Lichtenstein L (1972) Bone tumours, 4th edn. Mosby, St Louis

Lichtenstein L, Bernstein D (1959) Unusual benign and malignant chondroid tumors of bone. Cancer 12:1142–1157

Lichtenstein L, Jaffe HL (1943) Chondrosarcoma of bone. Am J Pathol 19:553–589

Lindenbaum S, Alexander H (1984) Infections simulating bone tumors. Clin Orthop 184:193–203

Llombart-Bosch A, Blache R, Pedro-Olaya A (1978) Ultrastructural study of 28 cases of Ewing's sarcoma. Cancer 41:1362–1373

Lowbeer L (1968) Multifocal osteosarcomatosis, a rare entity. Bull Pathol 9:52–53

Matsuno T, Unni KK, McLeod RA, Dahlin DC (1976) Telangiectatic osteogenic sarcoma. Cancer 38:2538–2547

McCarthy EF, Matsuno T, Dorfman HD (1979) Malignant fibrous histiocytoma of bone: a study of 35 cases. Human Pathol 10:57–70

McKenna RJ, Schwinn CP, Seong KY, Higinbotham NL (1964) Osteogenic sarcoma arising in Paget's disease. Cancer 17:42–66

McLeod RA, Beabout JW (1973) The roentgenographic features of chondroblastoma. Am J Roentgenol Radium Ther Nucl Med 118:464–471

McLeod RA, Dahlin DC, Beabout JW (1976) The spectrum of osteoblastoma. Am J Roentgenol Radium Ther Nucl Med 126:321–335

Milch RA, Changus GW (1956) Response of bone to tumour invasion. Cancer 9:340–351

Milgram JW (1983) The origins of osteochondromas and enchondromas. A histopathologic study. Clin Orthop 174:264–284

Mirra JM (1980) Bone tumours. Diagnosis and treatment. Lippincott, Philadelphia

Mirra JM, Marcove RC (1974) Fibrosarcomatous dedifferentiation of primary and secondary chondrosarcoma. Review of five cases. J Bone Joint Surg [Am] 56:285–296

Murphy FD, Blount WP (1962) Cartilaginous exostoses following irradiation. J Bone Joint Surg [Am] 44:662–668

Murphy WR, Ackerman LV (1956) Benign and malignant giant cell tumours of bone. A clinical pathological evaluation of thirty-one cases. Cancer 9:317–339

Murray RO, Jacobson HG (1971) The radiology of skeletal disorders: exercises in diagnosis. Williams and Wilkins, Baltimore.

Navas-Palacios JJ, Aparicio-Duque R, Valdes MD (1983) On the histogenesis of Ewing's sarcoma. An ultrastructural, immunohistochemical and cytochemical study. Cancer 53:1882–1901

Netherlands Committee on Bone Tumours (1973) Radiological atlas of bone tumours, vols 1 and 2. Williams & Wilkins, Baltimore

Pardo-Mirdan FJ, Ayala J, Joly M, Gimeno E, Vazquez JJ (1981) Primary liposarcoma of bone; light and electron microscopic study. Cancer 48:274–280

Paschall HA, Paschall MM (1975) Electron microscopic observations of 20 human osteosarcomas. Clin Orthop 111:42–56

Pochachevsky R, Yen YM, Sherman RS (1960) The roentgen appearance of benign osteoblastoma. Radiology 75:429–437

Porretta CA, Dahlin DC, Janes JM (1957) Sarcoma in Paget's disease of bone. J Bone Joint Surg [Am] 39:741–757

Reddick RL, Michelitch HJ, Levine AM, Triche TJ (1980) Osteogenic sarcoma. A study of the ultrastructure. Cancer 45:64–71

Revell PA (1981) Diseases of bones and joints. In: Berry CL (ed) Paediatric pathology. Springer, Berlin Heidelberg New York, pp 451–485

Revell PA, Scholtz CL (1979) Aggressive osteoblastoma. J Pathol 127:195–198

Roessner A, Grundmann E (1982) Electron microscopy in bone tumour diagnosis. In: Berry CL (ed) Bone and joint disease. Springer, Berlin Heidelberg New York, pp 153–198 (Current topics in pathology, vol 71)

Sabanas AO, Dahlin DC, Childs DS, Ivins JC (1956) Postradiation sarcoma of bone. Cancer 9:528–542

Sanerkin NG (1979) Primary leiomyosarcoma of the bone and its comparison with fibrosarcoma. A cytological, histological and ultrastructural study. Cancer 44:1375–1387

Sanerkin NG (1980) Definitions of osteosarcoma, chondrosarcoma and fibrosarcoma of bone. Cancer 46:178–185

Sanerkin NG, Jeffree GM (1980) Cytology of bone tumours: Colour atlas with text. Wright, Bristol, pp 51–84

Schajowicz F (1955) Aspiration biopsy in bone lesions. Cytological and histological techniques. J Bone Joint Surg [Am] 77:465–471

Schajowicz F (1959) Ewing's sarcoma and reticulum cell sarcoma of bone with special reference to the histochemical demonstration of glycogen as an aid to differential diagnosis. J Bone Joint Surg [Am] 41:349–356

Schajowicz F (1961) Giant cell tumors of bone (osteoclastoma): a pathological and histochemical study. J Bone Joint Surg [Am] 43:1–29

Schajowicz F (1981) Tumors and tumorlike lesions of bone and joints. Springer, Berlin Heidelberg New York

Schajowicz F (1983) Current trends in the diagnosis and treatment of malignant bone tumours. Clin Orthop 180:220–252

Schajowicz F, Derqui JC (1968) Puncture biopsy in lesions of the locomotor system. Review of results in 4050 cases, including 941 vertebral punctures. Cancer 21:531–548

Schajowicz F, Lemos C (1976) Malignant osteoblastoma. J Bone Joint Surg [Br] 58:202–211

Schajowicz F, Ackerman LV, Sissons HA (1972) Histologic typing of bone tumours. In: International histological classification of tumours No 6. World Health Organization, Geneva

Sim FH, Cupps RE, Dahlin DC, Ivins JC (1972) Postradiation sarcoma of bone. J Bone Joint Surg [Am] 54:1479–1489

Spanier SS, Enneking WF, Enriquez P (1975) Primary malignant fibrous histiocytoma of bone. Cancer 36:2084–2098

Spjut HJ, Dorfman HD, Fechner RE, Ackerman LV (1971) Tumors of bone and cartilage. In: Atlas of tumor pathology (fascicle 5). Armed Forces Institute of Pathology, Washington DC

Steiner GC (1964) Postradiation sarcoma of bone. Cancer 18:603–612

Stevens GM, Pugh DG, Dahlin DC (1957) Roentgenographic recognition and differentiation of parosteal osteogenic sarcoma. Am J Roentgenol 78:1–12

Strickland B (1959) The value of arteriography in the diagnosis of bone tumours. Br J Radiol 32:705–713

Turcotte B, Pugh DG, Dahlin DC (1962) The roentgenologic aspects of chondromyxoid fibroma of bone. Am J Roentgenol Radium Ther Nucl Med 87:1085–1095

Unni KK, Dahlin DC, Beabout JW, Sim JH (1976a) Chondrosarcoma: clear cell variant: a report of sixteen cases. J Bone Joint Surg [Am] 58:676–683

Unni KK, Dahlin DC, Beabout JW, Ivins JC (1976b) Parosteal osteogenic osteosarcoma. Cancer 37:2466–2475

Unni KK, Dahlin DC, Beabout JW (1976c) Periosteal osteogenic sarcoma. Cancer 37:2476–2485

Van der Heul RO, Von Ronnen JR (1967) Juxtacortical osteosarcoma: diagnosis, differential diagnosis, treatment and analysis of eighty cases. J Bone Joint Surg [Am] 49:415–439

Voutsinas S, Wynne-Davies R (1983) The infrequency of malignant disease in diaphyseal aclasis and neuro-fibromatosis. J Med Genet 20:345–349

Wick MR, McLeod RA, Siegal GP, Greditzer HG, Unni KK (1981) Sarcomas of bone complicating osteitis deformans (Paget's disease). Fifty years experience. Am J Surg Pathol 5:47–59

Williams AH, Schwinn CP, Parker JW (1976) The ultrastructure of osteosarcoma: a review of twenty cases. Cancer 37:1293–1301

Wold LE, Beabout JW, Unni KK, Pritchard DJ (1984) High-grade surface osteosarcomas. Am J Surg Pathol 8:181–186

Subject Index